Surgery
SOURCEBOOK

Fourth Edition

Health Reference Series

Fourth Edition

Surgery

SOURCEBOOK

Basic Consumer Health Information about Common Surgical Techniques and Procedures, including Appendectomy, Breast Biopsy, Carotid Endarterectomy, Cataract Removal, Cesarean Section, Coronary Artery Bypass, Cosmetic Surgery, Dilation and Curettage, Gallbladder Surgery, Hemorrhoidectomy, Hysterectomy, Hernia Repair, Low Back Surgery, Mastectomy, Prostatectomy, Tonsillectomy, and Weight-Loss (Bariatric) Surgery

Along with Facts about Emergency Surgery and Critical Care and Tips on Preparing for Surgery, Getting a Second Opinion, Managing Pain and Surgical Complications, and Recovering from Surgery, a Glossary of Related Terms, and a Directory of Resources for More Information

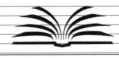

OMNIGRAPHICS

615 Griswold, Ste. 901, Detroit, MI 48226

NOV 2 0 2017

Bibliographic Note

Because this page cannot legibly accommodate all the copyright notices, the Bibliographic Note portion of the Preface constitutes an extension of the copyright notice.

* * *

Health Reference Series
Keith Jones, *Managing Editor*
***

OMNIGRAPHICS
A PART OF RELEVANT INFORMATION
***

Library of Congress Cataloging-in-Publication Data

Names: Omnigraphics, Inc., issuing body.

Title: Surgery sourcebook: basic consumer health information about common surgical techniques and procedures, including appendectomy, breast biopsy, carotid endarterectomy, cataract removal, cesarean section, coronary artery bypass, cosmetic surgery, dilation and curettage, gallbladder surgery, hemorrhoidectomy, hysterectomy, hernia repair, low back surgery, mastectomy, prostatectomy, tonsillectomy, and weight-loss (bariatric) surgery ; along with facts about emergency surgery and critical care and tips on preparing for surgery, getting a second opinion, managing pain and surgical complications, and recovering from surgery, a glossary of related terms, and a directory of resources for more information.

Description: Fourth edition. | Detroit, MI: Omnigraphics, [2017] | Series: Health reference series | Includes bibliographical references and index.

Identifiers: LCCN 2017015100 (print) | LCCN 2017018555 (ebook) | ISBN 9780780815667 (eBook) | ISBN 9780780815650 (hardcover: alk. paper)

Subjects: LCSH: Surgery--Popular works. | Consumer education--Popular works.

Classification: LCC RD31.3 (ebook) | LCC RD31.3.S87 2017 (print) | DDC 617--dc23

LC record available at https://lccn.loc.gov/2017015100

Table of Contents

Part II: Preparing for Surgery

Part III: Common Types of Surgery and Surgical Procedures

Part VI: Additional Help and Information

Preface

About This Book

According to the Agency for Healthcare Research and Quality (AHRQ), almost 15 million people undergo surgery each year at hospitals or same-day surgery centers in the United States. Whether it is done to relieve pain, prevent or treat a serious health condition, or repair trauma, surgery carries significant risks, such as infection, anesthesia reactions, and bleeding. Fortunately, new developments in surgical techniques, including lasers and laparoscopic surgery, have enabled surgeons to better control surgical complications and minimize patient risks.

Surgery Sourcebook, Fourth Edition describes the most common surgical procedures, including appendectomy, breast surgery, carotid endarterectomy, cataract, cesarean section, coronary artery bypass, cosmetic surgery, dilation and curettage, gallbladder surgery, hemorrhoidectomy, hysterectomy, hernia repair, low back surgery, tonsillectomy, and weight-loss (bariatric) surgery. The book discusses preparations patients may want to make prior to undergoing surgery, including choosing a surgeon, getting a second opinion, and donating blood, as well as postsurgical physical discomforts, nutrition and exercise considerations, and strategies for facilitating recovery. The book concludes with a glossary of related terms and a directory of resources for additional help and information.

How to Use This Book

This book is divided into parts and chapters. Parts focus on broad areas of interest. Chapters are devoted to single topics within a part.

Part I: Introduction to Surgery provides basic information about surgical specialties, including general surgery, neurosurgery, obstetrics and gynecology, ophthalmology, orthopedic surgery, otolaryngology, plastic surgery, and urology. It discusses specific types of surgical techniques including laparoscopic, laser, and robotic-assisted surgeries. The part concludes with the latest research on surgery.

Part II: Preparing for Surgery offers patients information on finding a qualified surgeon, obtaining a second opinion, and preparing for surgery. Services provided by ambulatory surgical centers are also detailed. The part also discusses blood donation, anxiety before surgery, tips on ensuring patient safety and preventing medical errors, financial planning facts, medical tourism, and the use of advance directives.

Part III: Common Types of Surgery and Surgical Procedures provides details about head and neck, eye, dental, breast, lung, heart and vascular, joint and spine, gastrointestinal, weight-loss (bariatric), gynecologic and obstetric, and urological surgeries. The part also highlights cosmetic and reconstructive surgical procedures, such as liposuction and surgery for skin. The part also offers information about organ transplants and emergency, critical care, and traumatic surgeries.

Part IV: Managing Pain and Surgical Complications focuses on the postoperative period and discusses methods for controlling pain, managing blood loss, and preventing surgical site and healthcare-associated infections that may develop during hospitalization, such as catheter-associated urinary tract infections, *Clostridium difficile* infections, *Pseudomonas aeruginosa*, methicillin-resistant *Staphylococcus aureus* (MRSA). The part also identifies other complications that may affect surgical patients, including abdominal adhesions, deep vein thrombosis, pneumonia, sepsis, and breast implant complications.

Part V: Recovering from Surgery offers insight into the process of recovering from surgery. Hospital discharge planning, postsurgical nutrition, and strategies for caring for incisions, surgical drains, and ostomy bags are discussed, along with information about blot clot risks and traveling after surgery.

Part VI: Additional Help and Information provides a glossary of important terms related to surgery and a directory of organizations that offer information to people undergoing surgery or their caregivers.

Bibliographic Note

This volume contains documents and excerpts from publications issued by the following U.S. government agencies: Agency for Healthcare Research and Quality (AHRQ); Centers for Disease Control and Prevention (CDC); Centers for Medicare and Medicaid Services (CMS); *Eunice Kennedy Shriver* National Institute of Child Health and Human Development (NICHD); Federal Bureau of Prisons (BOP); Health Resources and Services Administration (HRSA); National Cancer Institute (NCI); National Eye Institute (NEI); National Heart, Lung, and Blood Institute (NHLBI); National Institute of Arthritis and Musculoskeletal and Skin Diseases (NIAMS); National Institute of Biomedical Imaging and Bioengineering (NIBIB); National Institute of Dental and Craniofacial Research (NIDCR); National Institute of Diabetes and Digestive and Kidney Diseases (NIDDK); National Institute of General Medical Sciences (NIGMS); National Institute of Neurological Disorders and Stroke (NINDS); National Institute on Aging (NIA); National Institute on Deafness and Other Communication Disorders (NIDCD); National Institute on Drug Abuse (NIDA) for Teens; National Institutes of Health (NIH); National Science Foundation (NSF); *NIH News in Health*; NIHSeniorHealth; Office of Disease Prevention and Health Promotion (ODPHP); Office on Women's Health (OWH); U.S. Department of Health and Human Services (HHS); U.S. Department of Veterans Affairs (VA); and U.S. Food and Drug Administration (FDA).

In addition, this volume contains copyrighted documents from the following organizations: The American College of Surgeons; American Pregnancy Association; American Society of Anesthesiologists (ASA); and American Society of PeriAnesthesia Nurses (ASPAN).

It may also contain original material produced by Omnigraphics and reviewed by medical consultants.

About the Health Reference Series

The *Health Reference Series* is designed to provide basic medical information for patients, families, caregivers, and the general public. Each volume takes a particular topic and provides comprehensive coverage. This is especially important for people who may be dealing with a newly diagnosed disease or a chronic disorder in themselves or in a family member. People looking for preventive guidance, information about disease warning signs, medical statistics, and risk factors for health problems will also find answers to their questions in the *Health Reference Series*. The *Series*, however, is not intended to serve as a tool for diagnosing illness, in prescribing treatments, or as a substitute for the physician/patient relationship. All people concerned about medical symptoms or the possibility of disease are encouraged to seek professional care from an appropriate healthcare provider.

A Note about Spelling and Style

Health Reference Series editors use *Stedman's Medical Dictionary* as an authority for questions related to the spelling of medical terms and the *Chicago Manual of Style* for questions related to grammatical structures, punctuation, and other editorial concerns. Consistent adherence is not always possible, however, because the individual volumes within the *Series* include many documents from a wide variety of different producers, and the editor's primary goal is to present material from each source as accurately as is possible. This sometimes means that information in different chapters or sections may follow other guidelines and alternate spelling authorities.

Medical Review

Omnigraphics contracts with a team of qualified, senior medical professionals who serve as medical consultants for the *Health Reference Series*. As necessary, medical consultants review reprinted and originally written material for currency and accuracy. Citations including the phrase, "Reviewed (month, year)" indicate material reviewed by this team. Medical consultation services are provided to the *Health Reference Series* editors by:

Dr. Vijayalakshmi, MBBS, DGO, MD
Dr. Senthil Selvan, MBBS, DCH, MD
Dr. K. Sivanandham, MBBS, DCH, MS (Research), PhD

Our Advisory Board

We would like to thank the following board members for providing initial guidance on the development of this series:

- Dr. Lynda Baker, Associate Professor of Library and Information Science, Wayne State University, Detroit, MI

- Nancy Bulgarelli, William Beaumont Hospital Library, Royal Oak, MI

- Karen Imarisio, Bloomfield Township Public Library, Bloomfield Township, MI

- Karen Morgan, Mardigian Library, University of Michigan-Dearborn, Dearborn, MI

- Rosemary Orlando, St. Clair Shores Public Library, St. Clair Shores, MI

Health Reference Series *Update Policy*

The inaugural book in the *Health Reference Series* was the first edition of *Cancer Sourcebook* published in 1989. Since then, the *Series* has been enthusiastically received by librarians and in the medical community. In order to maintain the standard of providing high-quality health information for the layperson the editorial staff at Omnigraphics felt it was necessary to implement a policy of updating volumes when warranted.

Medical researchers have been making tremendous strides, and it is the purpose of the *Health Reference Series* to stay current with the most recent advances. Each decision to update a volume is made on an individual basis. Some of the considerations include how much new information is available and the feedback we receive from people who use the books. If there is a topic you would like to see added to the update list, or an area of medical concern you feel has not been adequately addressed, please write to:

Managing Editor
Health Reference Series
Omnigraphics
615 Griswold, Ste. 901
Detroit, MI 48226

Part One

Introduction to Surgery

Chapter 1

Overview of Surgical Specialties

Colon and Rectal Surgery

A colon and rectal surgeon is trained to diagnose and treat patients with various diseases of the intestinal tract, colon, rectum, anal canal, and perianal area through medical and surgical means. This specialist may also deal with the liver, urinary, and female reproductive systems if they are involved with primary intestinal disease. A colon and rectal surgeon has expertise in diagnosing and managing anorectal conditions such as hemorrhoids, fissures (painful tears in the anal lining), abscesses, and fistulae (infections located around the anus and rectum). Training in colon and rectal surgery also provides the specialist with in-depth knowledge of intestinal and anorectal physiology required for the treatment of problems such as constipation and incontinence. They also treat problems of the intestine and colon and perform endoscopic procedures to detect and treat conditions of the bowel lining, such as cancer, polyps (precancerous growths), and inflammatory conditions. A colon and rectal specialist also performs abdominal surgical procedures involving the colon, rectum, and small bowel for the treatment of cancer, diverticulitis, and inflammatory bowel disease (such as chronic ulcerative colitis and Crohn's disease).

These operations may be performed with traditional (open) or minimally invasive (laparoscopic) techniques.

General Surgery

A general surgeon is a specialist who is trained to diagnose, treat, and manage patients with a broad spectrum of surgical conditions affecting almost any area of the body. The surgeon establishes the diagnosis and provides the preoperative, operative, and postoperative care to patients and is often responsible for the comprehensive management of the trauma victim and the critically ill patient. The general surgeon has the knowledge and technical skills to manage conditions that relate to the head and neck, breast, skin and soft tissues, abdomen, extremities, and the gastrointestinal, vascular, and endocrine systems.

Surgeons may further specialize in an additional board certification from the American Board of Surgery in the following areas:

Pediatric Surgery

A pediatric surgeon is a specialist who is trained to diagnose, treat, and manage the preoperative, operative, and postoperative care of the child. They care for and operate on children whose development ranges from the newborn through the teenage years. All pediatric surgeons are board certified in general surgery and then complete two years of additional training before they are eligible to be certified in pediatric surgery. As a result of this additional training, pediatric surgeons have expertise in the following areas of responsibility: neonatal surgery (specialized knowledge in the surgical repair of birth defects in the newborn); prenatal surgery (detect abnormalities and plan for surgical corrections during the fetal stage of development); trauma (knowledge in the surgical care and prevention of traumatic injuries); pediatric surgical oncology (knowledge of the diagnosis and surgical care of children with tumors and growths); and surgical problems of the gastrointestinal tract, such as inflammatory bowel disease, appendicitis, gastroesophageal reflux (reflux of food from the stomach to the esophagus or trachea). Pediatric surgeons are also trained to care for certain surgical problems of the neck, skin and soft tissues, and vascular and endocrine systems.

Vascular Surgery

A vascular surgeon is a surgical specialist who cares for patients with diseases that affect the arteries, veins, and lymphatic systems exclusive of the heart and intracranial (within the brain) circulations. Hardening of the arteries or atherosclerosis is a common cause of vascular disease. Specialists in this field perform open operations, endovascular catheter-based procedures, and noninvasive vascular testing and interpretations. Common problems treated include stroke prevention by managing arterial blockages in the neck and upper chest, revascularization of upper and lower limbs for poor circulation, management of aneurysms such as occur in the abdomen and elsewhere, vascular trauma, and varicose veins. Treatment also includes angioplasty—stenting of arterial blockages, repair of abdominal aneurysms by less-invasive endovascular techniques—as well as medical management of vascular disorders. Vascular surgeons are board certified in general surgery and then complete additional training and testing in vascular surgery.

Surgery of the Hand

This specialty focuses on the investigation and treatment of patients with diseases, injuries, or abnormalities affecting the upper extremities. This specialty includes the performance of microvascular surgery, which is necessary for reattachment of amputated fingers or limbs. All hand surgeons are certified in general surgery and then complete additional training and testing in hand surgery.

Critical Care Surgery

This specialty focuses on the surgical and medical diagnosis and treatment of critically ill and injured patients, particularly the trauma victim. Specialists have the knowledge, skills, and compassion to provide timely, safe, effective, and efficient patient-centered care and manage the patient with multiple organ problems. They also coordinate the teams of doctors and nurses needed for the care of the critically ill and injured patient. Surgeons in this discipline are board certified in general surgery and then complete additional training and testing in critical care surgery.

Neurologic Surgery

A neurological surgeon provides operative and nonoperative management (prevention, diagnosis, evaluation, treatment, critical care, and rehabilitation) of patients with disorders of the brain, spinal cord, spinal column, and peripheral nerves, including their support structures and blood supply. They also evaluate and manage disorders

5

that affect the function of the nervous system and the operative and nonoperative management of certain types of pain. Common conditions managed by neurologic surgeons include disorders of the brain, meninges (membranes covering the brain and spinal cord), skull, spinal cord, and vertebral column. This also includes the carotid and vertebral arteries, the pituitary gland, spinal fusion or instrumentation, and disorders of the cranial and spinal nerves. Pediatric neurosurgeons manage children with head injuries, brain and spinal tumors, vascular malformation, seizures disorders, and hydrocephalus.

Obstetrics and Gynecology

Obstetrician/gynecologists provide medical and surgical care of the female patient. The focus for this specialty is on the female reproductive system, including performing surgical procedures, managing the care of pregnant women, delivering babies, and rendering gynecologic care, oncology care, and primary healthcare for women.

Specialty certification in obstetrics and gynecology includes:

Gynecology Oncology

This type of surgeon is an obstetrician/gynecologist who is certified in ob/gyn and then has an additional three to four years of specialized training in the treatment of gynecologic cancers including special surgical training and has subspecialty certification through the American Board of Obstetrics and Gynecology for the comprehensive management of patients with cancer unique to women. This specialist provides comprehensive management of women with precancerous and cancerous conditions of the female reproductive system. Expertise in surgery, chemotherapy, and indications for radiation therapy supports continuity of care of the gynecologic cancer patient.

Maternal Fetal Medicine

This specialist is an obstetrician/gynecologist who is certified in ob/gyn and has additional training in obstetrics and has subspecialty certification through the American Board of Obstetrics and Gynecology. This individual cares for patients with complications of pregnancy and has advanced knowledge of the obstetrical, medical and surgical complications of pregnancy and their effect on both mother and their fetuses. This specialist has expertise in the current diagnostic techniques and treatments for woman with complicated pregnancies. Special expertise also exists in the use of sonography in pregnancy.

Reproductive Endocrinology and Infertility

A surgeon with this specialty is an obstetrician/gynecologist who is certified in ob/gyn and has additional training in reproductive medicine and has subspecialty certification through the American Board of Obstetrics and Gynecology. This individual manages patients with complex problems related to reproductive medicine, including assisted reproductive technology, in vitro fertilization, reproductive surgery, infertility, menopause, contraception, endometriosis, and other reproductive disorders.

Female Pelvic Medicine and Reconstructive Surgery

This type of specialist is an obstetrician/gynecologist who is certified in ob/gyn and has additional training in the management of the female bladder and pelvic floor. Disorders managed by this subspecialty include disorders requiring advanced vaginal and laparoscopic surgery, female urinary incontinence, pelvic organ prolapse, vesico-vaginal fistula, and female anal incontinence.

Ophthalmologic Surgery

An ophthalmologist specializes in the comprehensive care of patients with disorders of their eyes and vision. Ophthalmologists are medically trained to diagnose and medically and surgically treat all ocular and visual disorders, including prescribing glasses and contact lenses. These specialists also treat problems affecting the eye and its structures, the eyelids, the orbit, the visual pathway, and acquired onset of double vision in adults and children from neurological and endocrine conditions such as stroke with cranial nerve palsies and thyroid-related eye disease. Cataract operations and basic glaucoma procedures are commonly performed by these specialists. Ophthalmologists may also have additional expertise in the following areas: adult strabismus, cornea and external disease, glaucoma, neuro-ophthalmology, ophthalmic pathology, ophthalmic plastic surgery, pediatric ophthalmology, and vitreoretinal diseases.

Oral and Maxillofacial Surgery

An oral and maxillofacial surgeon specializes in dentistry which includes the diagnosis and surgical and adjunctive treatment of patients with disease, injuries, and defects involving both the function and appearance of the oral and maxillofacial region. This specialty includes care of the oral cavity and face, removal of diseased and impacted teeth, anesthesia for dental procedures, dental implants, facial trauma, pathologic conditions (tumors or cysts), reconstructive and cosmetic surgery, facial pain including temporomandibular joint disorders, correction of dentofacial (Bite) deformities, and birth defects. Certification requires completion of training in an accredited residency program, evidence of posttraining experience, and successful completion of written and oral examinations on the entire scope of the specialty.

Orthopaedic Surgery

An orthopaedic surgeon is trained in the preservation, investigation, and restoration of the form and function of the extremities, spine, and associated structures by medical, surgical, and physical means. Specialized care is provided for patients with musculoskeletal problems including congenital deformities, trauma, infections, tumors, metabolic disturbance of the musculoskeletal system, deformities, injuries, and degenerative disease of the spine, hands, feet, knee, hip, shoulder, and elbow in children and adults. An orthopaedic surgeon also is involved with treatment of secondary muscular problems in patients who suffer from various central or peripheral nervous system lesions such as cerebral palsy, paraplegia, or stroke, as well as conditions that are treated medically or physically through the use of braces, casts, splints, or physical therapy.

Specialty certification in orthopaedics includes:

Orthopaedic Sports Medicine

An Orthopaedic Sports Medicine specialist provides care for all structures in the musculoskeletal system directly affected by participating in sporting events. The specialist is proficient in the conditioning, training, and fitness of the body as it relates to athletic performance and the effects of athletic performance and the impact of dietary supplements, pharmaceuticals, and nutrition on athletes' short- and long-term health and performance.

Surgery of the Hand

A specialist in this area is trained in the investigation, preservation and medical surgical and rehabilitation treatment of patients with diseases, injuries, or abnormalities affecting the upper extremities. This specialty includes the performance of microvascular surgery, which is necessary for reattachment of amputated fingers or limbs.

Otolaryngology—Head and Neck Surgery

An otolaryngologist—head and neck surgeon—provides medical and surgical care for patients with diseases and disorders that affect the ears, nose, throat, the respiratory and upper alimentary systems, and related structures of the head and neck. They diagnose and provide medical and surgical treatment of diseases and have skills and knowledge in audiology and speech-language pathology; the chemical senses; allergy, endocrinology, and neurology as they relate to the head and neck. Operations are performed on the head and neck, and face. Head and neck oncology, facial plastic and reconstructive procedures, and the treatment of disorders of hearing and voice are fundamental areas of expertise for the otolaryngologist.

Specialty certification in otolaryngology—head and neck surgery includes:

Neurotology

A neurotologist is an otolaryngologist—head and neck surgeon—who treats patients with diseases of the ear and temporal bone, including disorders of hearing and balance.

Pediatric Otolaryngology

An otolaryngologist—head and neck surgeon—has completed specialty training in the management of infants and children with congenital or acquired disorders of the head and neck, nose, paranasal sinuses, ear, and aerodigestive tract.

Plastic Surgery within the Head and Neck

An otolaryngologist—head and neck surgeon—has completed additional training in plastic cosmetic and reconstructive procedures within the head, face, and neck. This area includes skin, head and neck oncology and reconstruction, management of maxillofacial trauma, soft tissue repair, and neural surgery.

Plastic Surgery

Plastic surgeons specialize in the care of patients requiring repair, replacement, and reconstruction of defects of the form and function of the body covering and its underlying musculoskeletal system, with emphasis on the craniofacial structures, the oropharynx, the upper

9

and lower limbs, the breast, and the external genitalia. This surgical specialty also focuses on the aesthetic surgery of structures with undesirable form. Special knowledge and skill in the design and transfer of skin flaps, in the transplantation of tissues, and in the replantation of structures are vital to the performance of plastic surgery.

Specialty certification in plastic surgery includes:

Surgery of the Hand

This specialty focuses on the investigation and treatment of patients with diseases, injuries, or abnormalities affecting the upper extremities. This specialty includes the performance of microvascular surgery, which is necessary for reattachment of amputated fingers or limbs. All hand surgeons are certified in plastic surgery and then complete additional training and testing in hand surgery.

Plastic Surgery within the Head and Neck

A surgeon with this specialty is a plastic surgeon with additional training in cosmetic and reconstructive procedures within the head, face, and neck. This area includes skin, head and neck oncology and reconstruction, management of maxillofacial trauma, soft tissue repair, and neural surgery.

Thoracic and Cardiovascular Surgery

Thoracic surgeons specialize in management of patients with conditions of the chest and heart. This specialty includes providing surgical care of patients for coronary artery disease; cancers of the lung, esophagus, and chest wall; abnormalities of the heart, great vessels and heart valves; congenital anomalies; tumors of the mediastinum; and diseases of the diaphragm. The management of the airway and injuries to the chest are also areas of surgical practice for the thoracic surgeon. They have specialized knowledge of cardiorespiratory physiology and oncology, as well as capability in the use of extracorporeal circulation, cardiac assist devices, management of cardiac dysrhythmias, pleural drainage, respiratory support systems, endoscopy, and other invasive and noninvasive diagnostic technique.

Urology Surgeon

A surgeon who specializes in urology manages patients with benign and malignant (cancerous) medical and surgical disorders of the adrenal gland and of the genitourinary system. Urologists have comprehensive knowledge of, and skills in, endoscopic, percutaneous, and open surgery of congenital and acquired conditions of the reproductive and urinary systems.

Chapter 2

Types and Approaches to Surgery

Based on descriptions of discovered Egyptian papyri, surgeries were performed by the ancient Egyptians. The tools they used for surgery included knives, drills, saws, hooks, forceps, and pinchers. Some of these tools, somewhat modified, are still used for surgical purposes. In contrast with the role played by surgery in the past, surgery is more important now than ever. Surgical technology and techniques are so advanced that surgery is able to accomplish what ancient surgeons never dreamed of. Surgery is used for a great variety of diseases, including cancer treatment. Sometimes, surgeries for different purposes may take place simultaneously. For example, curative surgery may be performed right after a diagnostic surgery or a curative surgery may be followed by a reconstructive surgery.

Generally, surgery involves cutting into the body (incision) to explore or remove tissue while the patient is under anesthesia. Surgical techniques used for surgery include cryosurgery, electrocauterization surgery, laser surgery, gamma knife, and en bloc resection.

Types of Surgery

This chapter provides an overview of four types of surgery and details the purpose, benefits, and risks.

This chapter includes text excerpted from "Surgery," Surveillance, Epidemiology, and End Results Program (SEER), National Cancer Institute (NCI), September 8, 2016.

- Diagnostic surgery

- Preventive surgery

- Curative surgery

- Palliative and reconstructive surgery

Diagnostic Surgery

There are many ways to detect or confirm a suspicion of the presence of a cancer. Microscopic examination of biopsy samples is the ideal way that a positive diagnosis of cancer can be made. This procedure involves physically removing all or part (tissue, cells, or fluid) of a suspected tumor and examining this material under a microscope. The purpose of a biopsy is to identify the histologic type of cancer and possibly stage of disease.

Any organ in the body can be biopsied utilizing a variety of techniques. Some may require major surgery, while others may not even require local anesthesia. Types of biopsies include incisional biopsy, excisional biopsy, endoscopic biopsy, colposcopic biopsy, bone marrow biopsy, fine needle aspiration biopsy, stereotactic biopsy, and core biopsy, to name a few. Biopsies typically leave gross tumor in the body.

A pathologist performs the microscopic examination of the biopsied material. After careful evaluation, a benign or malignant diagnosis can usually be established. A written report prepared by the pathologist is sent to the doctor who treats the cancer patient. This doctor will then make decisions regarding treatment based on the information found in this report.

Take breast cancer for example: If a breast abnormality is detected with mammography or physical exam, the patient will typically be referred for additional breast imaging with diagnostic mammography, ultrasound, or other imaging tests. While all of these methods of diagnosis can help detect a breast abnormality, biopsy followed by pathological (microscopic) analysis is really the only definitive way to determine if cancer is present.

The method of biopsy chosen will depend on:

- How suspicious the abnormality appears

- The size, shape, and location of the abnormality

- The number of abnormalities present

- The patient's medical history

- The patient's preference

- The training of the physician who is performing the biopsy

- The breast imaging center or surgical center where the biopsy is performed

Side effects and risks of biopsy do exist, depending on the type of biopsy performed and certain biopsy techniques. Cytology procedures, needle biopsies, and core biopsies, sometimes may not even come up with a positive cancer diagnosis due to inadequate quantities of cells or tissue removed from the patient. In rare cases, an incorrect diagnosis could be made in the situation where the needle misses the tumor and removes only healthy or noncancerous tissue. As with the case of preventive surgery, patients are strongly encouraged to discuss the advantages and disadvantages of the different biopsy methods with their physician(s) prior to undergoing the procedure(s).

A biopsy that removes only a fragment or portion of the tumor, primary or metastatic, is recorded in the abstract as noncancer-directed treatment.

Preventive Surgery

In a preventive surgery, the surgeon removes tissue that does not yet contain cancer cells, but has the probability of becoming cancerous in the future. This may also be referred to as prophylactic surgery. For example, with the consent of the patient, the surgeon sometimes removes the ovaries of a woman to avoid the risk of ovarian cancer if the person has a very strong family history of ovarian cancer. Based on studies, a woman whose mother or sister had ovarian cancer has a higher than average risk of developing ovarian cancer. The procedure is called prophylactic oophorectomy (removal of both ovaries).

Preventive mastectomy is another example of a surgery with a preventive purpose. In the past, the surgeon may have removed the breast tissue but spared the nipple (subcutaneous mastectomy). Total mastectomy (removal of the entire breast and nipple) is considered in an effort to prevent or reduce the risk of breast cancer. In addition to women who have already had one breast removed due to cancer, preventive mastectomy may also be an option for women with a strong family history of breast cancer, especially if several close relatives developed the disease before age 50. Women in families with hereditary breast cancer who test positive for a known cancer-causing gene alteration (for example, *BRCA1* and *BRCA2*) may also consider prophylactic mastectomy surgery, as may women who have had lobular carcinoma in situ, a condition that increases their risk of developing breast cancer in the same breast and/or in the opposite breast.

Those patients who have a congenital or genetic trait that creates a high risk of developing cancer may benefit from preventive surgery. For example, studies have shown that half of the patients with familial polyposis of the colon, without a preventive colectomy, would develop cancer of the colon by age 40, and all would develop the disease by age 70.

Pros and cons exist for preventive surgeries. Some patients may not choose preventive mastectomy or oophorectomy due to their concerns about with sexual and reproductive function and self-image, even if the procedure may add years to their life expectancy. Due to unique risk factors for cancer of each individual patient, a preventive surgery does not guarantee the patient will never develop cancer. Therefore, the decision of a preventive surgery should only be considered after a careful discussion between the surgeon and the patient.

Curative Surgery

Surgery plays a vital role in the cancer treatment plan, especially in patients with solid tumors. Surgery is often used to attempt to cure patients whose tumors are localized at the time of the diagnosis. After definite cancer diagnosis, curative surgical operations are conducted to remove or destroy cancerous tissue. Unlike diagnostic surgeries which may remove a small amount of tissue to confirm the existence and the stage of the disease, curative surgeries take a much more radical surgical approach, typically resulting in partial or total removal of the organ of origin.

In a curative procedure, a certain amount of normal tissue as well as cancerous tissue may be removed to obtain adequate margins. The purpose is to minimize the risk of any cancer cells being left behind, which may result in a recurrence of the cancer. For the same purpose, the surgeon may also remove the lymph nodes that are adjacent to the tumor.

Resection of isolated metastases (removal of solitary metastases) may be performed in some cases, especially if there has been a disease-free interval of more than one year after the surgery. Second-look operations are sometimes performed following adjuvant therapies, but they have little effect on the final outcome in the great majority of cancer patients.

Scalpels or other instruments are used in excisional surgeries to eradicate the malignant tumor. Many types of excisional surgeries exist, each named for the particular area of the body in which they are performed. For example, laryngectomy involves removal of a large tumor of the larynx which may include removing part of the tongue or oropharynx. Similarly, parathyroidectomy refers to a surgery to remove parathyroid glands or tumors.

In addition to the more traditional surgical instruments such as scalpels, new technologies are employed in cancer curative surgeries depending on such factors as the patient's age and general health condition, location of tumor, and so on.

Laser surgery uses a powerful beam of light, which can be directed to specific parts of the body, without making a large incision, to destroy cancer cells. Laser also can be used in cancer treatment as well as preventive surgeries. For example, in the digestive system, laser is often used to remove colon polyps, which may later become cancerous. Laser has been used to treat abnormal tissue, carcinoma in situ, and early cancer of the cervix, vagina, and vulva, to name a few. Many women with breast cancer choose laser as the surgical tool because it is less painful and requires a shorter stay in the hospital.

Laser, as a tumor removal tool, has several advantages over scalpels. It is more precise and takes less operating time. Healing time is often shortened because laser heat seals blood vessels so there is less bleeding, swelling, and scarring involved in the surgical procedure. The downside of laser surgery is its cost and proper training of the cancer surgeons. The equipment can be bulky and technologically complicated compared with the more traditional surgical tools such as scalpels.

Working on a similar biological principle, electrosurgery uses high-frequency electrical currents to cut and destroy cancer cells. In electrosurgery, the high density of the radio-frequency current applied by the active electrosurgical electrode causes a cutting action, which can act like a fine micro-needle, a lancet, a knife, a snare, or even an energized scalpel or scissors.

Another innovative surgical technique to remove cancer is cryosurgery. Liquid nitrogen, or a probe that is very cold, is used to freeze and kill cancer cells. Traditionally, it has been used to treat external tumors, but now the technique is being employed as a treatment for tumors that occur internally.

Similar to laser, cryosurgery, incurs minimal blood loss, little discomfort, and shorter recovery time and shorter hospital stays. While researchers are still studying the effectiveness of cryosurgery as a treatment for other types of cancer, the technique has been used

17

successfully in treating prostate cancer. Just as with the laser techniques, cryosurgery has proven to be effective in preventive surgeries. For example, precancerous skin growths known as actinic keratosis and cervical intraepithelial neoplasia can be treated successfully with cryosurgery.

According to cancer specialists, the stage of the cancer plays an important role in opting for cryosurgery as a cancer surgical tool. Cryosurgery is most effective for younger patients whose disease is contained entirely within the prostate.

One frequently asked question is: "Can the surgeon cure the cancer after the surgery?" Unfortunately, there is not a definite answer to this question. In many cases, cancer cells can break away from the primary tumor site and spread (metastasize) to other parts of the body by the time of the diagnosis. These patients may not only receive surgery, but may also receive adjuvant treatment such as chemotherapy to destroy the metastases.

The decision of a curative surgery is often made based on such factors as the patient's age and general health condition, location of tumor, stage of tumor, presence or absence of enlarged nodes, and the patient's desire for preservation.

Each of the surgical procedures described above is recorded in the abstract as cancer-directed treatment.

Palliative and Reconstructive Surgeries

In addition to diagnostic, curative, and preventive surgeries, surgical procedures are also performed to improve the patient's quality of life. They can restore the function or appearance of organs or tissues that were either removed or changed by cancer treatment.

Palliative Surgery

Cancer causes pain to most cancer patients as does the treatment. It is estimated that 80 percent of cancer patients have two or more episodes of pain. More patients experience pain with advanced disease. The quality of life of those patients in great pain, resulting from either the disease or the treatment, is greatly compromised. Under such circumstances, palliative surgery may be performed. For example, the procedure may involve the removal of a painful primary or metastatic tumor mass such as a solitary spinal metastasis.

The purpose of palliative surgery is mainly to reduce pain for the patient. The surgery may not necessarily aim to eradicate cancer tissue in the patient. In fact, palliative surgery is often deemed as worthwhile and feasible by cancer specialists when the disease is not responsive to any type of curative treatment. A successful palliative surgery may not only make the patient's life more comfortable, but it may also prolong the cancer patient's life in some cases. Palliative surgery which removes cancer tissue is recorded as cancer-directed surgery. Palliative surgery such as a nerve block procedure to interrupt pain signals in the nervous system, or a stent placement to alleviate obstruction, etc., which does not remove cancer tissue is not recorded as cancer-directed surgery. Palliative procedures are recorded as non-cancer directed surgery.

Reconstructive Surgery

Reconstructive surgeries are performed on patients with physical deformities and abnormalities caused by traumatic injuries, birth defects, developmental abnormalities, or disease.

The goals of reconstructive surgery differ from those of cosmetic surgery; while cosmetic surgery is performed to reshape normal structures of the body to improve the patient's appearance and self-esteem, reconstructive surgery is performed on abnormal or damaged structures of the body. In many cases, the reason for the surgery is to repair the damage caused by the curative surgery, as well as to improve functions of certain anatomic parts of the body. In cancer treatment, if curative surgical procedures cause any disfigurement, dysfunction, or deformity, reconstructive surgery may be necessary. Breast reconstruction following surgical treatment for breast cancer is perhaps the most common example of reconstructive surgery.

For many simple or modified radical mastectomy patients, breast reconstruction may be possible during the same surgical procedure. In this type of reconstructive surgery, additional surgery is avoided and patients do not wake up to the "shock" of losing a breast. While a mastectomy is performed by the cancer surgeon, reconstructive surgery is usually performed by the plastic surgeon. Breast reconstruction may interfere with adjuvant treatment such as chemotherapy or radiation therapy. In these cases, reconstructive surgery may be delayed.

Sometimes, a one-stage reconstruction may not be enough; multiple stages may be necessary for optimal results when delayed tissue transfer is required. As with all other types of surgeries in cancer treatment, careful discussions between cancer patients and their doctors and plastic surgeons are encouraged so that the decisions regarding cancer surgery and reconstructive surgery can be made in the best interest of the patient.

Approaches of Surgery

Open Surgery

An "open" surgery is one in which the patient is cut open. A typical open surgery involves the use of a scalpel to make an incision into the skin and cut through the various layers of the dermis and subdermal layers and tissues to get to the desired tissue or organ. Some open surgeries use a laser to make the incision.

Endoscopic Surgery

Endoscopy is a surgical technique that involves the use of an endoscope, a special viewing instrument that allows a surgeon to see images of the body's internal structures through very small incisions.

Endoscopic surgery has been used for decades in a number of different procedures, including; gallbladder removal, tubal ligation, and knee surgery.

The Endoscope

An endoscope consists of two basic parts: A tubular probe fitted with a tiny camera and bright light, which is inserted through a small incision; and a viewing screen, which magnifies the transmitted images of the body's internal structures. During surgery, the surgeon watches the screen while moving the tube of the endoscope through the surgical area.

It's important to understand that the endoscope functions as a viewing device only. To perform the surgery, a separate surgical instrument—such as a scalpel, scissors, or forceps—must be inserted through a different point of entry and manipulated within the tissue.

Advantages of Endoscopy

All surgery carries risks and every incision leaves a scar. However, with endoscopic surgery, scars are likely to be much smaller and some of the after effects of surgery may be minimized.

In a typical endoscopic procedure, only a few small incisions, each less than one inch long, are needed to insert the endoscope probe and other instruments. For some procedures, such as breast augmentation, only two incisions may be necessary. For others, such as a forehead lift, three or more short incisions may be needed. The tiny "eye" of the endoscope's camera allows a surgeon to view the surgical site almost as clearly as if the skin were opened from a long incision.

Because the incisions are shorter with endoscopy, the risk of sensory loss from nerve damage is decreased. Also, bleeding, bruising and swelling may be significantly reduced. With the endoscopic approach, recovery may be quicker than that of an open surgery.

Endoscopic surgery may also allow you to avoid an overnight hospital stay. Many endoscopic procedures can be performed on an outpatient basis under local anesthesia with sedation. Patients should discuss this possibility with their doctor.

Surgical Techniques

Scalpel

The scalpel is the traditional cancer surgery tool. Other tools such as needles, forceps, or scissors are involved in cancer diagnostic surgeries. However, these traditional cancer surgery tools are being replaced by new and more effective cancer surgical tools such as laser and radiation. These new surgical tools often result in less operative time, cause less pain to cancer patients, and reduce complications, such as scarring that sometimes occur with surgeries performed with traditional surgical tools.

"Smart Scalpel," a dime-sized biological laser device, can quickly identify a cell population that has abnormal protein content (as cancer cells usually do). This device should assist surgeons in cutting away malignant tissue while minimizing the amount of healthy tissue removed.

Cryosurgery

Cryosurgery (also called cryotherapy) is the use of extreme cold to destroy cancer cells. Traditionally, it has been used to treat external tumors, such as those on the skin, but recently some physicians have begun using it as a treatment for tumors that occur inside the body. Cryosurgery for internal tumors is increasing in popularity as a result of developments in technology over the past several years.

For external tumors, liquid nitrogen (-196°C, -320.8°F) is applied directly to the cancer cells or tissue with a cotton swab or spraying device. For internal tumors, liquid nitrogen is circulated through an instrument called a cryoprobe, which is placed in contact with the tumor. To guide the cryoprobe and to monitor the freezing of the cells, the physician uses ultrasound (computerized moving pictures of the body generated by high-frequency sound waves). By using ultrasound, physicians hope to spare nearby healthy tissue.

21

Cryosurgery often involves a cycle of treatments in which the tumor is frozen, allowed to thaw, and then refrozen.

Advantages of cryosurgery:

- Minimally invasive—no blood loss, no surgical incision, and can be done as an outpatient.

- Favorable success rates and less complications—less complications than open surgery.

- Short recuperation period.

- Procedure can be repeated if the first cryosurgery has failed.

- Radiation therapy or radical surgery is still an option if the cryosurgery fails.

- Cost is less than traditional treatment.

Electrocauterization Surgery

Cauterization is the process of destroying tissue by using chemical corrosion, electricity, or heat. Electrocautery is done using a small probe, which has an electric current running through it, to cauterize (burn or destroy) the tissue.

Electrocautery is a safe procedure and is routinely used in surgery to burn unwanted or harmful tissue. It is also effectively used to reduce or stop hemorrhaging by "burning" the bleeding blood vessels (seals them off). Various types, shapes, and sizes of tips (probes) are available for specific treatments.

A specific type of electrocautery is fulguration, sometimes called electrodesiccation. Electrodesiccation is the destruction of tissue with a diathermy instrument. Electrodesiccation is particularly useful inside the bladder. Bladder electrodesiccation is performed via the urethra and viewed through a cystoscope.

Laser Surgery

L-A-S-E-R stands for Light Amplification by Stimulated Emission of Radiation. Through a complicated electronic process, a beam of light is produced which has special properties. This light is all one wavelength; that is, it is all one color of the spectrum. The light is focused so that all of its rays are traveling in the same direction. In a similar fashion, you might use the lens of a magnifying glass to focus rays of sunlight to a point.

Lasers are used for many reasons. In many instances, lasers can improve the precision of the surgeon with finely focused beams of light. Some lasers can reduce bleeding by coagulating blood vessels as they cut tissue. Others can be aimed down narrow passages or sent down fiber-optic channels in endoscopes to reach areas that are otherwise inaccessible.

Laser surgery uses the special properties of different wavelengths of laser light to selectively treat different problems. For instance, a yellow laser light absorbed by the red blood cells of a birthmark called a "portwine stain" can result in the selective destruction of the birthmark without affecting the skin cells around it. The result is that scarring of the remaining normal skin is lessened or avoided. In another instance of selective laser treatment, drugs that are retained by tumors are infused into the body and activated by lasers to destroy only the tumor, preserving normal structures.

In many instances, the cost of medical care can be reduced by lasers. Through their use, many procedures that previously required hospital admission can be done on an outpatient basis.

Photodynamic Therapy (PDT)

Photodynamic therapy (PDT) is a revolutionary medical technology that uses lasers to activate light-sensitive pharmaceuticals to treat cancer (and other diseases) in a minimally-invasive manner.

PDT is considered to be cancer-directed surgery, and there are specific codes in the surgery data fields for PDT of various primary sites.

PDT works as follows:

1. The patient is injected intravenously with a light-sensitive drug (most often, "photofrin").

2. The drug is retained by malignant tissue, remaining inactive until exposed to a specific wavelength of laser light.

3. Laser energy is directed to the site through a flexible fiberoptic device that allows the laser to be targeted precisely at the site.

4. When activated by the lasers' light energy, the drug creates a toxic form of oxygen that destroys the cancerous cells with minimal damage to surrounding healthy cells.

En Bloc Resection

An en bloc resection is a surgical procedure in which a lesion and surrounding tissues are removed. "En bloc" or "in continuity with" means that all of the tissues were removed during the same procedure, but not necessarily in a single specimen.

Chapter 3

Specialized Surgical Techniques

Chapter Contents

25

Section 3.1

Minimally Invasive Surgery (Laparoscopic Surgery)

This section contains text excerpted from the following sources:
Text in this section begins with excerpts from "Having Surgery?
What You Need to Know," Agency for Healthcare Research and
Quality (AHRQ), U.S. Department of Health and Human Services
(HHS), October 2005. Reviewed June 2017; Text under the heading
"Scope of Laparoscopic Surgery" is excerpted from "SBIR Phase II:
Enhanced Dexterity Minimally Invasive Surgical Platform," National
Science Foundation (NSF), October 26, 2016; Text beginning with
the heading "Instructions for Care after Outpatient Laparoscopic
Surgery" is excerpted from "Instructions for Care after Outpatient
Laparoscopic Surgery (Gynecology)," U.S. Department of Veterans
Affairs (VA), May 2005. Reviewed June 2017.

Is there more than one way of doing the operation? One way may
require more extensive surgery than another. Some operations that
once needed large incisions (cuts in the body) can now be done using
much smaller incisions. Some surgeries require that you stay in the
hospital for one or more days. Others let you come in and go home on
the same day.

Minimally Invasive Procedure

Usually, you will recover from this type of surgery more quickly.
These incisions let doctors insert a thin tube with a camera (a laparoscope) into the body to help them see. Then they use small tools to
do the surgery. This type of surgery is called laparoscopic surgery.
Removing the gallbladder, for example, is now mostly done with this
type of surgery.

Scope of Laparoscopic Surgery

In addition to patient benefits of less postsurgical pain, less scarring,
and quicker recovery, minimally invasive surgery also reduces healthcare cost due to shorter hospital stays and lower risk of postoperative

complications. Minimally invasive surgery impacts all surgical specialties, including gynecology, general, bariatric, urologic, and cardiothoracic. Although more than 1.5 million such procedures are performed
in the United States each year, wider adoption is limited by the high
cost of current surgical robots, training burden of traditional hand-held
instruments, and complexity of certain minimally invasive procedures.

Instructions for Care after Outpatient Laparoscopic Surgery

You have just had laparoscopic surgery in the outpatient surgery
unit. Self-care will be important for healing. You will want to understand and follow these directions:

1. You may well feel the effects of the anesthesia for the first 24
   hours after surgery. You can return to your regular diet if you
   feel up to it. If you feel nauseated (sick to your stomach) gradually work your way back to your regular diet over the next 24
   to 48 hours.

2. Do not drive for 24 hours after your surgery.

3. You will be given pain medicine. Be sure you know how often
   you can take it before you go home.

4. You can return to your regular activities after 48 hours, unless
   your doctor tells you something else.

5. You may remove the dressing (bandaid) after 48 hours. You
   need to keep the wound clean and dry. If your clothes will rub
   your wound or if you might get dirt or dust on it at work, put
   on a clean bandaid.

6. You may shower 24 hours after surgery. Remove the bandaid
   first. When drying the area, pat dry or dry with a hair dryer.
   Do not rub the wound with the towel or washcloth. Do not
   leave a wet bandaid on the wound.

7. Check your wound at least once a day for these signs of
   infection:

   - Increased pain

   - Increased swelling

   - Increased redness or warmth

- Any drainage (oozing)

- Fever (a temperature higher than 100.4°F) or chills

8. If you have any bleeding that soaks through the bandaid from the skin edges, put pressure on the wound for five minutes, then put on the wound for 15 minutes out of every hour for eight hours. If you have been given medicine or ointment, be sure you understand the instructions you were given before you leave. Follow all instructions carefully. If you have stitches that must be removed, you will be given an appointment to return in five to seven days to have them removed.

At this time, the doctor will also see how well you are healing. Self-dissolving stitches are usually used to close the incision (cut). If you have self-dissolving stitches, you will be scheduled for a follow-up appointment about two weeks after your surgery.

If you notice any of the signs of infection listed above, have any bleeding or oozing, or have any questions before your appointment, call the doctor.

Section 3.2

Robotic-Assisted Surgical Systems

This section contains text excerpted from the following sources: Text in this section begins with excerpts from "Computer-Assisted Surgical Systems," U.S. Food and Drug Administration (FDA), July 29, 2015; Text beginning with the heading "Background and Prevalence of Robotics in Surgery" is excerpted from "Robotic Surgery: Risks vs. Rewards," Agency for Healthcare Research and Quality (AHRQ), U.S. Department of Health and Human Services (HHS), February 2016.

Different types of computer-assisted surgical systems can be used for preoperative planning, surgical navigation, and to assist in performing surgical procedures. Robotically-assisted surgical (RAS) devices are one type of computer-assisted surgical system. Sometimes referred to as robotic surgery, RAS devices enable the surgeon to use computer and software technology to control and move surgical instruments through one or more tiny incisions in the patient's body (minimally invasive) for a variety of surgical procedures.

The benefits of a RAS device may include its ability to facilitate minimally invasive surgery and assist with complex tasks in confined areas of the body. The device is not actually a robot because it cannot perform surgery without direct human control.

RAS devices generally have several components, which may include:

- A console, where the surgeon sits during surgery. The console is the control center of the device and allows the surgeon to view the surgical field through a 3D endoscope and control movement of the surgical instruments;

- The bedside cart that includes three or four hinged mechanical arms, camera (endoscope), and surgical instruments that the surgeon controls during surgical procedures; and

- A separate cart that contains supporting hardware and software components, such as an electrosurgical unit (ESU), suction/irrigation pumps, and light source for the endoscope.

Most surgeons use multiple surgical instruments and accessories with the RAS device, such as scalpels, forceps, graspers, dissectors, cautery, scissors, retractors, and suction irrigators.

Common Uses of Robotic-Assisted Surgical (RAS) Devices

The U.S. Food and Drug Administration (FDA) has cleared robotically-assisted surgical (RAS) devices for use by trained physicians in an operating room environment for laparoscopic surgical procedures in general surgery cardiac, colorectal, gynecologic, head and neck, thoracic, and urologic surgical procedures. Some common procedures that may involve RAS devices are gall-bladder removal, hysterectomy, and prostatectomy (removal of the prostate).

Recommendations for Healthcare Providers and Patients about RAS

Patients

Robotically-assisted surgery is an important treatment option but may not be appropriate in all situations. Talk to your physician about the risks and benefits of robotically-assisted surgeries, as well as the risks and benefits of other treatment options.

Patients who are considering treatment with robotically-assisted surgeries should discuss the options for these devices with their healthcare provider, and feel free to inquire about their surgeon's training and experience with these devices.

Healthcare Providers

Robotically-assisted surgery is an important treatment option that is safe and effective when used appropriately and with proper training. The FDA does not regulate the practice of medicine and therefore does not supervise or provide accreditation for physician training nor does it oversee training and education related to legally marketed medical devices. Instead, training development and implementation is the responsibility of the manufacturer, physicians, and healthcare facilities. In some cases, professional societies and specialty board certification organizations may also develop and support training for their specialty physicians. Specialty boards also maintain certification status of their specialty physicians.

Physicians, hospitals, and facilities that use RAS devices should ensure that proper training is completed and that surgeons have appropriate credentials to perform surgical procedures with these devices. Device users should ensure they maintain their credentialing. Hospitals and facilities should also ensure that other surgical staff that use these devices complete proper training.

Users of the device should realize that there are several different models of robotically-assisted surgical devices. Each model may operate differently and may not have the same functions. Users should know the differences between the models and make sure to get appropriate training on each model.

If you suspect a problem or complications associated with the use of RAS devices, the FDA encourages you to file a voluntary report through MedWatch, the FDA Safety Information and Adverse Event Reporting Program (www.accessdata.fda.gov/scripts/medwatch/index.cfm?action=reporting.home). Healthcare personnel employed by facilities that are subject to FDA's user facility reporting requirements should follow the reporting procedures established by their facilities. Prompt reporting of adverse events can help the FDA identify and better understand the risks associated with medical devices.

Background and Prevalence of Robotics in Surgery

The use of robotic assistance in surgery has expanded exponentially since it was first approved in 2000. It is estimated that, worldwide, more than 570,000 procedures were performed with the da Vinci robotic surgical system in 2014, with this figure growing almost 10 percent each year. Robotic-assisted surgery (RAS) has found its way into almost every surgical subspecialty and now has approved uses in urology, gynecology, cardiothoracic surgery, general surgery, and otolaryngology. RAS is most commonly used in urology and gynecology; more than 75 percent of robotic procedures performed are within these two specialties. Robotic surgical systems have the potential to improve surgical technique and outcomes, but they also create a unique set of risks and patient safety concerns.

RAS is a derivative of standard laparoscopic surgery and was developed to overcome the limitations of standard laparoscopy. Like traditional laparoscopy, RAS uses small incisions and insufflation of the anatomical operative space with carbon dioxide. The robotic camera and various instruments are placed through the ports into the body and can be manipulated by the surgeon performing the operation. In the case of RAS, though, the surgeon, seated at a computer console in the operating room, uses robot assistance to utilize the tools (instead of doing it himself or herself directly at the bedside). In RAS, a bedside assistant exchanges the instruments and performs manual tasks like retraction and suction. There are three major components of the system including:

- The robot, which is a mobile tower with four arms, including a camera arm and three instrument arms.

- The bedside cart, consisting of the image processing equipment and light source, which is transmitted to monitors in the operating suite and sends the image to the surgeon console.

- The console, at which the surgeon sits to operate; there are two binocular lenses that magnify and create a three-dimensional image for the surgeon. Two hand pieces transmit the surgeon's hand movements to the instruments within the patient, manipulating the surgical instruments to perform the operation. A built-in motion filtration system minimizes tremor, and foot pedals at the console control different types of energy and also allow for movement of the different robotic components within the patient.

Benefits of RAS

In theory, RAS marries the benefits of laparoscopic surgery with that of open techniques by combining a minimally invasive approach with the additional benefit of a three-dimensional, magnified image. In addition, RAS offers improved ergonomics and dexterity compared to traditional laparoscopy, and these advantages may lead to a shorter learning curve for surgeons. The purported benefits of RAS also include smaller incisions, decreased blood loss, shorter hospital stays, faster return to work, improved cosmesis, and lower incidence of some surgical complications.

While we appreciate these advantages of RAS, most of these benefits are short term and limited to the acute perioperative period. In fact, there is little evidence demonstrating that robotic surgery provides any long-term benefits over open techniques. Taking the above case as an example, robotic-assisted laparoscopic prostatectomy (RALP) has been one of the most commonly adopted robotic procedures; more than 85 percent of all prostatectomies are now performed with robotic assistance in the United States. Multiple, well-validated studies have shown that RALP has significantly less blood loss, with much lower transfusion rates, and shorter hospital stays than with open approaches.

In addition, the rates of some complications—deep vein thrombosis, wound infections, lymphoceles and hematomas, anastomotic leaks, and ureteral injuries—appear to be slightly lower than with open approaches. RALP appears to have similar advantages over laparoscopic prostatectomy, although the difference is less pronounced. When compared to standard laparoscopic prostatectomy, robotic assistance has been shown to have decreased blood loss, lower rates of blood transfusion, and slightly shorter hospital stays. Like with robotic assistance, pure laparoscopic techniques share a significant learning curve. While some studies have also suggested that robotic surgery may be more effective at total removal of cancerous tissue in prostate surgery (i.e., lower positive surgical margin rates) than with open and pure laparoscopic procedures, large systematic reviews and well-validated meta-analyses have shown similar rates of oncologic control.

Interestingly, the proponents of RALP frequently boast improved urinary continence and sexual function after surgery (or at least equivalent rates) when compared to open prostatectomy. The data has generally been equivocal in this area; standardized, comparable, long-term data are lacking.

A study using surveillance, epidemiology, and end results Medicare claims data compared open to minimally invasive prostatectomy (laparoscopic and robotic). Their results supported previous findings of lower transfusion rates, shorter hospital stays, similar oncologic control, and fewer miscellaneous complications. On the other hand, they discovered that men who had undergone robotic prostatectomy had higher rates of postprostatectomy incontinence and erectile dysfunction than men who had an open procedure.

It may be a matter of experience: Many of RALP proponents have performed thousands of procedures, which may lead to improved outcomes in their hands but may not be generalized to other, less experienced, urologists.

Risks of RAS

RAS shares the same risks of open and laparoscopic surgery, including the potential for infection, bleeding, and the cardiopulmonary risks of anesthesia. On top of that, there are additional risks that are unique to the robotic system. Not only is there potential for human error in operating the robotic technology, but an added risk of mechanical failure is also introduced. Multiple components of the system can malfunction, including the camera, binocular lenses, robotic tower, robotic arms, and instruments. The energy source, which is prone to electric arcing, can cause unintended internal burn injuries from the cautery device. Arcing occurs when electrical current from the robotic instrument leaves the robotic arm and is misdirected to surrounding tissue.

This can cause sparks and burns leading to tissue damage which may not always be immediately recognized. There is a small risk of temporary, and even permanent, nerve palsies from the extreme body positioning needed to dock the robot and access the pelvis adequately to perform RALP. Direct nerve compression from the robotic arms can also lead to nerve palsies. RAS has also been shown to take significantly longer than nonrobotic procedures when performed at centers with lower robotic volume and by surgeons with less experience, and, overall, it is more expensive than open surgery.

As mentioned earlier, the outcomes in RAS seem to correlate with individual surgeon experience. For example, in cancer surgery, surgeons with more experience are more likely to have clean margins. Other studies have documented lower complication rates with an increasing number of procedures. These findings of practice makes perfect are not specific to robotic surgery; such findings have been seen in many procedures. There are varying reports of exactly how many cases are required to master the robotic learning curve, and the number varies by surgical procedure. For RALP, the range has been reported from as low as 40 to as many as 250. For hysterectomies, the literature reports a range of 20–50 cases to master the operation and reports that less experienced surgeons have significantly longer operative times.

Notwithstanding the concerns, RAS has been accepted as generally safe. RALP has reported complication rates (including all grades of perioperative complications, from minor to life-threatening) of around 10 percent. Multiple risk factors can increase the possibility of complications and errors: patient factors (i.e., obesity or underlying comorbidities), surgeon factors (training and experience), and robotic factors (i.e., mechanical malfunction). The reported complication rate related directly to robotic malfunction is very low, approximately 0.1%–0.5%.

However, when robotic errors do occur, the rates of permanent injury have been reported anywhere from 4.8%–46.6%, and this literature may suffer from underreporting. Although fewer than 800 complications directly attributable to the robotic operating system have been reported to the U.S. Food and Drug Administration (FDA) over the past 10 years, in a web-based survey among urologists performing RALP, almost 57 percent of respondents had experienced an irrecoverable intraoperative malfunction of the robot. The most common areas of complications were malfunction of the robotic arms, joint setup and camera, followed by power error, instrument malfunction, and breakage of the handpiece.

Preventing Complications of RAS

Standardized Credentialing and Training

There are no universal standard guidelines on appropriate training or credentialing for robotic surgery. Some organizations have made progress in this area. The American Urological Association (AUA) has made recommendations for training and credentialing procedures consisting of specific online curriculum, testing, caseload requirements, and also recommendations that all physicians complete the da Vinci online robotic safety training course on set-up, draping, specific safety features, and troubleshooting. Training in robotics is still a relatively new field, and there is not a strong body of evidence to support a specific training and credentialing model. Various authors have developed different curriculums and simulation models, but an ideal model has yet to be found, as this is a new and developing field.

Until well-validated credentialing and training models can be developed, hospitals should require a basic robotic safety curriculum, such as provided by the AUA, for any surgeons using the surgical robot, and require case logs be supplied or case proctoring prior to granting robotic privileges.

Stricter Reporting Guidelines

Developing a more uniform system of error reporting and tougher penalties for noncompliance may potentially help capture a more accurate representation of the true incidence of adverse events. It is important to determine the true incidence of different complications and the surrounding circumstances. The goal should be to identify key risk factors for errors and complications with a focus on those that are modifiable. This ideally would lead to improved outcomes and fewer complications. There are clearly gaps with the current FDA device tracking system, as many more robotic errors are experienced than are ever reported to the FDA. There needs to be a more rigorous reporting effort by individual hospitals to capture the true incidence of robotic malfunction. These institutional reports can be submitted to the FDA so that recurrent mechanical problems can be more easily and rapidly recognized and addressed by the manufacturer.

Appropriate Risk Disclosure to Patients

The idea of robotic surgery is very enticing to patients and has influenced the growth of robotics in the United States. However, Schroeck and colleagues found that men undergoing robotic prostatectomy were more likely to express "regret" and "dissatisfaction" than men undergoing open surgery, which was attributed to unrealistic patient expectations associated with the robot. Kaushik and colleagues found that less than 70 percent of patients were appropriately counseled preoperatively on the potential risks specific to robotic surgery, including possible robotic malfunction or potential conversion to an open procedure. The direct-to-consumer marketing phenomenon could be used to improve safety in robotics by appropriately educating patients. Institutions should ensure appropriate patient counseling and informed consent for RAS is happening consistently. This tracking could be accomplished through auditing of informed consent materials as well as intermittent patient interviews.

While RAS has many potential benefits for patients and providers, the case above clearly demonstrates that the technology itself may place patients at risk. National organizations and individual institutions should ensure appropriate training and credentialing, accurate and timely error reporting, and consistent informed consent for patients. Discussions about robotic surgery—both with individual patients and at the policy level—should appropriately balance the advantages and potential with the real risks and limited evidence of major advantages in terms of long-term outcomes.

Section 3.3

Laser Surgery

This section contains text excerpted from the following sources: Text beginning with the heading "Laser" is excerpted from "Frequently Asked Questions about Lasers," U.S. Food and Drug Administration (FDA), February 27, 2017; Text beginning with the heading "Medical Lasers" is excerpted from "Surgical and Therapeutic Products— Medical Lasers," U.S. Food and Drug Administration (FDA), November 30, 2016.

Laser

Laser stands for Light Amplification by the Stimulated Emission of Radiation. One basic type of laser consists of a sealed tube, containing a pair of mirrors, and a laser medium that is excited by some form of energy to produce visible light, or invisible ultraviolet or infrared radiation.

There are many different types of lasers and each uses a different type of laser medium. Common laser media include gases such as argon or a helium and neon mixture, solid crystals such as ruby, and liquid dyes or chemicals. When energy is applied to the laser medium, it becomes excited and releases energy as particles of light (photons).

A pair of mirrors at either end of the sealed tube either reflects or transmits the light (see illustration below) in the form of a concentrated stream called a laser beam. Each laser medium produces a beam of a unique wavelength and color.

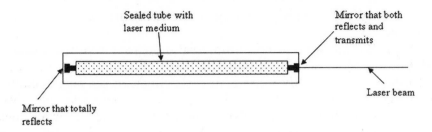

Figure 3.1. *Laser*

Uses of Lasers

Lasers are used for a variety of purposes including pointing out objects during a presentation, aligning materials at construction sites and in the home, and by doctors for cosmetic and surgical procedures. Many items you encounter on a daily basis use lasers, including CD and DVD players; bar code scanners; dental drills; laser-guided tools, such as levels; and laser pointers.

Lasers Are Uniquely Hazardous

Two characteristics of laser light contribute to the hazard:

- Laser light can be emitted in a tight beam that does not grow in size at a distance from the laser. This means that the same degree of hazard can be present both close to and far from the laser.

- The eye can focus a laser beam to a very small, intense spot on its retina, which can result in a burn or blind spot.

Laser Radiation

Some lasers emit radiation in the form of light. Others emit radiation that is invisible to the eye, such as ultraviolet or infrared radiation. In general, laser radiation is not in itself harmful, and behaves much like ordinary light in its interaction with the body. Laser radiation should not be confused with radio waves, microwaves, or the ionizing X-rays or radiation from radioactive substances such as radium.

Lasers and Their Legal Usage

Are all lasers legal for consumer use? No. Some lasers are strictly for use by medical, industrial, or entertainment professionals and should only be used by a person with appropriate training and licenses.

The U.S. Food and Drug Administration (FDA) requires labels on most laser products that contain a warning about the laser radiation and other hazards, and a statement certifying that the laser complies with FDA safety regulations. The label must also state the power output and the hazard class of the product. Consumer laser products are generally in classes I, II, and III a, while lasers for professional use may be in classes III b and IV.

Medical Lasers

Medical lasers are medical devices that use precisely focused light sources to treat or remove tissues. Laser light has a specific wavelength. It is focused in a narrow beam and creates a very high-intensity light. Because lasers can focus very accurately on tiny areas, they can be used for very precise surgical work or for cutting through tissue (in place of a scalpel).

Procedures Using Laser

Lasers are used in many types of surgical procedures. Some examples include:

- Cosmetic surgery (to remove tattoos, scars, stretch marks, sun spots, wrinkles, birthmarks, spider veins, or hair)

- Refractive eye surgery (to reshape the cornea in order to correct or improve vision as in laser-assisted in situ keratomileusis (LASIK) or PRK)

- Dental procedures (such as endodontic/periodontic procedures, tooth whitening, and oral surgery)

- General surgery (such as tumor removal, cataract removal, breast surgery, plastic surgery, and most other surgical procedures)

Risks and Benefits of Using Laser

With proper use, lasers allow the surgeon to accomplish more complex tasks, reduce blood loss, decrease postoperative discomfort, reduce the chance of wound infection, and achieve better wound healing.

As with any type of surgery, laser surgery has potential risks. Risks of laser surgery include incomplete treatment of the problem, pain, infection, bleeding, scarring, and skin color changes.

Laser surgery uses nonionizing radiation, so it does not have the same long-term risks as X-rays or other types of ionizing radiation.

Chapter 4

Understanding Pediatric Surgery

The understanding that children are not merely small adults paved way for the evolution of pediatric surgery as a specialty nearly 82 years ago. Children need a different approach for their medical treatment. They cannot always clearly explain their symptoms and are generally incapable of answering medical questions. Medical examination of children can also be difficult due to their inability or refusal to cooperate.

Who Is a Pediatric Surgeon?

A pediatric surgeon is a specialist who is trained to perform surgical procedures on newborns, children, and adolescents. They have the proficiency to treat a range of congenital, oncologic, gastrointestinal, thoracic, vascular, infectious, and traumatic disorders specific to children, and they are skilled in negotiating with sick children and their anxious parents. Offices for pediatric surgical practices often have interiors decorated and designed specifically for children. The waiting and examination rooms may have toys, books, and videos to make the atmosphere conducive and nonthreatening.

"Understanding Pediatric Surgery," © 2017 Omnigraphics. Reviewed June 2017.

What Role Does a Pediatric Surgeon Play in Treating Children?

Pediatric surgeons are involved in the diagnosis and management of all operative stages during surgery for children. They often consult with neonatologists, pediatricians, and other specialists to determine if surgery can improve the quality of life for a child. Pediatric surgeons also play a major role in treating congenital deformities that will hamper a child's quality of life if not surgically corrected.

What Expertise Do Pediatric Surgeons Possess?

Pediatric surgery can be subdivided into several different specialties:

Neonatal: Focused on treating life-threatening birth defects and conditions in newborns such as tracheoesophageal fistula, imperforate anus, etc.

Pediatric Oncology: The diagnosis and surgery of malignant tumors and benign growths in children.

Prenatal: Prenatal pediatric surgeons consult radiologists and use diagnostic techniques such as ultrasound to detect and correct developmental anomalies in fetuses.

Trauma: Pediatric trauma surgeons attend to a large number of children who have sustained traumatic injuries that require surgical intervention, such as gunshot wounds or injuries are skilled in a car accident. Pediatric surgeons play an important role in preventing traumatic injuries in children by participating in community prevention programs.

What Are the Surgeries Done by Pediatric Surgeons?

Pediatric surgeons perform many of the same procedures as general surgeons, including

- Surgery for congenital abdominal wall defects.
- Surgical care for abnormalities of the groin which include undescended testes, hernias, hydroceles and varicoceles.
- Surgical removal of congenital obstructions of the gastrointestinal tract.

- Surgical repair of birth defects.

- Surgical treatment of injuries like gunshot wounds, knife cuts, and lacerations in the liver.

- Cancer surgeries

- Transplantations

- Appendectomy

- Endoscopic procedures such as bronchoscopy and colonoscopy.

What Kind of Training Do Pediatric Surgeons Undergo?

Pediatric surgeons complete regular medical school and have at least 5 years of experience in general surgery in an accredited residency program. They have to practice pediatric surgery for two more years in a fellowship program to ensure the highest level of surgical knowledge for treating infants and children before becoming certified by the American Board of Surgery (ABS). The certificate is renewable every 10 years to ensure competency and requires up to date knowledge in pediatric surgery.

References

1. "What is a Pediatric Surgeon?" American Pediatric Surgical Association, n.d.

2. "What is a Pediatric Surgeon?" American Academy of Pediatrics, November 21, 2015.

3. "Pediatric Surgery," Association of Women Surgeons, n.d.

4. "What is a Pediatric Surgeon?" Actforlibraries.org, n.d.

Chapter 5

Surgery in Older Adults

Have you been told by your doctor that you need surgery? If so, you're not alone. Millions of older Americans have surgery each year.

For most surgeries, you will have time to find out about the operation, talk about other treatments with your surgeon (medical doctor who does the operation), and decide what to do. You also have time to get a second opinion.

Questions to Ask

Deciding to have surgery can be hard, but it may be easier once you know why you need surgery. Talk with your surgeon about the operation. It may help to take a member of your family or a friend with you. Don't hesitate to ask the surgeon any questions you might have. For example, do the benefits of surgery outweigh the risks? Risks may include infections, bleeding a lot, or a reaction to the anesthesia (medicine that puts you to sleep).

Your surgeon should be willing to answer your questions. If you don't understand the answers, ask the surgeon to explain more clearly. Answers to the following questions will help you make an informed decision about your treatment:

- What is the surgery? Do I need it now, or can I wait?

- Can another treatment be tried instead of surgery?

This chapter includes text excerpted from "Considering Surgery?" National Institute on Aging (NIA), National Institutes of Health (NIH), July 26, 2016.

- How will the surgery affect my health and lifestyle?

- What kind of anesthesia will be used? What are the side effects and risks of having anesthesia?

- Will I be in pain? How long will the pain last?

- When will I be able to go home after the surgery?

- What will the recovery be like? How long will it take to feel better?

- What will happen if I don't have the surgery?

- Is there anything else I should know about this surgery?

Choosing a Surgeon

Your primary care doctor may suggest a surgeon to you. Your state or local medical society can tell you about your surgeon's training. Try to choose a surgeon who operates often on medical problems like yours.

Getting a Second Opinion

Getting a second opinion means asking another doctor about your surgical plan. It is a common medical practice. Most doctors think it's a good idea. With a second opinion, you will get expert advice from another surgeon who knows about treating your medical problem. A second opinion can help you make a good decision.

You can ask your surgeon to send your medical records to the second doctor. This can save time and money since you may not have to repeat tests. When getting a second opinion, be sure to tell the doctor about all your symptoms and the type of surgery that has been suggested.

Medicare may help pay for a second opinion. If you have a private supplemental health insurance plan, find out if it covers a second opinion.

Informed Consent

Before having any surgery, you will be asked to sign a consent form. This form says that the surgeon has told you about the operation, the risks involved, and what results to expect. It's important to talk about all your concerns before signing this form. Your surgeon should be willing to take the time needed to make sure you know what is likely to happen before, during, and after surgery.

Outpatient Surgery

Outpatient surgery, sometimes called same-day surgery, is common for many types of operations. Outpatient surgery can be done in a special part of the hospital or in a surgical center. You will go home within hours after the surgery. Outpatient surgery can cost less than an overnight hospital stay. Your doctor will tell you if outpatient surgery is right for you.

Planning for Surgery

There are many steps you can take to make having surgery a little easier.

Before surgery:

- Make sure you have your preoperation tests and screenings, such as blood tests and X-rays.

- Be sure you have all your insurance questions answered.

- Make plans for any medical equipment or help with healthcare you will need when you go home.

- Arrange for an adult to drive you home and stay with you for the first 24 hours after surgery.

- Get written instructions about your care, a phone number to call if you have a problem, and prescription medicines you'll need at home.

The day of surgery:

- Leave your jewelry at home.

- Don't wear makeup or contact lenses to surgery.

Following surgery:

- Make sure you follow all your doctor's directions once you're home.

- Go for your scheduled postoperative check-up.

- Ask your doctor when you can return to your normal activities.

Paying for Surgery

The total cost of any surgery includes many different bills. Your surgeon can tell you how much he or she charges. You may also be billed by other doctors, such as the anesthesiologist. There will be hospital charges as well. To find out what the hospital will cost, call the hospital's business office.

For information about Medicare benefits, call the toll-free customer service line at 800-633-4227. If you have secondary or supplemental health insurance, check to see what part of the costs it will pay. Talk to your surgeon if you can't afford the surgery.

In Case of Emergency Surgery

An accident or sudden illness may result in emergency surgery. That's why you should always carry the following information with you:

- your doctor's name and phone number
- family names and phone numbers
- ongoing medical problems
- medicines you take, including prescription and over-the-counter drugs
- allergies to medicines
- health insurance information and policy numbers

Make copies of this information to keep in your wallet and glove compartment of your car—just in case you need emergency care.

Chapter 6

Surgery Statistics

Chapter Contents

Section 6.1

Ambulatory Surgery Data

This section includes text excerpted from "Ambulatory
Surgery Data from Hospitals and Ambulatory Surgery
Centers: United States, 2010," Centers for Disease
Control and Prevention (CDC), February 28, 2017.

Ambulatory surgery, also called outpatient surgery, refers to surgical and nonsurgical procedures that are nonemergency, scheduled in advance, and generally do not result in an overnight hospital stay.

Ambulatory surgery has increased in the United States since the early 1980s. Two factors that contributed to this increase were medical and technological advancements, including improvements in anesthesia and in analgesics for the relief of pain, and the development and expansion of minimally invasive and noninvasive procedures (such as laser surgery, laparoscopy, and endoscopy). Before these advances, almost all surgery was performed in inpatient settings. Any outpatient surgery was likely to have been minor, performed in physicians' offices, and paid for by Medicare and insurers as part of the physician's office visit reimbursement.

Ambulatory Surgery Procedure and Visit Overview

- In 2010, 28.6 million ambulatory surgery visits to hospitals and ambulatory surgery centers occurred. During these visits, an estimated 48.3 million surgical and nonsurgical procedures were performed.

- An estimated 25.7 million (53%) ambulatory surgery procedures were performed in hospitals and 22.5 million (47%) were performed in ambulatory surgery centers.

- Private insurance was the expected payment source for 51 percent of the visits for ambulatory surgery, Medicare payment was expected for 31 percent, and Medicaid for 8 percent. Only 4 percent were self-pay.

- Ninety-five percent of the visits with a specified discharge disposition had a routine discharge, generally to the patient's home. Patients were admitted to the hospital as inpatients during only 2 percent of these visits.

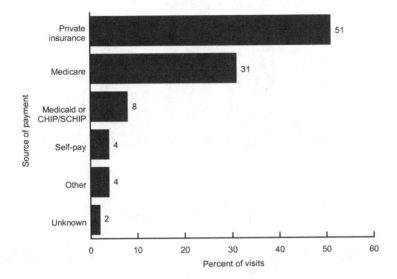

Figure 6.1. *Percent Distribution of Ambulatory Surgery Visits in Hospitals and Ambulatory Surgery Centers, by Principal Expected Source of Payment: United States, 2010.*

Note: CHIP is Children's Health Insurance Program and SCHIP is State Children's Health Insurance Program.
Source: NCHS, National Hospital Ambulatory Medical Care Survey, 2010

Ambulatory Surgery Procedures, by Sex and Age

- For both males and females, 39 percent of procedures were performed on those aged 45–64.

- For females, about 24 percent of procedures were performed on those aged 15–44 compared with 18 percent for males, whereas the percentage of procedures performed on those under 15 was lower for females than for males (4% compared with 9%).

- About 19 percent of procedures were performed on those aged 65–74, with about 14 percent performed on those aged 75 and over.

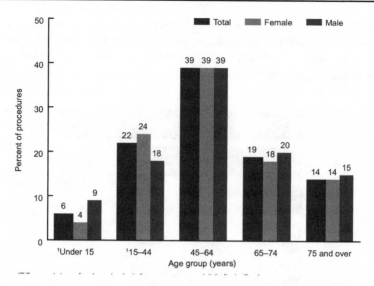

Figure 6.2. *Percent Distribution of Ambulatory Surgery Procedures in Hospitals and Ambulatory Surgery Centers, by Age and Sex: United States, 2010.*

[1]*Differences between females and males in these age groups are statistically significant.*

Notes: Numbers may not add to totals because of rounding.

Source: NCHS, National Hospital Ambulatory Medical Care Survey, 2010.

Types of Procedures

Seventy percent of the 48.3 million ambulatory surgery procedures were included in the following clinical categories:

- operations on the digestive system (10 million or 21%),
- operations on the eye (7.9 million or 16%),
- operations on the musculoskeletal system (7.1 million or 15%),
- operations on the integumentary system (4.3 million or 9%), and
- operations on the nervous system (4.2 million or 9%).

These procedure categories made up 72 percent of procedures performed on females and 67 percent of those performed on males. Within the above-mentioned categories, data on procedures performed more than 1 million times are presented below.

Under operations on the digestive system, endoscopy of large intestine—which included colonoscopies—was performed 4 million times, and endoscopy of small intestine was performed 2.2 million times. Endoscopic polypectomy of large intestine was performed an estimated 1.1 million times.

Eye operations included extraction of lens, performed 2.9 million times; insertion of lens, performed 2.6 million times for cataracts; and operations on eyelids, performed 1 million times.

Musculoskeletal procedures included operations on muscle, tendon, fascia, and bursa (1.3 million).

Operations on the integumentary system included excision or destruction of lesion or tissue of skin and subcutaneous tissue (1.2 million). Operations on the nervous system included injection of agent into spinal canal (2.9 million), including injections for pain relief.

Section 6.2

Benign Uterine Fibroids Surgery

This section includes text excerpted from "Procedures to Treat Benign Uterine Fibroids in Hospital Inpatient and Hospital-Based Ambulatory Surgery Settings, 2013," Agency for Healthcare Research and Quality (AHRQ), U.S. Department of Health and Human Services (HHS), January 2016.

By the age of 50, as many as 70–80 percent of women will develop uterine fibroids (leiomyomas)—typically benign tumors of the uterus. For many women, uterine fibroids pose no health risks and women are asymptomatic. For others, uterine fibroids may cause symptoms such as heavy bleeding, pain, and frequent urination, and they are associated with an increased risk of pregnancy complications. Some women are more likely than others to develop uterine fibroids. For instance, uterine fibroids are more common in Black than in White women, and Black women tend to have more severe symptoms. Research also indicates that, compared with White women, Black women develop uterine fibroids at a younger age and have more severe fibroids (e.g., larger size, number, and growth rate).

For women with symptomatic fibroids, a variety of treatment options are available. Women with mild symptoms may choose medical treatments such as pain relievers and hormonal drugs. Those with moderate to severe symptoms may need surgery to treat uterine fibroids. Common surgical treatment options include hysterectomy (removing the uterus), myomectomy (removing the fibroids), uterine fibroid embolization (blocking the blood supply to the fibroids), and endometrial ablation (removing the lining of the uterus, which controls bleeding without directly affecting the fibroids).

This chapter focuses on four common surgical treatments of benign uterine fibroids: hysterectomy, myomectomy, uterine fibroid embolization, and endometrial ablation. An overview of characteristics of women with benign uterine fibroids who underwent one of these surgical treatments in 2013 is provided by hospital setting. It also presents trends in the four surgical procedures to treat benign uterine fibroids by hospital setting from 2005 through 2013. The distribution of these four procedures by patient race/ethnicity and expected primary payer in each hospital setting is provided for 2013. Only differences of at least 10 percent are noted in the text.

Highlights

- In 2013, four surgical procedures for benign uterine fibroids were about as common in the hospital-based ambulatory surgery (AS) setting as in the inpatient setting (47.8 versus 52.2%). Compared with inpatient stays, AS visits had a shorter average length of stay (0.6 versus 2.3 days) and lower average hospital charges ($25,200 versus $28,000).

- Between 2005 and 2013, the overall rate of hysterectomy decreased by 20 percent, from 210.8 to 168.0 per 100,000 women aged 18–54 years. This change was driven by a 52 percent decrease in the rate of inpatient hysterectomy. The rate of AS hysterectomy increased by over 400 percent during this time period.

- The rate of inpatient myomectomy decreased by 29 percent, and the rate of AS myomectomy remained relatively constant. The rate of both inpatient and AS uterine fibroid embolization increased by approximately 170 percent. The rate of endometrial ablation decreased in both the inpatient and AS settings (40 and 19% decrease, respectively).

- To treat benign uterine fibroids, Black and Hispanic women more commonly had inpatient surgery whereas White women more commonly had AS.

- Private insurance was the predominant expected payer for both inpatient stays and AS visits involving procedures to treat benign uterine fibroids. Medicaid paid for more inpatient stays than AS visits.

Characteristics of hospitalization for benign uterine fibroids by setting, in 13 States, 2013

- Four surgical procedures for benign uterine fibroids were about as common in the hospital-based ambulatory surgery setting as in the hospital inpatient setting, but the length of stay and hospital charges were lower in the ambulatory surgery setting.

In 2013, 47.8 percent of benign uterine fibroids were treated in the hospital-based ambulatory surgery setting compared with 52.2 percent in the hospital inpatient setting using the four surgical procedures. The outpatient length of stay was substantially shorter than the inpatient length of stay (0.6 versus 2.3 days), and mean hospital charges were lower in the ambulatory surgery setting ($25,200 versus $28,000).

- White women, privately insured patients, and those in higher income quartiles were a larger proportion of patients treated for benign uterine fibroids in the hospital-based ambulatory surgery setting than in the inpatient setting.

Black women represented the largest proportion (40.3%) of hospital inpatient stays involving the four surgical procedures for benign uterine fibroids in 2013. White women were the largest proportion (51.4%) of hospital-based ambulatory surgery visits for these procedures.

Private insurance was the expected primary payer for the majority of hospitalizations involving the four surgical procedures for benign uterine fibroids. Privately insured women were a higher proportion of ambulatory surgery visits than inpatient stays (80.4 versus 70.1%), whereas women covered by Medicaid and uninsured women were a lower proportion of ambulatory surgery visits than inpatient stays (Medicaid: 10.6 versus 17.7%; uninsured: 3.2 versus 6.3%).

Patients living in communities in the lowest income quartile were a higher proportion of inpatient stays than ambulatory surgery visits (24.8 versus 21.2%).

Ninety percent of women with the four surgical procedures for benign uterine fibroids were aged 35–54 years in both the hospital-based ambulatory surgery and inpatient settings.

- A majority of the four surgical procedures for benign uterine fibroids were hysterectomies.

In 2013, hysterectomy constituted more than three-fourths of the inpatient surgeries and two-thirds of the hospital-based ambulatory surgery visits for benign uterine fibroids involving the four surgical procedures (76.5 and 66.8%, respectively). Myomectomy represented approximately 22 percent of surgeries in both the inpatient and ambulatory surgery settings. Uterine fibroid embolization and endometrial ablation were a higher proportion of the four surgical procedures in the ambulatory surgery setting than in the inpatient setting (uterine fibroid embolization: 6.7 versus 1.6%; endometrial ablation: 4.3 versus 0.1%).

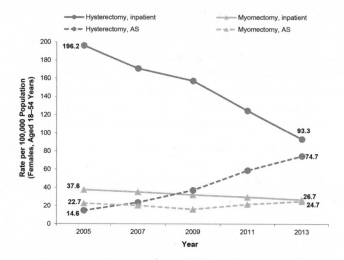

Figure 6.3. *Rate of Hysterectomy and Myomectomy to Treat Benign Uterine Fibroids by Hospital Setting, in 13 States, 2005–2013.*

Abbreviations: AS, ambulatory surgery
Source: Agency for Healthcare Research and Quality (AHRQ), Center for Delivery, Organization, and Markets, Healthcare Cost and Utilization Project (HCUP), State Inpatient Databases (SID) and State Ambulatory Surgery and Services Databases (SASD) from 13 States, 2005, 2007, 2009, 2011, 2013

Rate of hysterectomy and myomectomy to treat benign uterine fibroids by hospital setting, in 13 States, 2005–2013

- Between 2005 and 2013, the rates of hysterectomy and myomectomy decreased in the hospital inpatient setting; the rate of hysterectomy increased in the hospital-based ambulatory surgery setting.

Overall, the population rate of hysterectomy for benign uterine fibroids decreased 20 percent between 2005 and 2013, from 210.8 to

168.0 per 100,000 women aged 18–54 years. This decrease was driven by a 52 percent decrease in the rate of hysterectomy in the hospital inpatient setting, from 196.2 to 93.3 per 100,000 women in 2013. At the same time, the rate of hysterectomy increased 410 percent in the hospital-based ambulatory surgery setting, from 14.6 to 74.7 per 100,000 women. The rate of myomectomy also decreased 29 percent in the inpatient setting (from 37.6 to 26.7 per 100,000 women) but remained relatively constant in the hospital-based ambulatory surgery setting.

Rate of uterine fibroid embolization and endometrial ablation to treat benign uterine fibroids by hospital setting, in 13 States, 2005–2013

- Between 2005 and 2013, the rate of uterine fibroid embolization increased in the hospital inpatient and ambulatory surgery settings; the rate of endometrial ablation decreased in both settings.

Overall, the rates of uterine fibroid embolization and endometrial ablation were much lower than the rates of hysterectomy and

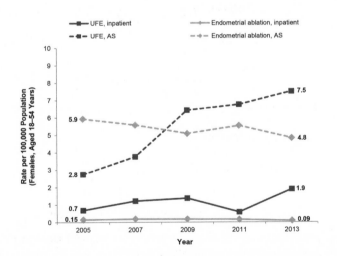

Figure 6.4. *Rate of Uterine Fibroid Embolization and Endometrial Ablation to Treat Benign Uterine Fibroids by Hospital Setting, in 13 States, 2005–2013.*

Abbreviations: AS, ambulatory surgery; UFE, uterine fibroid embolization
Source: Agency for Healthcare Research and Quality (AHRQ), Center for Delivery, Organization, and Markets, Healthcare Cost and Utilization Project (HCUP), State Inpatient Databases (SID) and State Ambulatory Surgery and Services Databases (SASD) from 13 States, 2005, 2007, 2009, 2011, 2013

myomectomy. Between 2005 and 2013, the rate of uterine fibroid embolization increased approximately 170 percent in both the hospital inpatient and ambulatory surgery settings (inpatient: from 0.7 to 1.9 per 100,000 women; AS: from 2.8 to 7.5 per 100,000 women). The rate of endometrial ablation decreased in both settings during this same time period (inpatient: 40% decrease, from 0.15 to 0.09 per 100,000 women; AS: 19% decrease, from 5.9 to 4.8 per 100,000 women).

Distribution of surgical procedures to treat benign uterine fibroids by hospital setting, in 13 States, 2013

- Most open hysterectomy and myomectomy procedures were performed in the hospital inpatient setting, whereas most laparoscopic hysterectomy and myomectomy procedures were performed in the hospital-based ambulatory surgery setting.

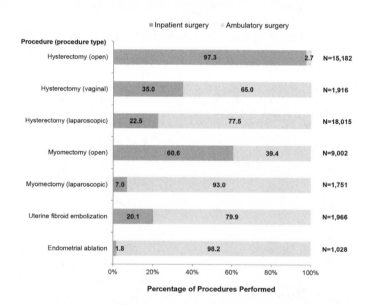

Figure 6.5. *Distribution of Surgical Procedures to Treat Benign Uterine Fibroids by Hospital Setting, in 13 States, 2013.*

Notes: Open hysterectomy and myomectomy involve removing the uterus or fibroids through an abdominal incision. Laparoscopic hysterectomy and myomectomy utilize a telescopic camera and surgical tools inserted through small abdominal incisions. Vaginal hysterectomy is performed through the vagina.

Source: Agency for Healthcare Research and Quality (AHRQ), Center for Delivery, Organization, and Markets (CDOM), Healthcare Cost and Utilization Project (HCUP), State Inpatient Databases (SID) and State Ambulatory Surgery and Services Databases (SASD) from 13 States, 2013

In 2013, nearly all open hysterectomies (97.3%) and the majority of open myomectomies (60.6%) were performed in the hospital inpatient setting. In contrast, laparoscopic or vaginal procedures occurred more commonly in the hospital-based ambulatory surgery setting (laparoscopic hysterectomy: 77.5%; vaginal hysterectomy: 65.0%; laparoscopic myomectomy: 93.0%). Uterine fibroid embolization and endometrial ablation were performed primarily in the hospital-based ambulatory surgery setting (79.9 and 98.2%, respectively).

Distribution of hospital setting for three surgical procedures to treat benign uterine fibroids by patient race/ethnicity, in 13 States, 2013

- White women more commonly had hysterectomy and myomectomy in the hospital-based ambulatory surgery setting, whereas Black and Hispanic women more commonly had inpatient surgery for these procedures.

In 2013, White women more commonly had hysterectomy and myomectomy for benign uterine fibroids in the hospital-based ambulatory

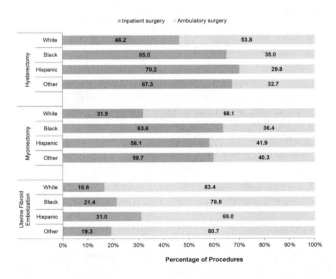

Figure 6.6. *Distribution of Hospital Setting for Three Surgical Procedures to Treat Benign Uterine Fibroids by Patient Race/Ethnicity, in 13 States, 2013.*

Source: Agency for Healthcare Research and Quality (AHRQ), Center for Delivery, Organization, and Markets, Healthcare Cost and Utilization Project (HCUP), State Inpatient Databases (SID) and State Ambulatory Surgery and Services Databases (SASD) from 13 States, 2013

surgery setting than in the inpatient setting (hysterectomy: 53.8%; myomectomy: 68.1%). In contrast, it was more common for Black and Hispanic women to have these procedures performed in the hospital inpatient setting. Although all women more commonly had uterine fibroid embolization performed in the ambulatory surgery setting, regardless of race/ethnicity, having this procedure performed in the ambulatory surgery setting was somewhat more common among White women (83.4%) than among Black (78.6%) and Hispanic (69.0%) women.

Distribution of hospital setting for three surgical procedures to treat benign uterine fibroids by expected primary payer, in 13 States, 2013

- Women covered by Medicaid and uninsured women more commonly had hysterectomy and myomectomy in the hospital inpatient setting, whereas privately insured women had outpatient surgery about as often as inpatient surgery for these two procedures.

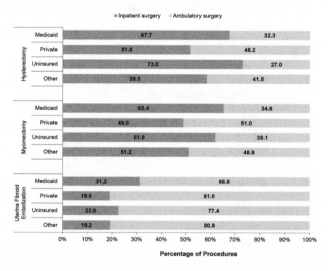

Figure 6.7. *Distribution of Hospital Setting for Three Surgical Procedures to Treat Benign Uterine Fibroids by Expected Primary Payer, in 13 States, 2013.*

Note: Other expected primary payer includes Medicare.
Source: Agency for Healthcare Research and Quality (AHRQ), Center for Delivery, Organization, and Markets, Healthcare Cost and Utilization Project (HCUP), State Inpatient Databases (SID) and State Ambulatory Surgery and Services Databases (SASD) from 13 States, 2013

In 2013, it was more common for women covered by Medicaid to have hysterectomy and myomectomy for benign uterine fibroids in the hospital inpatient setting than in the ambulatory surgery setting (hysterectomy: 67.7%; myomectomy: 65.4%). Uninsured women also more commonly had inpatient stays than ambulatory surgery visits for hysterectomy (73.0%) and myomectomy (61.9%). In contrast, privately insured women had these two procedures performed in the ambulatory surgery setting about as often as in the inpatient setting. Although uterine fibroid embolization was more commonly performed in the ambulatory surgery setting across payers, it was less common among women covered by Medicaid (68.8%) than among privately insured (81.0%) and uninsured (77.4%) women.

Section 6.3

Knee Replacement Surgery

This section includes text excerpted from "Hospitalization for Total Knee Replacement among Inpatients Aged 45 and Over: United States, 2000–2010," Centers for Disease Control and Prevention (CDC), September 2, 2015.

Key Findings

In 2010, total knee replacement was the most frequently performed inpatient procedure on adults aged 45 and over. In the 11-year period from 2000 through 2010, an estimated 5.2 million total knee replacements were performed. Adults aged 45 and over comprised 98.1 percent of those surgeries. This chapter uses data from the National Hospital Discharge Survey (NHDS) to present trends in the rate of hospitalizations for total knee replacement, mean age at hospitalization, and discharge status for inpatients aged 45 and over from 2000 through 2010.

- The rate of total knee replacement increased for both men (86%) and women (99%) aged 45 and over from 2000 through 2010.

- For both 2000 and 2010, women had a higher rate of total knee replacement (33.0 and 65.5 per 10,000 population, respectively) than men (24.3 and 45.3 per 10,000, respectively).

- The mean age at total knee replacement decreased from 2000 through 2010 for both men and women aged 45 and over.

- Higher percentages of men and women aged 45 and over who were hospitalized for total knee replacement were discharged home in 2010 (69.8% and 54.1%) than in 2000 (53.5% and 40.8%).

- In both 2000 and 2010, a lower percentage of women aged 45 and over (40.8% and 54.1%, respectively) were discharged home after total knee replacement than men aged 45 and over (53.5% and 69.8%, respectively).

Total Knee Replacement in the Population Aged 45 and over by Sex

- The rate of total knee replacement increased for both men and women. Among men, the rate increased from 24.3 per 10,000 population in 2000 to 45.3 per 10,000 in 2010 (an 86% increase). Among women, the rate almost doubled from 33.0 per 10,000 in 2000 to 65.5 per 10,000 in 2010 (a 99% increase).

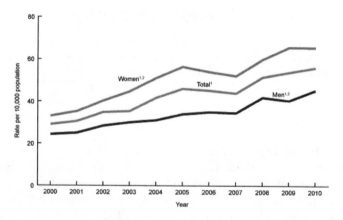

Figure 6.8. *Total Knee Replacement among Inpatients Aged 45 and over, by Sex: United States, 2000–2010.*

[1]*Significant linear trend from 2000 through 2010 (p< 0.05).*
[2]*Significant difference in rates between men and women in each year.*
Notes: Total knee replacement is defined as code 81.54 of the International Classification of Diseases, Ninth Revision, Clinical Modification (ICD–9–CM) for any of four collected procedures. Rates were calculated using U.S. Census Bureau 2000-based postcensal civilian population estimates.
Source: Centers for Disease Control and Prevention (CDC)/NCHS, National Hospital Discharge Survey, 2000–2010.

- The rate of total knee replacement was higher for women compared with men for each year of the 11-year period. In 2000, the rate of total knee replacement for women was 35.8 percent higher than for men (33.0 and 24.3, respectively). In 2010, the rate of total knee replacement for women was 45.6 percent higher than for men (65.5 and 45.3, respectively).

Total Knee Replacement, by Sex and Age

- Women aged 45–64 had higher rates (16.4 and 46.6) than men aged 45–64 (8.7 and 28.6) in both 2000 and 2010.

- In 2000, there was no difference in the rate of total knee replacement between men and women aged 65 and over, while in 2010, women had a higher rate (99.3) than men (82.6).

- Those aged 65 and over had higher rates of total knee replacement than those aged 45–64 in both 2000 and 2010 (58.0 and 92.1, respectively for those aged 65 and over compared with 12.7 and 37.8 for those aged 45–64).

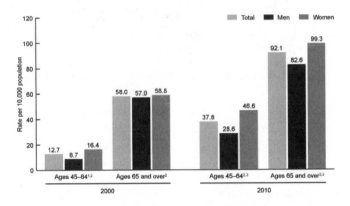

Figure 6.9. *Total Knee Replacement among Inpatients Aged 45 and over, by Sex and Age Group: United States, 2000 and 2010.*

[1]*Significant difference in 2000 between men and women within age group (p< 0.05).*
[2]*Significant difference between 2000 and 2010 within sex and age group (p< 0.05).*
[3]*Significant difference in 2010 between men and women within age group (p< 0.05).*
Notes: Total knee replacement is defined as code 81.54 of the International Classification of Diseases, Ninth Revision, Clinical Modification (ICD–9–CM) for any of four collected procedures. Rates were calculated using U.S. Census Bureau 2000-based postcensal civilian population estimates.
Source: CDC/NCHS, National Hospital Discharge Survey, 2000 and 2010.

- Higher rates of total knee replacement were found for both men and women aged 65 and over compared with those aged 45–64 in both 2000 and 2010.

Mean Age at Which Inpatients Aged 45 and over Have Total Knee Replacement

- Overall, the mean age for having a total knee replacement was lower in 2010 compared with 2000, by 3.9 percent, decreasing from 68.9 in 2000 to 66.2 in 2010.

- Among men, the mean age decreased from 69.3 to 66.5, and among women, the mean age decreased from 68.7 to 66.0.

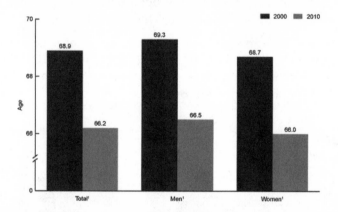

Figure 6.10. *Mean Age at Total Knee Replacement among Inpatients Aged 45 and over, by Sex: United States, 2000 and 2010.*

[1] Significant difference in mean age between 2000 and 2010 (p< 0.05).
Notes: Total knee replacement is defined as code 81.54 of the International Classification of Diseases, Ninth Revision, Clinical Modification (ICD–9–CM) for any of four collected procedures. Percentages are calculated only for inpatients aged 45 and over.
Source: CDC/NCHS, National Hospital Discharge Survey, 2000 and 2010.

Discharged Home after a Total Knee Replacement, by Sex and Age

- The percentages of men and women aged 45 and over discharged home after hospitalization for total knee replacement were higher in 2010 (69.8% and 54.1%, respectively) than in 2000 (53.5% and 40.8%, respectively).

- In both 2000 and 2010, lower percentages of women than men were discharged home after total knee replacement.

- In 2010, nearly two-thirds of men aged 65 and over (62.3%) were discharged home, while less than one-half of women aged 65 and over (42.5%) were discharged home.

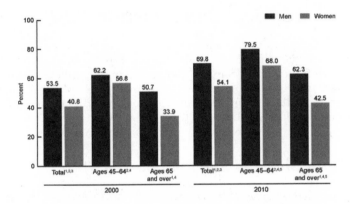

Figure 6.11. *Inpatients Aged 45 and over with Total Knee Replacement Discharged Home, by Sex and Age Group: United States, 2000 and 2010.*

[1]*Significant difference between men and women (p< 0.05).*
[2]*Significant difference between 2000 and 2010 for men (p< 0.05).*
[3]*Significant difference between 2000 and 2010 for women (p< 0.05).*
[4]*Significant difference between age groups for women (p< 0.05).*
[5]*Significant difference between age groups for men (p< 0.05).*
Notes: Total knee replacement is defined as code 81.54 of the International Classification of Diseases, Ninth Revision, Clinical Modification (ICD–9–CM) for any of four collected procedures. Percentages are calculated only for inpatients aged 45 and over.
Source: CDC/NCHS, National Hospital Discharge Survey, 2000 and 2010.

Section 6.4

Surgical Site Infection (SSI)

This section contains text excerpted from the following sources: Text under the heading "Facts about Surgical Site Infection (SSI)" is excerpted from "NHSN Surgical Site Infection Surveillance in 2016," Centers for Disease Control and Prevention (CDC), March 2, 2016; Text under the heading "Prevalence Study on SSIs" is excerpted from "Surgical Site Infection (SSI) Event," Centers for Disease Control and Prevention (CDC), January 2017.

Facts about Surgical Site Infection (SSI)

- Surgical site infection (SSI) and pneumonia are two most common healthcare-associated infections (HAIs)

- Estimated HAI SSI infections in United States 157,500 per year

- Estimated 8,205 deaths associated with SSI each year.

- Estimated 11 percent of all deaths in intensive care units are associated with SSI.

- SSI are the most common healthcare associated infection and account for $3.2 billion in attributable cost per year in acute care hospitals.

- Estimated additional 11 days of hospitalization for each SSI per patient.

- SSI are the most frequent cause (20%) of unplanned readmissions after surgery.

Prevalence Study on SSIs

In 2010, an estimated 16 million operative procedures were performed in acute care hospitals in the United States. A prevalence study found that SSIs were the most common healthcare-associated infection, accounting for 31 percent of all HAIs among hospitalized patients. The Centers for Disease Control and Prevention (CDC) healthcare-associated infection (HAI) prevalence survey found that there were an estimated 157,500 surgical site infections associated with inpatient surgeries in 2011. National Healthcare Safety Network (NHSN) data included 16,147 SSIs following 849,659 operative procedures in all groups reported, for an overall SSI rate of 1.9 percent between 2006–2008. A 19 percent decrease in SSI related to 10 select procedures was reported between 2008 and 2013.

While advances have been made in infection control practices, including improved operating room ventilation, sterilization methods, barriers, surgical technique, and availability of antimicrobial prophylaxis, SSIs remain a substantial cause of morbidity, prolonged hospitalization, and death. SSI is associated with a mortality rate of 3 percent, and 75 percent of SSI associated deaths are directly attributable to the SSI.

Chapter 7

Recent Research and Trends in Surgery and Patient Outcomes

Chapter Contents

Section 7.1

Anesthesia: Is It Safe for Young Brains?

This section includes text excerpted from
"Anesthesia: Is it Safe for Young Brains?" U.S. Food and
Drug Administration (FDA), April 20, 2017.

When infants or young children need surgery, does anesthesia affect their developing brains?

With more than 1 million children under age 4 requiring anesthesia for surgery in the United States each year, the U.S. Food and Drug Administration (FDA) and other health organizations are working together to answer this question.

Previous scientific studies in young animals have shown that commonly used anesthetics can be harmful to the developing brain. However, results have been mixed in children. Some studies of infants and young children undergoing anesthesia have reported long-term deficits in learning and behavior; other studies have not.

These conflicting results show that more research is needed to fully understand the risks anesthesia may pose to very young patients.

To close these research gaps, FDA and the International Anesthesia Research Society (IARS) started an initiative called SmartTots (Strategies for Mitigating Anesthesia-Related neuroToxicity in Tots). SmartTots seeks to ensure that children under age 4 will be as safe as possible when they need anesthesia during surgery. Studies have shown that this is a period of significant brain development in young children.

"Our hope is that research funded through SmartTots will help us design the safest anesthetic regimens possible," says Bob Rappaport, M.D., director of the Division of Anesthesia, Analgesia and Addiction Products at FDA. "This research can potentially foster the development of new and safer anesthetic drugs for use in pediatric medicine."

According to SmartTots steering committee co-chair James Ramsay, M.D., young children usually do not undergo surgery unless the procedure is vital to their health. "Therefore, postponing a necessary procedure may itself lead to significant health problems and may not be an option for the majority of children," Ramsey says.

Ongoing Research

SmartTots was launched in 2010 in part to fund research that would build on the work done at FDA and several universities.

Merle Paule, Ph.D., director of the Division of Neurotoxicology at FDA's National Center for Toxicological Research (NCTR), and colleagues have been exploring the effects of ketamine—an anesthetic commonly used on children-on the brains and learning ability of young rhesus monkeys.

"Earlier research has shown that exposing young rat pups to ketamine caused learning problems when they became adults, but we wanted to see what would happen with primates," said Paule. Primates, such as the rhesus monkey used in this research, more closely resemble humans in physiology and behavior. All animal procedures were approved by the National Center for Toxicological Research's (NCTR) Institutional Animal Care and Use Committee (IACUC), and conducted in accordance with the Public Health Service (PHS) Policy on the Humane Care and Use of Laboratory Animals.

"The learning of concepts such as matching (see a triangle, match it with another triangle from among other symbols) took much longer in the ketamine-treated monkeys and even after basic concepts were learned, the ketamine-exposed animals performed less accurately than animals in the control group," Paule says.

The same holds true for the test monkeys even today, Paule says. Six years after their ketamine treatment, they're still showing below-normal brain function.

What might that mean for young children who have been exposed to ketamine or other anesthetics during surgery?

"We can't know with certainty at this time," says Rappaport, a member of the steering committee that coordinates, manages and oversees the SmartTots initiative. "We need to definitively answer the questions of whether anesthetic use in children poses a risk to their development and, if so, under what circumstances."

FDA and other health-related organizations recognize the importance of learning more on this topic. For example, do other forms of anesthesia similarly affect the brain's ability to, learn and remember? How long might these deficits last?

SmartTots Paves the Way

The SmartTots partnership seeks to mobilize the scientific community around this issue, stimulate dialogue among leaders in the anesthesia community and work to raise funding for the necessary research ahead.

As part of these efforts, SmartTots issued a consensus statement, endorsed by organizations including the FDA, American Academy of Pediatrics (AAP), the American Society of Anesthesiologists (ASA) and the European Society of Anesthesiology (ESA) in December 2012. The statement acknowledged that, in the absence of conclusive evidence, it would be unethical to withhold sedation and anesthesia when necessary.

SmartTots is funding research underway at Columbia University and the University of Iowa on the effects of anesthesia on infant brain development, and on cognitive and language ability. All research first undergoes approval by an Institutional Review Board (IRB), a committee formally designated to approve, monitor, and review biomedical and behavioral research involving humans. The number one priority of IRBs is to protect human subjects from physical or psychological harm.

In the meantime, Ramsay says that parents and other caretakers must talk to their pediatrician or other healthcare professionals about the risks and benefits of procedures requiring anesthetics and weigh them against the known health risks of not treating certain conditions.

Section 7.2

Imaging Technique for Analysis of Brain Tumor Tissue during Surgery

This section includes text excerpted from "New Imaging Technique Allows Quick, Automated Analysis of Brain Tumor Tissue during Surgery," National Institute of Biomedical Imaging and Bioengineering (NIBIB), February 9, 2017.

Brain surgery for removing cancerous tissue is a delicate and high-stakes task. Now researchers funded by the National Institute of Biomedical Imaging and Bioengineering (NIBIB) have created a way to improve tumor removal surgery by distinguishing cancerous tissue from healthy tissue faster. The method makes brain tumor surgery more precise, improving safety.

Surgeons tread a fine line when removing a brain tumor, wanting to be sure to remove as much tumor as possible while sparing healthy brain. During surgery, a pathologist may look at a piece of tissue to better inform decisions, but prepping the tissue sample to be examined under the microscope can take 30 minutes, extending surgery time, upping the cost, and increasing risks to the patient. Furthermore, many hospitals performing brain tumor removal don't have easy access to a neuropathologist. The new method not only decreases tenfold the time needed to examine a tissue sample, it also allows for automatic processing, enabling pathologists to confirm diagnoses from afar.

"This technology reduces tissue processing time and could significantly increase the accuracy of brain tumor surgery in operating room," said Behrouz Shabestari, Ph.D., director of the NIBIB program in Optical Imaging and Spectroscopy. "It basically optimizes the surgical result and has the potential to improve patient outcomes by increasing safety and survival rates."

The team from the University of Michigan Medical School, led by Daniel Orringer, M.D., a neurosurgeon and lead author of the paper, used stimulated Raman scattering (SRS), a type of microscopy that does not require tissue processing, or slicing the tissue and staining it. They adapted the procedures so they could be performed in the operating room. Previously, microscopes capable of SRS were too big and expensive for a clinical setting. But by switching to a fiber-laser microscope, which uses the same type of fiber optics as Internet and phone cables, and devising a way to decrease background signals common to fiber-laser images, the team created a portable, safe, high-resolution system and validated its use in more than 100 patients.

They also created a way to quickly process the resulting images, called stimulated Raman histology (SRH). The new method takes advantage of intrinsic chemical properties of the tissue, making proteins and deoxyribonucleic acid (DNA) appear purple and lipids appear pink. The resulting image is strikingly similar to the widely used hematoxylin and eosin (H&E) staining, so pathologists don't need to be specially trained to interpret it. By eliminating the time-consuming process of sectioning and staining, SRH takes about three minutes, 10 times less than standard techniques used during surgery. When tested on 30 samples, pathologists came to similar conclusions using SRH as when using conventional techniques.

"It really provides a new vision for how pathology might be implemented in the operating room, eliminating the need for a frozen section procedure, which many surgeons rely so much on to make decisions while they're taking care of their patients," Orringer said.

The researchers also demonstrated that the images can be automatically classified by a computer program. In their initial study, the algorithm was able to predict the subtype of brain tumor with 90 percent accuracy. Orringer is hopeful that, in the future, an SRH machine will make a preliminary diagnosis that can be confirmed by a remote pathologist, assisting those surgical centers without pathologists on staff. "In this current era where we're increasingly connected, this system might be the linchpin that brings the expertise to the center where the surgery is being performed," he added.

Since the SRH method provides for quicker assessment of tissue as either cancerous or healthy, surgeons can make better informed decisions about how much tissue to remove and how much to leave behind. The method may also be extended to other types of tumors, such as breast or neck cancer, in which the tumor margins are unclear.

The combination of better accuracy and speed means safer surgeries and better outcomes for patients, decreasing the time they spend on the operating table. "We've never had a system which makes that information available in a rapid fashion for surgeons," Orringer said. "We're arming surgeons with the microscopic information about the tissue that they're operating on."

Section 7.3

Contaminated Devices Putting Open-Heart Surgery Patients at Risk

This section includes text excerpted from "Contaminated Devices Putting Open-Heart Surgery Patients at Risk," Centers for Disease Control and Prevention (CDC), October 13, 2016.

The Centers for Disease Control and Prevention (CDC) is warning healthcare providers and patients about the potential risk of infection from certain devices used during open heart (open-chest) surgery.

Patients who have had open heart surgery should seek medical care if they are experiencing symptoms associated with infections, such as night sweats, muscle aches, weight loss, fatigue, or unexplained fever. This advice follows new information indicating that some LivaNova

PLC (formerly Sorin Group Deutschland GmbH) Stöckert 3T heater-cooler devices, used during many of these surgeries, might have been contaminated during manufacturing which could put patients at risk for life-threatening infections.

More than 250,000 heart bypass procedures using heater-cooler devices are performed in the United States every year. Heater-cooler units are an essential part of these life-saving surgeries because they help keep a patient's circulating blood and organs at a specific temperature during the procedure. Approximately 60 percent of heart bypass procedures performed in the United States utilize the devices that have been associated with these infections. CDC estimates that in hospitals where at least one infection has been identified, the risk of a patient getting an infection from the bacteria was between about 1 in 100 and 1 in 1,000. While these infections can be severe, and some patients in this investigation have died, it is unclear whether the infection was a direct cause of death. Available information suggests that patients who had valves or prosthetic products implanted are at higher risk of these infections.

CDC also released a Health Alert Network (HAN) advisory to help hospitals and healthcare providers identify and inform patients who might have been put at risk.

"It's important for clinicians and their patients to be aware of this risk so that patients can be evaluated and treated quickly," said Michael Bell, M.D., deputy director of CDC's Division of Healthcare Quality Promotion (DHQP). "Hospitals should check to see which type of heater-coolers are in use, ensure that they're maintained according to the latest manufacturer's instructions, and alert affected patients and the clinicians who care for them."

CDC and the U.S. Food and Drug Administration (FDA) initially published information and alerts about these potentially contaminated heater-cooler devices in 2015. CDC's Morbidity and Mortality Weekly Report details laboratory tests by CDC and National Jewish Health that show bacteria from the 3T heater-cooler devices match bacteria found in patients in several states. These results build on previous evidence from Europe that suggests the bacteria contaminated these devices during manufacturing in Germany.

The bacteria, *Mycobacterium chimaera*, is a species of *nontuberculous mycobacterium* (NTM) often found in soil and water. In the environment, *M. chimaera* rarely makes healthy people sick. Patients who have been exposed to the bacteria through open-heart surgery can develop general and nonspecific symptoms that can often take months to develop. As a result, diagnosis of these infections can be missed or delayed, sometimes for years, making these infections more difficult to treat. There is no test to determine whether a person has been exposed to the bacteria. Infections can be diagnosed by detecting the bacteria by laboratory culture; the slow growing nature of the bacteria can require up to two months to rule out infection.

Patients who have had open-heart surgery and are concerned about symptoms they may be experiencing should contact their healthcare providers. Clinicians or patients with questions should contact CDC Info at 800-CDC-INFO (800-232-4636) or wwwn.cdc.gov/dcs/ContactUs/Form.

Section 7.4

Aortic Valve Replacement Surgery for High Risk Patients

This section includes text excerpted from "New Method for Performing Aortic Valve Replacement Proves Successful in High Risk Patients," National Heart, Lung, and Blood Institute (NHLBI), October 31, 2016.

Researchers at the National Institutes of Health (NIH) have developed a new, less invasive way to perform transcatheter aortic valve replacement (TAVR), a procedure widely used to treat aortic valve stenosis, a lethal heart condition. The new approach, called transcaval access, will make TAVR more available to high risk patients, especially women, whose femoral arteries are too small or diseased to withstand the standard procedure.

Aortic valve stenosis involves the narrowing of the heart's aortic valve which reduces blood flow through the heart. For about 85 percent of patients with this condition, doctors typically perform TAVR through the femoral artery in the leg. But for the other 15 percent, doctors must find a different access route. The most common alternative routes are through the chest, which requires surgery and are associated with significantly more complications.

Transcaval access, which can be performed in awake patients, involves electrifying a small wire so that it crosses between neighboring blood vessels in the abdomen. The technique calls for making large holes in both the abdominal aorta and the inferior vena cava, which physicians previously considered dangerous because of the risk of fatal bleeding.

The new method was developed by researchers at the National, Heart, Lung and Blood Institute (NHLBI) and tested in a trial on 100 patients at 20 hospitals across the United States. Researchers said it proved successful in 99 of the patients.

"This is a seminal study," said the lead author, cardiologist Adam B. Greenbaum, M.D., co-director of the Henry Ford Hospital Center for Structural Heart Disease, Detroit. "It challenged conventional wisdom, objecting to the idea of safe passage between the vena cava and the aorta. More important, it is the first of many nonsurgical minimally-invasive tissue-crossing, or so-called transmural catheter procedures developed at NIH that can be applied to diverse fields of medicine."

Robert J. Lederman, M.D., a senior investigator in National Heart, Lung, and Blood Institute's (NHLBI) Division of Intramural Research (DIR) who led the study, said researchers developed the method to address a specific clinical need, even though they knew it would be a challenging proposition for most surgeons and physicians to accept. The proposed and counterintuitive mechanism of action is that bleeding from the aorta spontaneously decompresses into a corresponding hole the physician makes in the vein, because the surrounding area behind the peritoneum has higher pressure than the vein.

The results of the research, which were independently confirmed by a committee of outside cardiologists, show the procedure not only has a high success rate, but also an acceptable rate of bleeding and vascular complications, particularly in the high-risk patients studied. The study builds on the access technique that Lederman's NHLBI team developed and first tested in animals in 2012 and first applied with Henry Ford physicians to help patients in 2013. NHLBI and its collaborators are now working to find ways to train more specialists to perform the procedure.

Section 7.5

Tissue Engineering and Surgery for Fixing Flawed Body Parts

This section includes text excerpted from "Fixing Flawed Body Parts," *NIH News in Health*, National Institutes of Health (NIH), February 2015.

How can you mend a broken heart? Or repair a damaged liver, kidney, or knee? National Institutes of Health (NIH)-funded scientists are exploring innovative ways to fix faulty organs and tissues or even grow new ones. This type of research is called tissue engineering. Exciting advances continue to emerge in this fast-moving field.

Tissue engineering could allow doctors to repair or replace worn-out tissues and organs with living, working parts. Most important, tissue engineering might help some of the 120,000 people on the waitlist to receive donated kidneys, livers, or other organs.

Doctors have long used tissue-engineered skin to heal severe burns or other injuries. But most tissue engineering methods are still experimental. They've been tested only in laboratory dishes and sometimes in animals, but only a few new approaches have been tested in people. Several clinical studies (involving human volunteers) are in the early stages of testing newly developed tissues.

"With this approach, scientists are combining engineering and biology to restore a damaged organ or tissue, whether it's been damaged by disease or injury or something else," says Dr. Martha Lundberg, NIH expert in heart-related tissue engineering.

Some scientists are creating special net-like structures, or scaffolds, in desired shapes and then coaxing cells to grow within them. Some use a mixture of natural substances called growth factors, which direct cells to grow and develop in certain ways.

"Other scientists are using different 3-D bioprinting technologies—some are like fancy inkjet printers—to create new tissues or organs," Lundberg says. They've printed 3-D kidneys and other organs that look like the real thing. But while most of these printed body parts have the right shape, they're not fully functional.

"Scientists haven't yet figured out how to print an organ that includes the correct blood vessel patterns, nerve connections, and other components that come together in a mature organ," Lundberg says. "When creating a new organ, if it can perform the right job and functions, it may not need to look like the real thing."

Many tissue engineering methods use stem cells, which can be nudged to turn into different cell types. One research team guided human stem cells to become a 3-D structure that can respond to light. The method might one day lead to new therapies for eye disorders. Other stem cell approaches may lead to improved treatment for spinal cord injuries, diabetes, and more.

Another approach, called decellularization, involves removing all the cells from an organ. What's left behind is a thin, pale framework that contains the organ's natural structural proteins, including the pathways for tiny blood vessels and nerves. By infusing new cells into this mesh-like matrix, some researchers have successfully created working animal kidneys, livers, hearts, lungs, and other organs.

The decellularization technique was used by Dr. Martin Yarmush and his colleagues to create a functional rat liver that included a network of working blood vessels. Yarmush is a biomedical engineer at Rutgers University and the Massachusetts General Hospital. The engineered livers his team created were kept alive in the laboratory for days and functioned for several hours after transplantation into rats. The researchers are now working to help those transplanted livers survive even longer. They're also scaling up the methods to create a decellularized human liver that can be repopulated with functional cells.

"A parallel effort we are pursuing involves taking a donated organ that is not considered transplantable for a particular reason, and then using a reconditioning solution and perhaps even stem cells to revitalize the organ so it becomes transplantable," Yarmush says.

Other researchers are working to repair damaged body parts that are still in the body. At the University of Washington in Seattle, Dr. Charles Murry and colleagues are searching for ways to fix injured hearts. One of their latest studies used human stem cells to repair damaged hearts in monkeys. The stem cells were coaxed to become early-stage heart cells, which were then infused near the heart injury.

The new cells made their way into the damaged heart muscle and organized into muscle fibers in all of the treated monkeys. The infused stem cells replaced nearly half of the damaged heart tissue and began beating in sync with the heart. Still, the scientists note, they need years of research before this type of therapy might be tried in people.

Some methods are already being tested in humans. Dr. Martha Murray, a surgeon at Boston Children's Hospital, is exploring new ways to heal a common knee injury known as a torn ACL (anterior cruciate ligament). Athletes who do a lot of twisting and turning, as in basketball or soccer, are at risk for damaging the ACL.

"Typical treatment today, called ACL reconstruction, works well, and it gets patients back to the playing field at a relatively high rate," Murray says. But the surgery involves removing a piece of tendon from elsewhere in the body and using that to replace the ACL. "So it involves making 2 injuries that the body has to heal from. And even with this treatment, patients still develop arthritis in the knee 15 to 20 years later," Murray adds. "We wanted to find a better therapy—something less invasive."

After testing several biomaterials, Murray's team found that stitching a bioengineered sponge between the torn ends of an injured ACL allows blood to clot and collect around the damaged ligament. Because blood naturally contains stem cells and growth factors, the blood-soaked sponge acts as a "bridge" that encourages ACL healing. The sponge is made of some of the same proteins normally found in ligaments, and it dissolves after a few weeks.

Studies in large animals showed that the bioengineered sponge was much less likely to lead to arthritis, and it healed ACL injuries as well as standard reconstruction surgery. The U.S. Food and Drug Administration (FDA) approved human safety testing of the sponge in 10 people with ACL injuries.

Metal, plastic, and other nonbiological devices can also replace or enhance malfunctioning body parts. One promising possibility still in development is an artificial kidney that could be implanted in the body and used in place of dialysis to treat end-stage kidney disease. Scientists are also studying a synthetic glue modeled after a natural adhesive that might help to repair tissues in the body.

Section 7.6

Technologies Enhance Tumor Surgery

This section includes text excerpted from "Technologies
Enhance Tumor Surgery," *NIH News in Health*, National
Institutes of Health (NIH), February 2016.

For surgeons, removing a tumor is a balancing act. Cut out too much
and you risk removing healthy tissues that have important functions.
Remove too little and you may leave behind cancer cells that could
grow back into a tumor over time.

The National Institutes of Health (NIH)-funded researchers are
developing new technologies to help surgeons determine exactly where
tumors end and healthy tissue begins. Their ultimate goal is to make
surgery for cancer patients safer and more effective.

"Currently, surgeons view MRI and CT scans taken prior to an
operation to establish where a tumor is located and to plan a surgical
approach that will minimize damage to healthy tissues," says Dr. Steven Krosnick, an NIH expert in image-guided surgery. "But once the
operation has begun, surgeons generally rely only on their eyes and
sense of touch to distinguish tumor from healthy tissue."

Surgeons go through many years of training to understand the
subtle cues that can distinguish tumor from normal surroundings.
Sometimes the tumor is a slightly different color than healthy tissue,
or it feels different. It might also bleed more readily or could contain calcium deposits. Even with these cues, however, surgeons don't
always get it right.

"In a lot of cases, we leave tumor behind that could be safely
removed if only we were able to better visualize it," says Dr. Daniel
Orringer, a neurosurgeon at the University of Michigan.

In operating rooms, pathologists can often help surgeons determine
if all of a tumor has been taken out. A pathologist may view the edges
of the tissue under a microscope and look for cancer cells. If they're
found, the surgeon will remove more tissue from the patient and send
these again to the pathologist for review. This process can occur repeat-
edly while the patient remains on the operating table and continue
until no cancer cells are detected.

81

"Each time a pathologist analyzes tissue during an operation, it can take up to 30 minutes because the tissue has to be frozen, thinly sliced, and stained so it can be viewed under the microscope," Krosnick says. "If multiple rounds of tissue are taken, it can greatly increase the length of the surgery."

In the days following an operation, the pathologist conducts a more thorough review of the tissue. If cancer cells are found at the margins, the patient may undergo a second surgery to remove cancer that was left behind.

Orringer is part of a research team that's testing a new technology that could help surgeons tell the difference between a tumor and healthy brain tissue during surgery. The team developed a special microscope with National Institutes of Health (NIH) support that shoots a pair of low-energy lasers at the tissue. That causes the chemical bonds in the tissue's molecules to vibrate. The vibrations are then analyzed by a computer and used to create detailed images of the tissue.

From a molecular point of view, the components of a tumor differ from those in healthy tissue. This specialized microscope can reveal differences between the tissues that can't be seen with the naked eye.

"Our technology enables us to get a microscopic view of human tissues without taking them out of the body," Orringer says. "We can see cells, blood vessels, the connections between brain cells...all of the microscopic components that make up the brain."

Orringer and colleagues developed a computer program that can quickly analyze the images and assess whether or not cancer cells are present. This type of analysis could help surgeons decide whether all of a tumor has been cut out. To date, Orringer has used the specialized microscope to help remove cancer tissue in nearly 100 patients with brain tumors.

Other researchers are taking different approaches. For example, Dr. Quyen Nguyen—a head and neck surgeon at the University of California, San Diego—has developed a fluorescent molecule that's currently being tested in clinical trials. The patient receives an injection of the molecules before surgery. When exposed to certain types of light, these molecules cause cancer cells to glow, making them easier to spot and remove. The surgeon then uses a near-infrared camera to visualize the glowing tumor cells while operating.

Nguyen is also developing a fluorescent molecule to light up nerves. Accidental nerve injury during surgery can leave patients with loss of movement or feeling. In some cases, sexual function may be impaired.

"Nerves are really, really small, and they're often buried in soft tissue or encased within bone. When we have to do cancer surgery, they can be encased in the cancer itself," Nguyen says. The fluorescent molecule could help surgeons detect hard-to-spot nerves, so they can be protected. The nerve-tagging molecule is now being tested in animal studies.

Other NIH-funded researchers are focusing on ways to speed up cancer surgeries. Dr. Milind Rajadhyaksha, a researcher at Memorial Sloan Kettering Cancer Center, has developed a microscope technique to reduce the amount of time it takes to perform a common surgery for removing nonmelanoma skin cancers.

Each year about 2 million people in the United States undergo Mohs surgery, in which a doctor successively removes suspicious areas until the surrounding skin tissue is free of cancer. The procedure can take several hours, because each time more tissue is removed, it has to be prepared and reviewed under a microscope to determine if cancer cells remain. This step can take up to 30 minutes.

The technique developed by Rajadhyaksha shortens the time for assessing removed tissue to less than 5 minutes, which greatly reduces the overall length of the procedure. Tissue is mounted in a specialized microscope that uses a focused laser line to do multiple scans of the tissue. The resulting image "strips" are then combined, like a mosaic, into a complete microscopic image of the tissue.

About 1,000 specialized skin surgeries have already been performed guided by this technique. Rajadhyaksha is currently developing an approach that would allow doctors to use the technology directly on a patient's skin, before any tissue has been removed. This would allow doctors to identify the edges of tumors before the start of surgery and reduce the need for several presurgical "margin-mapping" biopsies.

There are many types of cancer surgeries, and researchers continue to work hard to develop better techniques.

Section 7.7

Bariatric Surgery for Obesity

This section includes text excerpted from "New
Insights into Bariatric Surgery for Obesity," National
Institutes of Health (NIH), April 7, 2014.

Researchers found that a bariatric surgical procedure reduces obesity and improves glucose tolerance in mice by increasing bile acids and altering gut microbes. The finding hints at new targets for nonsurgical interventions to treat obesity.

Bariatric surgeries—operations that alter the stomach, intestines, or both—are among the most effective treatments for severe obesity. The surgeries are thought to lead to weight loss and improvements in related health conditions, such as type 2 diabetes, by reducing the size of the stomach so that less food can be consumed. There are several different types of bariatric operations. Some also alter how food is digested, further decreasing the absorption of calories and nutrients.

Many of the metabolic improvements seen after bariatric operations occur before substantial weight loss, suggesting that other processes may be involved. A team of researchers led by Drs. Karen Ryan and Randy Seeley at the University of Cincinnati set out to investigate how bariatric procedures lead to health benefits. The research was funded in part by NIH's National Institute of Diabetes and Digestive and Kidney Diseases (NIDDK) and National Heart, Lung, and Blood Institute (NHLBI). Results appeared online on March 26, 2014, in Nature.

In vertical sleeve gastrectomy (VSG), about 80 percent of the stomach is removed. This creates a gastric "sleeve" that connects the esophagus and small intestine. VSG is known to increase circulation of bile acids. The bile acids bind to farsenoid-X receptor (FXR), a receptor in the nuclei of cells that regulates gene expression.

To test whether the effects of VSG surgery are mediated by FXR, the team created mice that lacked the receptor. These mice and their normal littermates were fed a high-fat diet to induce obesity. They then underwent VSG or sham surgery.

The researchers found that after VSG, the obese mice lost weight and had improved glucose tolerance, as expected. These mice also

84

exhibited a change in the composition of microbes in their gut. In mice that lacked FXR, however, the ability of bariatric surgery to reduce body weight and improve glucose tolerance was substantially reduced.

The findings suggest that the beneficial effects of VSG didn't result just from the mechanical restriction imposed by a smaller stomach. The surgery also increased circulating bile acids and induced changes in the gut microbial community via FXR signaling pathways.

"There are not enough surgery tables or surgeons to treat the obesity epidemic, so we need to understand how bariatric surgery works so that we can offer more scalable solutions," Seeley says. "Manipulating the gut bacteria is another way we think that we might be able to mimic how surgery works without having to do the cutting and stapling."

Part Two

Preparing for Surgery

Chapter 8

How to Find a Qualified Surgeon

Whether you are referred to a physician for surgical care, or you make the choice yourself, don't take your surgeon's qualifications for granted. Make sure your operation is performed by a competent physician whose specialty is surgery. It could be the most important decision you make.

Here are some qualifications to look for:

1. **Board certification**

   A good sign of a surgeon's competence is certification by a surgical board that is approved by the American Board of Medical Specialties (ABMS). When you choose a surgeon who is board certified in a surgical specialty, you are assured that he or she has completed years of residency training in his or her specialty and has demonstrated knowledge and competence by successfully completing a rigorous examination.

2. **Fellowship in the American College of Surgeons**

   The letters F.A.C.S. (Fellow of the American College of Surgeons) after a surgeon's name are an indication to the patient that the surgeon has passed a thorough evaluation of both professional competence and ethical fitness. Fellows are

---

Text in this chapter is from "Surgeon Qualifications and Certifications," © 1996-2017 American College of Surgeons, Chicago, IL 60611-3211. Reprinted with permission.

board-certified surgeons or, in unusual circumstances, have met other standards comparable to board certification. A Fellow has committed herself unequivocally to place the welfare of her patients above any other consideration; to avoid division of fees with other physicians; to make her fees commensurate with the services she renders; and to refrain from performing unjustified operations. In instances where a Fellow has been found to violate these principles, she has been subjected to disciplinary action and even has been expelled from Fellowship.

3. Practice in an accredited healthcare facility

Your surgeon will arrange for your operation to be performed in a hospital or ambulatory surgery center where he has been approved for practice. It is a good idea to make sure that the hospital is accredited by the Joint Commission on Accreditation of Healthcare Organizations (JCAHO), a professionally sponsored program to stimulate a higher quality of patient care in hospitals and other healthcare facilities.

There is also an accreditation option that is available for ambulatory or outpatient surgery centers. If your operation is scheduled to be performed in one of these facilities, you can check to see if the center has been accredited by a nationally recognized organization such as the Joint Commission or the Accreditation Association for Ambulatory Health Care. When a hospital or ambulatory surgery center has voluntarily sought accreditation, it is a good indication that the facility is committed to providing the best possible care for its patients.

If you are unsure of a surgeon's qualifications, don't hesitate to ask her about them or direct your inquiries to your local or state medical society, to the hospital or facility where your operation will be performed, to the surgical department of the nearest medical school, or to your family physician. They will be able to tell you if a surgeon is board certified and/or a Fellow of the American College of Surgeons.

To determine if a hospital or ambulatory surgery center is accredited, contact your local or state hospital association, or call the facility and ask if it is accredited by the Joint Commission or the Accreditation Association for Ambulatory Health Care.

In some instances, such as during an emergency or in areas where fully trained surgeons in all specialties are not available, the performance of certain operations by physicians who are not surgical specialists may be in the best interest of patients.

Surgery by Surgeons

A fully trained surgeon is a physician who, after medical school, has gone through years of training in an accredited residency program to learn the specialized skills of a surgeon. One good sign of a surgeon's competence is certification by a national surgical board approved by the American Board of Medical Specialties. All board-certified surgeons have satisfactorily completed an approved residency training program and have passed a rigorous specialty examination.

The letters F.A.C.S. (Fellow of the American College of Surgeons) after a surgeon's name are a further indication of a physician's qualifications. Surgeons who become Fellows of the College have passed a comprehensive evaluation of their surgical training and skills; they also have demonstrated their commitment to high standards of ethical conduct. This evaluation is conducted according to national standards that were established to ensure that patients receive the best possible surgical care.

Chapter 9

How to Get a
Second Opinion

Second Opinion

A second opinion is when a doctor other than your regular doctor gives his or her view about your health problem and how it should be treated. Getting a second opinion can help you make a more informed decision about your care.

Medicare Part B (Medical Insurance) helps pay for a second opinion before surgery. When your doctor says you have a health problem that needs surgery, you have the right to:

- Know and understand your treatment choices.

- Have another doctor look at those choices with you (second opinion).

- Participate in treatment decisions by making your wishes known.

When to Get a Second Opinion

If your doctor says you need surgery to diagnose or treat a health problem that isn't an emergency, you should consider getting a second

This chapter includes text excerpted from "Getting a Second Opinion before Surgery," Centers for Medicare and Medicaid Services (CMS), July 2016.

opinion. It's up to you to decide when and if you'll have surgery. You might also want a second opinion if your doctor tells you that you should have certain kinds of major nonsurgical procedures.

Medicare doesn't pay for surgeries or procedures that aren't medically necessary, like cosmetic surgery. This means that Medicare won't pay for second opinions for surgeries or procedures that aren't medically necessary.

Don't wait for a second opinion if you need emergency surgery. Some types of emergencies may require surgery right away, like:

• Acute appendicitis

• Blood clot or aneurysm

• Accidental injuries

Finding a Doctor for a Second Opinion

Make sure the doctor giving the second opinion accepts Medicare. To find a doctor for a second opinion, you can:

• Visit www.medicare.gov/physiciancompare to find doctors who accept Medicare.

• Call 1-800-MEDICARE (1-800-633-4227). TTY users should call 1-877-486-2048. Ask for information about doctors who accept Medicare.

• Ask your doctor for the name of another doctor to see for a second opinion. Don't hesitate to ask—most doctors want you to get a second opinion. You can also ask another doctor you trust to recommend a doctor.

Before Getting a Second Opinion

Before you visit the second doctor, you should:

• Ask the first doctor to send your medical records to the doctor giving the second opinion. That way, you may not have to repeat the tests you already had.

• Call the second doctor's office and make sure they have your records.

• Write down a list of questions to take with you to the appointment.

• Ask a family member or friend to go to the appointment with you.

During the visit with the second doctor, you should:

- Tell the doctor what surgery you're thinking about having.

- Tell the doctor what tests you already had.

- Ask the questions you have on your list and encourage your friend or loved one to ask any questions that he or she may have.

The second doctor may ask you to have additional tests performed as a result of the visit. Medicare will help pay for these tests just as it helps pay for other services that are medically necessary.

When the First and Second Opinions Are Different

If the second doctor doesn't agree with the first, you may feel confused about what to do. In that case, you may want to:

- Talk more about your condition with your first doctor.

- Talk to a third doctor. Medicare helps pay for a third opinion.

Getting a second or third opinion doesn't mean you have to change doctors. You decide which doctor you want to do your surgery.

Medicare and Paying for a Second Opinion

Medicare Part B helps pay for a second (or third) opinion and related tests just as it helps pay for other services that are medically necessary. If you have Part B and are in Original Medicare:

- Medicare pays 80 percent of the Medicare-approved amount.

- Your share is usually 20 percent of the Medicare-approved amount after you pay your yearly Part B deductible.

Medicare Advantage Plans and Second Opinion

If you're in a Medicare Advantage Plan, like a Health Maintenance Organizations (HMO) or Preferred Provider Organization (PPO), you have the right to get a second opinion. If the first two opinions are different, your plan will help pay for a third opinion.

Even though you have the right to get a second opinion, you should keep these things in mind:

- Some plans will only help pay for a second opinion if you have a referral (a written OK) from your primary care doctor.

- Some plans will only help pay for a second opinion from a doctor who's in your plan's provider network.

If you're in a Medicare Advantage Plan, call your plan for more information.

If you have Medicaid, it might also pay for second surgical opinions. To find out, call your Medicaid office. You can get the phone number by:

- Visiting www.medicare.gov/contacts

- Calling 1-800-MEDICARE (1-800-633-4227). TTY users should call 1-877-486-2048.

Chapter 10

How to Prepare for Surgery

If you are facing surgery, you are not alone. Every year, more than 15 million Americans have surgery. Popular TV shows would have you believe that surgery is always an immediate, life-or-death matter. In reality, most operations are not emergencies.

This means you have time to learn about the surgery your doctor has recommended so you understand what's involved and feel comfortable that it's the best treatment. It also means you have time to find the right surgeon and hospital and to ask your surgeon questions to make sure the operation is as safe as possible.

Most likely, the doctor you see for general medical care is your primary care doctor. He or she may be the doctor who recommends you have surgery and refers you to a surgeon. You may want to find an additional surgeon to get a second opinion to confirm an operation is the right treatment for you.

Ask your doctor to explain:

- **Why you need to have surgery.** There are many reasons to have surgery: to relieve or prevent pain, reduce a symptom of a problem, improve the way your body functions, or even save your life. Make sure you understand how the operation your doctor has suggested will improve your medical condition.

This chapter contains text excerpted from the following sources: Text in this chapter begins with excerpts from "Navigating the Healthcare System," Agency for Healthcare Research and Quality (AHRQ), U.S. Department of Health and Human Services (HHS), October 2014; Text beginning with the heading "Consent" is excerpted from "Preparing for Inpatient Surgery," Clinical Center, National Institutes of Health (NIH), November 2015.

- **What kind of operation he or she is recommending.** Ask your surgeon to explain the surgery and how it is done. Your surgeon can draw a picture or a diagram and explain the steps involved in the surgery. Ask if there is more than one way of doing the operation. For example, some operations that once required large incisions now can be performed using much smaller incisions. For some surgeries you need to stay in the hospital for 1 day or longer, but for others it is possible for you go home on the same day.

- **If there are alternatives to surgery.** Depending on your condition, surgery may not be the only answer to a medical problem. Medicines or treatments, such as special exercises or changes in diet, could give you the same—or even better—results as surgery.

- **The benefits of the operation.** Ask your surgeon to explain what you will gain by having the operation. If you need a hip replacement, for example, you may be able to walk without pain after the surgery. Ask how long the benefits will last. In some cases, you may need another operation after a short time for the benefits to continue. In other cases, the benefits of the surgery may last your lifetime.

- **The risks of the operation.** All operations have some risk. That's why it is important to balance the benefits of the operation with the risk of complications or side effects. Typical complications include infection, too much bleeding, accidental injury, or reaction to anesthesia. Ask your doctor to explain what side effects you might have, such as swelling or soreness around the incision. Find out what steps the doctors and nurses will take to control any pain you may feel after surgery.

- **What will happen if you don't have this operation.** Based on what you learn about the benefits and the risks of the operation, you may decide not to have it. Ask your surgeon what you stand to lose—or gain—by not having the operation now. Will you be in more pain in the future? Could your condition get worse? Could the condition get better on its own?

- **How much the operation will cost.** Call your health insurance company before you have the operation. Even with insurance, there may be costs that you will have to pay, depending on the hospital and surgeon you use. You will also get a bill from the hospital for your care and from the other doctors who took care of you during your hospital stay. If you don't have health insurance, talk to the hospital's billing staff and your surgeon to see if you can get a discount on the cost of the operation.

Even though millions of operations are performed each year, surgery is a big decision for every patient. Take the time you need to ask questions before you undergo surgery. When you are well-informed about your treatment, the chances are better that you will be more satisfied with the results.

Consent

Your surgeon will review your presurgery results and discuss the details of your surgery with you. Your surgeon will answer your questions and ask you to sign a consent for the surgery. You must give your written consent before any surgery can be performed.

You may also be asked to sign a blood transfusion consent. Not all surgeries require you to receive a blood transfusion. Your surgeon will decide based on your individual case. Please tell your provider if you have had reactions in the past to blood transfusions or if you have any religious prohibitions.

Night before Surgery

Hygiene

Please shower the night before surgery, and clean yourself thoroughly. Generally, soap and water will do, but, in some situations, you may be asked to use a special cleanser. Do not apply any fragranced soap, lotion, or spray during or after your shower. If you have an I.V. (intravenous line) or venous access device, please ask the nurse to cover it so that it will not get wet.

Fasting

Do not eat or drink anything after midnight the night before surgery. It is important to follow these instructions to decrease your risk of vomiting during the operation. The risk of vomiting increases with sedation and can cause serious complications. Your nurse will give you any medication(s) that you need to take the morning of your surgery.

Bowel Preparation Regimen

For some surgeries, your provider may order "bowel prep" (bowel preparation) to clean out your intestines so that they can see the walls of your intestines. Starting at lunch the day before your procedure, you will only be allowed to eat and drink clear liquids. After your clear-liquid dinner you must drink a laxative drink to cause bowel movements. Your bowel movements should be clear before your surgery. If they are not, inform your nurse. Drink plenty of water before midnight on the night before your surgery.

Belongings

It is recommend that your family takes responsibility for your valuables. You can also ask Admissions to lock up your belongings. The intensive care unit (ICU) does not have storage space. Your nurse can help you with this process.

Morning of Surgery

Preparation

Before your procedure/surgery, your nurse will ask you to put on TED stockings (compression stockings) to help prevent blood clots, a possible complication of surgery. Your nurse will apply a dressing(s) to protect your skin.

Antibiotics

Your provider may prescribe an antibiotic for you during and after your surgery to prevent infection. Some surgeries (for example, abdominal surgeries) put you at a higher risk for infection.

Preparing for the Surgery

Before your surgery, you will meet your surgical team, including your surgeon, operating room nurses, and postanesthesia care unit (PACU) nurses. If you are going to have anesthesia (sedation), you will also meet an anesthesiologist and/or a nurse anesthetist who will examine you and administer the anesthesia during the surgery. The surgical team will take care of you before and after the operation.

Before the operation, you will be brought into the preop room and helped onto a stretcher. The operating room nurse will ask for your name and date of birth as well as take your vital signs and ask several presurgery questions. Some of these will include questions about allergies, medications, and diet. Your provider will also make sure that you signed an operative consent and confirm today's surgery. An Intravenous (I.V.) line will be placed in one of the veins in your arm or hand. If you already have a venous access device, please let your nurse know.

After Surgery

Upon arrival in the postanesthesia care unit (PACU), your nurse will frequently check your vital signs and dressing. Your recovery time in the PACU depends on the type of surgery performed, the amount of medication given, and your status after the surgery.

Chapter 11

Choosing a Hospital

When you're sick, you may go to the closest hospital or the hospital where your doctor practices. But which hospital is the best for your individual needs? Research shows that some hospitals do a better job taking care of patients with certain conditions than other hospitals.

When you have a life-threatening emergency, always go to the nearest hospital. However, if you're planning to have surgery, or if you have a condition like heart disease and know you may need hospital care in the future, learn about your hospital choices. Understanding your choices will help you have a more informed discussion with your doctor or other healthcare provider.

Before You Get Started

Make the most of your appointments with your doctor or other healthcare provider to learn about your condition and healthcare needs:

- Before your appointment, make a list of things you want to talk about (such as recent symptoms, drug side effects, or other general health questions). Bring this list to your appointment.

This chapter includes text excerpted from "Guide to Choosing a Hospital," Centers for Medicare and Medicaid Services (CMS), May 2010. Reviewed June 2017.

- Bring any prescription drugs, over-the-counter drugs, vitamins, and supplements to your appointment and review them with your doctor or provider.

- During your appointment, take notes. Then, take a moment to repeat back to the doctor or provider what you were told. Ask any questions you may have.

- Consider bringing along a trusted family member or friend.

- Ask if there's any written information about your condition that you can take with you.

- Call the office if you have questions when you get home.

Steps to Choosing a Hospital

Step One: Learn about the Care You Need and Your Hospital Choices

Talk to your doctor/healthcare provider about the following:

- Find out which hospitals they work with.

- Ask which hospitals they think give the best care for your condition (for example, have enough staffing, coordinate care, promote medication safety, and prevent infection).

- Ask how well these hospitals check and improve their quality of care. Do the hospitals participate in Medicare?

Based on your condition, ask your doctor/healthcare provider questions such as:

- Which hospitals have the best experience with your condition?

- Should you consider a specialty hospital, teaching hospital (usually part of a university), community hospital, or one that does research or has clinical trials related to your condition?

- If you need a surgeon or other type of specialist, what is his or her experience and success treating your condition?

- Who will be responsible for your overall care while you're in the hospital?

- Will you need care after leaving the hospital and, if so, what kind of care? Who will arrange this care?

- Are there any alternatives to hospital care?

Step Two: Think about Your Personal and Financial Needs

Check your hospital insurance coverage:

- Do you need permission from your health plan (like a preauthorization or a referral) before you're admitted for hospital care?

- If you need care that's not emergency care, do you have to use certain hospitals? Do you have to see certain surgeons or specialists?

- Do you have to pay more to use a hospital (surgeon or specialist) that doesn't participate in your plan?

- Do you need to meet certain requirements to get care after you leave the hospital?

- If you don't have insurance, call the hospital before you're admitted, and ask to speak to someone about setting up a payment plan or other resources to help with payment.

Think about your preferences:

- Do you want a hospital near family members or friends?

- Does the hospital have convenient visiting hours and other rules that are important to you? For example, can a relative or someone helping with your care stay overnight in the room with you?

Step Three: Find and Compare Hospitals Based on Your Condition and Needs

Use the Hospital Compare Web tool at www.medicare.gov/hospitalcompare/search.html to do the following and more:

- Find hospitals by name, city, county, state, or ZIP code.

- Check the results of patient surveys (what patients said about their hospital experiences).

- Compare the results of certain measures of quality that show how well these hospitals treat certain conditions.

You can also call 1-800-MEDICARE (1-800-633-4227). TTY users should call 1-877-486-2048. Search online for other sources to compare the quality of the hospitals you're considering. Some states have laws that require hospitals to report data about the quality and cost of their care and post the data online.

Step Four: Discuss Your Hospital Options and Choose a Hospital

- Talk with family members or friends about the hospitals you're comparing.

- Talk to your doctor or healthcare provider how the hospital information you gathered applies to you.

- Choose the hospital that's best for you.

Hospital Quality Check

Here's a quick summary of what to look for when comparing hospitals:

Look for a hospital that:

- Has the best experience with your condition.

- Checks and improves the quality of its care.

- Performs well on measures of quality, including a national patient survey, that are published on the Hospital Compare Web tool (www.medicare.gov/hospitalcompare/search.html).

- Participate in Medicare.

- Meets your needs in terms of location and other factors, like visiting hours.

- Is covered by your health plan.

Chapter 12

Ambulatory Surgical Centers

What Are Ambulatory Surgical Centers (ASCs)?

Ambulatory surgical centers (ASCs), also known as surgicenters, are healthcare facilities where surgical procedures that do not require hospital admission are carried out within the same day.

Until the introduction of ASCs, all surgeries in the United States were carried out in a hospital setting. Waiting periods for a surgery ranging from weeks to months were not uncommon and patients spent weeks recovering from their treatment. The ambulatory surgical centers were pioneered in the 1970s when two physicians opened a facility offering a low-cost and high-quality alternative to inpatient surgical services in hospitals. They presented ASCs as a better option for routine surgeries after being frustrated with scheduling issues, waiting periods, operating room nonavailability, and limited equipment at traditional hospitals.

ASCs are not health clinics and do not provide diagnostic and primary healthcare services. They provide surgical intervention for patients whose physicians have recommended certain types of procedures for treatment.

How Do You Choose Quality Ambulatory Care?

Your physician can help you determine if an ambulatory surgical center is the best option for your procedure and, if so, which facility is best. Also, take into account the following information to help you make the best choice:

Questions Regarding Care

- Is this a state licensed facility? Is it accredited?
- Can your family members accompany and wait with you until you can go home?
- What are the risks and frequency of such surgeries at the facility?
- How is pain dealt with during surgery? Can you discuss this with the anesthesiologist?
- Ask for a copy or your legal rights and responsibilities and enquire if it will be explained to you in laymen terms.
- Will your treatment details remain confidential? What are the cases under which patient information is disclosed?
- Does this facility participate in your health insurance?

Questions Regarding Staff

- Are the doctors and nurses professionally qualified and do they have adequate experience?
- Are the healthcare staff trained in medical emergency procedures such as CPR (cardiopulmonary resuscitation)?

Questions Regarding Emergency Care Postsurgery

- Is a 24-hour emergency telephone number available in case of an emergency? Will it be answered by a doctor or nurse in case you have questions?
- Does the facility have a disaster readiness plan? Can the facility handle a power failure or natural disaster?
- Does the facility have a transfer agreement with a local hospital?

What Are Some Common Surgical Procedures Carried Out in ASCs?

Common surgical specialties in an ambulatory setting include the following:

- Plastic surgery of the neck

- Cosmetic and facial surgeries such as chin reconstruction, augmentation and reduction of facial bones, and revision of the eyelids and sockets
- Endoscopic procedures of the nose, sinus, vascular, upper GI, small bowel, kidney, and ureter
- Laryngoscopy
- Colonoscopy
- Arthroscopy of the wrist, shoulder, hip, and knee
- Ophthalmological surgeries such as corneal transplantation, glaucoma surgery, cataract surgery, and ocular implantation

Frequently carried out surgical procedures include tonsillectomy, lens and cataract procedures, myringotomy, adenoidectomy, and semilunar knee cartilage removal.

What Are the Advantages of ASCs?

Depending on the procedure and the individual facility, an ambulatory surgical center can have the following benefits:

Cost. Outpatient surgical procedures at ASCs can cost one-half to one-third of what is charged at hospitals. Medicare beneficiaries may also pay lesser at ASCs compared to hospitals. Be aware that the cost varies based on the procedure and patients must consult with Medicare before preparing for their surgery.

Convenience. Generally, there is less paperwork and administrative concerns at ASCs. Also, doctors are in charge of setting standards for staffing, safety, operative procedures, and patient care rather than managerial staff as is the case in hospitals.

Efficiency. ASCs are generally more efficient at scheduling surgeries, getting equipment and materials ready for surgery. This is an advantage that surgeons benefit from. Surgeons can in fact take care of multiple patients at the same time that they take to treat one patient in a hospital environment.

What Are the Federal Rules Governing Ambulatory Surgical Centers?

ASC facilities are governed by federal and state laws in the United States. The rules that apply to all other healthcare facilities apply to

ASCs as well. Adherence to standards of quality and safety in ASCs are governed by three processes. They are:

1. State licensure

2. Medicare certification

3. Voluntary accreditation.

The rules for licensure of ASCs in each state varies. ASCs serving Medicare beneficiaries must be certified by the program. Medicare standards must be complied with initially and on an ongoing basis. ASCs also choose to be accredited with independent bodies such as the Joint Commission on Accreditation of Healthcare Organizations (JCAHO), the Accreditation Association for Ambulatory Health Care (AAAHC), the American Association for the Accreditation of Ambulatory Surgery Facilities (AAAASF), and the American Osteopathic Association (AOA). Accrediting agencies conduct onsite inspections and ASCs benchmark themselves to stay competent.

References

1. "Ambulatory Surgery Centers: A Positive Trend in Healthcare," The American Society for Gastrointestinal Endoscopy, n.d.

2. "Helping You Choose: Quality Ambulatory Care," The Joint Commission, October 2013.

3. "Ambulatory Surgery Centers," Advameg, Inc., n.d.

4. "What Are the 5 Most Common Ambulatory Surgeries?" Medical Transcription Billing, Corp, September 19, 2016.

5. "Using the Ambulatory Surgery Rate Codes in APGs," New York State Department of Health, April 2, 2009.

Chapter 13

Anesthesia

Chapter Contents

Section 13.1

Anesthesia Basics

This section includes text excerpted from "Anesthesia
Fact Sheet," National Institute of General Medical
Sciences (NIGMS), June 22, 2016.

Anesthesia is a medical treatment that prevents patients from
feeling pain during surgery. Anesthesia has made possible countless
procedures that improve human health, longevity and quality of life.
Every year, millions of Americans safely undergo surgery with anesthesia, although some risks exist.

Anesthesia consists of several components, including sedation,
unconsciousness, immobility, analgesia (lack of pain) and amnesia
(lack of memory). Scientists have developed drugs called anesthetics
that target each of these elements.

Most anesthetics fall into one of two broad categories: general or
local/regional.

General Anesthesia

General anesthesia affects the entire body. It is used when it is
important for a patient to be unconscious. Many major, life-saving
procedures like open-heart surgery, brain surgery or organ transplantation would be impossible without general anesthesia.

General anesthetics are either delivered intravenously or breathed
in as a gas. Intravenous anesthetics act quickly and disappear rapidly
from the bloodstream, so patients can go home sooner after surgery.
Inhaled anesthetics may take longer to wear off.

Although general anesthetics are usually considered quite safe for
most patients, they can pose risks, particularly for elderly patients, those
with certain genetic variations, and those with some chronic, systemic
diseases, such as diabetes. In addition, some patients, especially the
elderly and children, may have lingering effects for several days after
general anesthesia. Fortunately, serious side effects—such as danger-
ously low blood pressure—are much less common than they once were.

Local and Regional Anesthesia

Doctors use local and regional anesthetics to block pain in a part of the body. Local anesthetics affect a small part of the body, such as a single tooth. Regional anesthetics affect larger areas, such as everything below the waist.

With local and regional anesthetics, patients can remain conscious and comfortable during surgery. But, like all drugs, these anesthetics can have side effects, and delivering them to the right spot is sometimes difficult.

How Anesthesia Works

For many decades after anesthetics became a routine part of surgery, practically nothing was known about how they work. Virtually all scientists believed that anesthetics blocked nerve cell signaling by disrupting fatty molecules in the membranes that envelop cells. This theory, first put forward in the early 1900s, dominated research on anesthetics for much of the 20th century. Anesthetics are difficult to work with in the laboratory, and the lack of tools to study them at the molecular level contributed to this period of slow scientific progress.

Advances in cell biology, genetics and molecular biology have transformed anesthesiology into an active area of research. Scientists no longer think that anesthetics work by acting on fatty molecules in cell membranes. The bulk of the evidence now supports the idea that the drugs interfere with nerve signals by targeting specific protein molecules embedded in nerve cell membranes. Researchers also believe that inhaled and intravenous anesthetics each act on a different set of molecules to bring about their characteristic effects.

Surgery before the Availability of Anesthesia

Prior to the 1840s, doctors and dentists did not routinely use anesthesia when operating on patients. Most doctors attempted surgery only when it was absolutely necessary to save a person's life, and operations were largely limited to amputations and removal of external growths. Although alcohol, opium or other botanicals sometimes helped alleviate the agony, most surgical patients remained conscious and endured excruciating pain.

Anesthesia: At the Beginning

In 1846, a dentist publicly demonstrated that ether, a colorless liquid that vaporizes quickly, would put patients to sleep during surgery. The practice began to spread. Doctors and dentists soaked a sponge or a cloth with ether and had patients breathe in the fumes through an inhaler.

The fumes knocked the person out, but there was no way to control the amount inhaled. If patients inhaled too little, they could wake up during surgery and flail about in pain; if they inhaled too much, they might never wake. To make matters worse, ether is highly flammable, and a spark in the operating room could cause a dangerous explosion. Despite the problems with ether, its use enabled surgeons to perform internal procedures that would have been too painful or complicated to conduct on conscious patients.

The introduction of less flammable anesthetic gases made operating rooms safer, and the discovery of intravenous anesthetic agents such as sodium thiopental made it possible for surgeons to control the dose. But well into the 1950s, doctors still usually sedated their patients using some type of anesthetic gas and monitored them with nothing more sophisticated than a stethoscope. Dangerous side effects were common and included heart rhythm and breathing problems, lowered blood pressure, nausea, and vomiting.

Training Anesthesiologists

Like all medical doctors, anesthesiologists earn an undergraduate degree (often in a life sciences field) and a medical degree (M.D. or D.O.). Then they must complete a four year residency program in anesthesiology. Many choose to complete an additional one year fellowship in a specialty such as pain management, pediatric anesthesiology or critical care medicine.

During Surgery

Anesthesiologists carefully monitor patients throughout surgery using electronic devices that continually display vital signs. Major advances in monitoring include the continuous measurement of blood pressure, blood oxygen levels, heart function and respiratory patterns. These advances have dramatically improved the safety of general anesthesia and make it possible to operate on many patients who were previously considered too sick to undergo surgery.

Role of Anesthesiologist outside the Operating Room

The role of the anesthesiologist has expanded to include caring for patients during postoperative recovery. Anesthesiologists also provide anesthesia for nonsurgical procedures such as endoscopy and various cardiac interventions, as well as during labor and delivery. As experts in pain management, anesthesiologists may manage pain clinics or advise other specialists on how to manage pain.

Advancements in Anesthesia

As scientists learn more about the molecular mechanisms by which anesthetics cause their various effects, they will be able to design agents that are more targeted, more effective and safer, with fewer side effects.

Observations of the short- and long-term effects of anesthetics on subsets of the population, such as the elderly or cancer survivors, will reveal whether certain anesthetics are better than others for members of those groups. Research on how a person's genetic makeup influences the way he or she responds to anesthetics will enable doctors to further tailor anesthesia to individual patients.

Research in Anesthesia

Knowledge of how anesthetics affect pain and consciousness helps scientists gain a better understanding of the mechanisms that underlie these physiological states. Understanding these mechanisms could lead to new ways to alleviate pain and to new treatments for conditions associated with a decrease or loss of consciousness, such as epilepsy and coma. Studies of anesthesia may also provide insights into the nature of consciousness itself.

Section 13.2

Regional Anesthesia for Postsurgical Pain

This section includes text excerpted from "Regional Anesthesia FAQs," U.S. Department of Veterans Affairs (VA), June 5, 2014.

What Is Regional Anesthesia?

"Regional anesthesia" is a targeted type of anesthesia. It involves injecting numbing medicine around nerves that provide sensation to specific regions or parts of your body (e.g., arm, leg, foot) and can be used instead of general anesthesia or in addition to general anesthesia as a way to control pain after surgery. Anesthesiologists can perform these procedures before surgery to prevent pain, or they can provide regional anesthesia as a "rescue" technique to relieve pain after surgery. Types of regional anesthesia procedures include spinal, epidural or peripheral nerve block. Depending on the type of numbing medicine (local anesthetic) used, a nerve block can last for a few hours or up to a whole day. For more painful surgeries, anesthesiologists can insert a tiny tube (also known as a "catheter") that can continuously bathe the nerves in numbing medicine for an additional 2–3 days.

There are many advantages to regional anesthesia. Because you will have decreased sensation, you need to take less opioid (narcotic) pain medicines even though you will commonly have these medications prescribed to you. Patients who receive regional anesthesia also have less nausea, recover more quickly immediately after surgery, and sleep better overnight compared to patients who do not have regional anesthesia.

Even if you choose regional anesthesia instead of general anesthesia, you don't have to be "awake" during surgery. Anesthesiologists often combine regional anesthesia with either intravenous sedation or general anesthesia, both of which can allow you to "sleep" during surgery. You should discuss your preferences with your anesthesiologist prior to surgery.

There are always risks associated with performing any procedure. Fortunately, serious complications associated with regional anesthesia are exceedingly rare. Anesthesiology practices that specialize in regional anesthesia commonly have systems in place to prevent complications and treat them quickly if or when they occur.

What Can I Expect on the Day of Surgery?

Before surgery (or on the day of surgery at the latest), you will meet with an anesthesiologist who will evaluate whether or not regional anesthesia is the right option for you. If you are eligible and desire regional anesthesia preoperatively, the anesthesiologist will perform your nerve block approximately 30–60 minutes before your surgery. Nerve blocks may be performed in a specialized area ("block room") outside of the operating room. After your intravenous (IV) is inserted, your anesthesiologist may provide you with sedating medication during the performance of your nerve block. Before the procedure starts, your anesthesiologist will perform a "time-out" with you to confirm the correct site and side of your surgical procedure. It has become increasingly common for anesthesiologists to use ultrasound to identify your unique anatomy and safely inject numbing medication around the nerves. After the nerve block, your affected limb will "go to sleep" over the next 10–20 minutes.

What Are My Regional Anesthesia Options for Hand, Wrist, Forearm, or Elbow Surgery?

For hand, wrist, forearm, or elbow surgeries (e.g., carpal tunnel release, fracture repair, or tendon transfer) there are a few different locations in which to place the nerve block depending on the site of surgery and expected placement of the tourniquet (if utilized). Most commonly, the nerve block is performed above the collarbone ("supraclavicular block") or below the collarbone ("infraclavicular block"). For extensive surgeries involving bones and/or joints, your anesthesiologist can place a catheter that will bathe the nerve in numbing medicine for an additional 2–3 days. An infraclavicular catheter may have advantages over the supraclavicular catheter in terms of pain control.

What Are My Regional Anesthesia Options for Upper Arm or Shoulder Surgery?

For surgeries involving the upper arm or shoulder, nerve blocks are most commonly performed in the neck ("interscalene block"). For extensive arthroscopic shoulder surgery and shoulder replacement, a catheter near the nerves that can deliver numbing medicine for 2–3 days is recommended. This type of pain relief helps you perform physical therapy and reduces your need for opioid (narcotic) pain medications.

What Are My Regional Anesthesia Options for Knee Surgery?

For surgeries involving the knee including total knee replacement, nerve blocks are routinely placed near the groin ("femoral nerve block") or on the inside part of the thigh where the nerves to the front of the knee are located ("adductor canal block"). For patients having total knee replacement, your anesthesiologist may place a catheter to deliver numbing medicine near the nerves for 2–3 days. This type of pain relief will help you perform physical therapy, reduce your need for opioid (narcotic) pain medications, and decrease the time it takes for you to achieve discharge criteria. An adductor canal catheter may help patients walk further immediately after total knee replacement surgery compared to a femoral nerve catheter although both provide effective pain relief.

It is important to realize that any nerve block may also cause weak muscles. Therefore, after your nerve block, you must realize that you are at increased risk of falling because your leg may not be strong enough to support your weight. Anesthesiology practices that provide regional anesthesia for pain relief after joint replacement are advised to have a comprehensive fall prevention program in place. However, in the immediate postoperative period it is important to always ask for assistance anytime you need to get out of bed. Do not attempt to walk by yourself.

What Are My Regional Anesthesia Options for Hip Surgery?

For hip surgery, nerve blocks are performed above the groin crease near the nerves that affect the front and side of the hip ("fascia iliaca block" or femoral nerve block) or in the back ("lumbar plexus block"); both approaches provide similar pain relief. Alternatively, a spinal block with numbing and/or opioid (narcotic) pain medication may be placed.

It is important to realize that any nerve block may also cause weak muscles. Therefore, after your nerve block, you must realize that you are at increased risk of falling because your leg may not be strong enough to support your weight. Anesthesiology practices that provide regional anesthesia for pain relief after joint replacement are advised to have a comprehensive fall prevention program in place. However, in the immediate postoperative period it is important to always ask for assistance anytime you need to get out of bed. Do not attempt to walk by yourself.

What Are My Regional Anesthesia Options for Foot or Ankle Surgery?

For surgeries involving the foot or ankle, nerve blocks are most commonly performed in the area behind your knee ("popliteal sciatic block") or at the level of the ankle ("ankle block"). For more invasive surgeries of this area (e.g., tendon/ligament repairs and fractures), your anesthesiologist may recommend a catheter near the nerves that can deliver numbing medicine into the area for 2–3 days. This type of pain relief helps you perform physical therapy and reduces your need for opioid (narcotic) pain medications.

What Are My Regional Anesthesia Options for Facial Surgery?

For surgeries involving the face and neck, it may be possible to perform specific nerve blocks to minimize your postoperative pain. These may be performed by your anesthesiologist or surgeon. Common procedures that are suitable for these nerve blocks include skin cancer excision, endoscopic sinus surgery, septoplasty, and rhinoplasty. Your anesthesiologist will discuss these options with you on the day of surgery and determine if you are a good candidate for regional anesthesia.

What Are My Regional Anesthesia Options for Chest or Abdominal Surgery?

For major surgeries involving the chest or abdomen, your anesthesiologist may offer you an epidural or spinal block in addition to general anesthesia. Alternatively, special types of nerve block procedures, paravertebral blocks and TAP blocks, have also been shown to provide effective pain relief after these surgeries. Your anesthesiologist will discuss these options with you on the day of surgery and determine if you are a good candidate for regional anesthesia.

How Long Will the Numbness from the Local Anesthetic Medication Last?

The intensity and duration of your block largely depends on the type of numbing medicine (local anesthetic) that was used, as well as whether you receive a single dose of medication or have a nerve block catheter in place. As a single dose, some local anesthetic medications provide a few hours of numbness while others can provide numbness that lasts up to a day.

What Should I Know about The "Nerve Block Catheter"?

A nerve block catheter is a skinny tube placed near your nerves in order to continuously bathe your nerves with local anesthetic (numbing) medication. The catheter is attached to a pump the size of a small grapefruit or a similar type of device. This pump is filled with local anesthetic (numbing) medication which is continuously delivered through the catheter to provide you with pain relief for 2–3 days. Once the medication runs out, the catheter should be removed. Removal is a simple procedure that you or a caretaker can do at home. Your anesthesiologist or another healthcare provider should follow up with you daily (by phone if you are at home) and be available for any questions that you may have regarding the catheter and pump.

Catheters are more suitable for certain surgeries and nerve sites than others. Your anesthesiologist will help you determine whether or not this is a good option for you.

Does It Hurt to Get a Nerve Block?

Getting a nerve block should be no more painful than getting an IV. The skin is numbed before placing the nerve block and mild sedation can also be provided prior to the procedure. Also, using ultrasound to locate the nerves during the procedure minimizes the amount of pain that you feel.

Is It Safe to Get a Nerve Block?

There are always risks associated with performing any procedure. Fortunately, serious complications associated with regional anesthesia are exceedingly rare. Anesthesiology practices that specialize in regional anesthesia commonly have systems in place to prevent complications and treat them quickly if or when they occur. This procedure is performed in a sterile manner to minimize the risk of infection. The possibility of trauma to the nerves exists, but your anesthesiologist may take special precautions, including the use of ultrasound, to decrease this risk. Most commonly, patients report mild bruising or soreness from the site of injection.

Section 13.3

Surgery Risks

Thanks to advances in science, research and modern medicine by physicians, surgery and anesthesia are safer than ever before. But this doesn't mean these procedures aren't without risks. Any number of things can go wrong in the operating room, which is why it is important to talk with your doctor in advance and have a highly trained physician anesthesiologist supervising your care.

Think of physician anesthesiologists as your seat belt during surgery: When there are emergencies or complications, they can save your life.

Thanks to advances in science, research and modern medicine, surgery and anesthesia are safer than ever. But this doesn't mean these procedures are without risks. To minimize your risk, it's important to speak with your physician in advance and have a highly trained physician anesthesiologist supervising your care.

Certain health conditions may increase the risks of surgery and the potential for complications from anesthesia. These cos include:

- high blood pressure

- heart disease (angina, valve disease, heart failure or a previous heart attack)

- diabetes
- stroke
- seizures or other neurological disorders
- obesity
- obstructive sleep apnea
- lung conditions (asthma and chronic obstructive pulmonary disease, or COPD)
- kidney problems
- allergies to anesthesia or a history of adverse reactions to anesthesia

Smoking, or drinking two or more alcoholic beverages a day, also can increase the risks of surgery and complications from anesthesia.

To determine your risk before any surgery or procedure, your physician anesthesiologist will take a complete medical history to find out if you have any of these conditions or other issues, as well as ask if you are taking any medications, supplements or vitamins. It's important for you to share all of your health information so your physician anesthesiologist can safely and effectively manage your care and treat any complications that might occur before, during or after surgery. For example, your physician anesthesiologist may choose a different type of anesthesia or method for providing it, which may be safer for you, based on your health conditions.

There also are simple steps you can take to ensure the best possible outcome.

Anesthesia Awareness

Very rarely—in only one or two out of every 10,000 medical procedures involving anesthesia—a patient may become aware or conscious. The condition—called anesthesia awareness—means the patient can recall the surroundings or an event related to the surgery while under general anesthesia. Although it can be upsetting, patients usually do not feel pain.

Certain surgeries or circumstances increase the risk of awareness during surgery because the usual dose of required anesthesia cannot be used safely. These include emergency surgeries—such as C-sections, heart surgery and trauma surgery—as well as when patients

122

have multiple medical conditions. Physician anesthesiologists closely monitor surgeries using sophisticated equipment to ensure that, even in the rare case when awareness occurs, a patient is safe and does not feel pain.

If you think you experienced anesthesia awareness during a procedure, tell your physician anesthesiologist or healthcare team as soon as possible.

It's not uncommon for patients to believe they were aware during surgery, when this was not the case. A patient typically remembers the time when the anesthesia has just begun to work but has not completely taken effect, or shortly after surgery, when the anesthesia has not yet worn off, but this is not considered awareness which would take place during the procedure.

Patients also are more likely to have awareness with procedures that do not involve general anesthesia. For example, you may recall all or part of your procedure if you have:

- Intravenous, or "twilight" sedation, often given during minor procedures such as a colonoscopy, a biopsy or a dental procedure

- Local or regional anesthesia, such as an epidural or spinal block, or a nerve block

To reduce your risk of experiencing awareness during procedures with general anesthesia, it is important to tell your physician anesthesiologist important health information, including:

- Previous problems with anesthesia, including a history of being aware during surgery

- All medications you are taking, both prescription, over-the-counter and herbal supplements

- Concerns you may have about surgery, including fear of being aware during surgery

Patients who have experienced anesthesia awareness during a procedure can get counseling to help ease any feelings of confusion, stress or trauma.

Obesity and Anesthesia

More than one-third of Americans are obese or significantly overweight and at increased risk for a number of health conditions, including heart disease, cancer, diabetes and stroke.

If you or a loved one are overweight or obese and planning to have surgery, you should be aware that excess weight can make it more challenging to safely administer anesthesia during surgery. Common challenges in administering anesthesia in overweight patients may include:

- Increasing difficulty in locating veins in order to deliver anesthesia and life-saving emergency medications intravenously
- Determining and providing the right dose of medications
- Ensuring you get enough oxygen and airflow. Obstructive Sleep Apnea, a chronic medical problem common with obesity, can present with serious breathing problems before, during, and after surgery
- Taking a longer time to regain consciousness
- Increasing the risk of affecting breathing with narcotics and other pain medicines
- Placing a breathing tube

Improving your health before surgery, including losing weight under a doctor's supervision, can help make surgery as safe as possible, decrease your chances of complications and help you get back on your feet faster. Your physician anesthesiologist will meet with you prior to surgery to discuss your overall health including your weight and any other medical issues you might have such as high blood pressure, diabetes or gastro-esophageal reflux disease (GERD). With an understanding of your current health conditions, your physician anesthesiologist can be fully prepared to provide you the safest, highest-quality care during surgery or a procedure.

Sleep Apnea and Anesthesia

Sleep apnea affects as many as 18 million Americans, and as many as 16 million don't realize they have it. The condition can lead to health issues, such as high blood pressure, and can cause complications during surgery. You might have sleep apnea if you:

- Are frequently tired when you wake in the morning and throughout the day
- Have trouble staying asleep at night
- Have been told that you snore or stop breathing during sleep
- Wake up throughout the night or constantly turn from side to side

- Have been told that your legs or arms jerk while you're sleeping

- Make abrupt snorting noises during sleep

The most common type of sleep apnea is obstructive sleep apnea which occurs when the soft tissue in the rear of the throat narrows and closes during sleep, causing you to stop breathing, which in turn wakes you up to take a breath. You may not remember waking up even though it may happen hundreds of times each night.

Anesthesia can make the condition worse, which is why it's extremely important to let your physician anesthesiologist know you may have obstructive sleep apnea if you're having surgery. Anesthesia also can cause the throat to relax and close up and sleep apnea can lead to breathing problems after surgery. It also can make it more difficult to regain consciousness after surgery and take a breath.

If you have or suspect you have obstructive sleep apnea and you need surgery, be sure to discuss your symptoms with your physician anesthesiologist prior to the procedure. While complications are rare, there are precautions that can be taken before, during and after your surgery to help ensure the best outcome.

Smoking and Anesthesia

Smoking can cause significant health problems, from heart disease to asthma to lung cancer. And if you are having surgery, it also can increase the risk of anesthesia-related complications like wound infections, pneumonia and heart attack. Here's how:

- If you smoke, your heart and lungs don't work as well as they should and you may have breathing and lung problems during or after surgery.

- After surgery, you are much more likely to need a ventilator—a machine that breathes for you—because of your increased risk of breathing and lung problems.

That's why it's important to quit smoking as soon as possible before surgery and for as long as possible after. Quitting at least a week before the procedure is ideal, but even quitting the day before surgery can help. Research shows the body begins to heal within hours of quitting smoking. The lungs begin to function better and blood flow improves which is important for getting through surgery safely and healing from it quickly.

Surgery might present the perfect time to kick the habit for good. Physician anesthesiologists are heart and lung specialists and during surgery, they see first-hand the heavy toll smoking takes on the body which is why they strongly encourage anyone who smokes to quit for good. Quitting improves your overall health and can:

- Add at least six to eight years to your life

- Reduce your risk of lung cancer and heart disease

- Save you an average of $1,400 a year

- Reduce your loved ones' exposure to second-hand smoke

Free help to quit smoking is available by calling 1-800-QuitNow, where you will be connected to trained specialists who can guide you and provide a customized plan to help you quit.

Chapter 14

Substance Use and Surgery

Chapter Contents

Section 14.1

Alcohol Use and Heart Surgery

"Alcohol Use and Heart Surgery," © 2017 Omnigraphics.
Reviewed June 2017.

It is important to disclose history of active alcohol use prior to heart surgery because it is associated with serious postsurgical complications. Alcohol use will likely impact planned recovery. It is crucial to let your surgeon know how many drinks you consume per day or per week. Excessive drinking is defined as having more than 3 drinks per day and is known to affect the outcome of surgery.

How Does Alcohol Use Affect Heart Surgery?

A standard drink is defined as 12 ounces of beer, 5 ounces of wine or 1.5 ounces of 80-proof liquor. Consuming more than three drinks a day could lead to complications after heart surgery. Alcohol withdrawal syndrome manifests when people stop drinking suddenly after consuming alcohol for an extended period of time. The central nervous system "overreacts" during withdrawal, causing shakiness, sweating, hallucinations, and other symptoms.

If left untreated, it results in life-threatening conditions such as tremors, seizures, delirium tremens and sometimes, even death. Ultimately, this leads to a longer stay in the intensive care unit (ICU) for recovery after heart surgery. Heavy drinking also causes organ systems to malfunction and interferes with biochemical controls. This might lead to conditions harmful to survival after heart surgery.

Why Are the Outcomes of Alcohol Withdrawal Treatment before Surgery?

Alcohol withdrawal treatment prior to surgery offers the following benefits.

- Strong doses of sedatives may not be needed.

- Restraining devices may not be required.

- Decrease in seizures and delirium tremens after surgery.
- Ventilator support may not be needed for a long-term.
- Reduction in complications in organs and biochemical processes.
- Reduction in falls and injuries.
- Shorter stay after surgery for recovery.

How to Understand That You Could Be at Risk for Alcohol Withdrawal?

Once heart surgery is finalized as the course of treatment, you will be interviewed and asked to answer a questionnaire. Make sure you answer honestly all the questions in it. This could facilitate better treatment and increase your chances of full recovery. The information you provide is kept confidential and should not be a cause of concern.

When Can I Drink Alcohol after Heart Surgery?

Consult with your doctor before you start drinking after surgery to be on the safer side. This way you can be assured that you will not be causing yourself any harm.

Will Alcohol Interact with Prescribed Medication?

Alcohol interacts with medication, potentially changing its effects depending on the type of medication you have been prescribed. Mixing alcohol with certain medications is possibly lethal, particularly painkillers and sleep medication. Excessive alcohol also affects coagulation of blood. And you should be careful if you've been prescribed anticoagulants such as Warfarin.

Is It Safe to Drink after Full Recovery?

It is fine to drink within recommended limits after recovery from heart surgery. However, check with your doctor to make sure it is indeed safe for you to drink. If you've been diagnosed with certain types of cardiomyopathy you will be advised to avoid drinking completely.

Some drinks known as caffeinated alcoholic drinks contain caffeine and overwork the heart. They are not advisable if you've been diagnosed with tachycardias and arrhythmias.

Does Drinking in Moderation Have Its Benefits?

Excessive drinkers statistically carry more risk of cardiovascular complications compared to teetotalers. On the other hand, some studies have indicated that moderate drinkers are at 25 percent lesser risk of complications postsurgery compared to patients who do not drink at all.

Men are advised not to have more than two drinks a day and women should restrict themselves to one a day.

References

1. "Alcohol & Heart Surgery," Cleveland Clinic, n.d.

2. "Advisory: Alcohol Screening and Management Protocols," Commonwealth of Massachusetts, Board of Registration in Medicine, July 2013.

3. "Heart Conditions and Alcohol," British Heart Foundation, n.d.

4. "Alcohol and Heart Health," American Heart Association, January 12, 2015.

Section 14.2

Smoking and Surgery

Did you know that before surgery is the best time to quit smoking?

- You will decrease your risk of complications.

- Hospitals are a smoke-free environment, so you won't be tempted.

- The quit rate is much higher when you quit before your operation.

Do your part and quit now! Your surgical team is here to help.

Smoking Increases Your Risk of Heart and Breathing Problems

Smoking increases the mucus in the airways and decreases your ability to fight infection. It also increases the risk of pneumonia and other breathing problems. Airway function improves if you quit 8 weeks before your procedure.

The nicotine from cigarettes can increase your blood pressure, heart rate, and risk of arrhythmias (irregular heart beat). The carbon monoxide in cigarettes decreases the amount of oxygen in your blood. Quitting at least 1 day before your operation can reduce your blood pressure and irregular heart beats.

Smokers have an increased risk of blood clots and almost twice the risk of a heart attack as nonsmokers. A smoker is 2.2 times more likely to get pneumonia than a nonsmoker. So if a nonsmoker has a 10 percent risk, a smoker has a 22 percent risk.

Smoking Increases Your Risk of Wound Complications

Oxygen is needed for your tissues to heal. Smoking can decrease the amount of blood, oxygen, and nutrients that go to your surgical site. A smoker has almost 4 times the risk of tissue damage at the surgical site.

Smoking interferes with all phases of wound healing. It also decreases the ability of the cells to kill bacteria and fight infection. Having a wound infection increases the average length of stay by 2 to 4 days. Quitting 4 weeks before a surgical procedure reduces postoperative complications by 20 to 30 percent.

Studies identify that patients who smoke have:

- Increased wound infection and splitting open of the wound in patients having general surgery or hip and knee replacements.

- Increased sternal (chest bone) wound infection after coronary bypass surgery.

- Increased wound necrosis (tissue death) after mastectomy and breast reconstruction.

- Increased incisional and recurrent inguinal hernias.

131

- Lack of bone healing after orthopaedic surgery.

- Delayed healing and tissue death in plastic surgery.

- Greater pain intensity and higher amounts of narcotics needed for pain control.

Smoking Cessation at the Time of Surgery May Be the Best Time to Quit

- Smoking cessation counseling before a surgical procedure increases the quit rate.

- Multiple approaches (counseling plus medication) work best to help you stay quit for life.

- You will most likely be receiving pain medication after surgery, which will decrease your withdrawal effects.

Smoking Increases Your Risk of Cancer Recurrence

In cancer survivors, continued smoking increases the risk of death from cancer and other diseases. It also increases your risk of developing another cancer. Secondhand smoke causes lung cancer in both children and adults who don't smoke.

Treatment

The following treatments are proven to be effective for smokers who want help to quit. Be sure to discuss with your doctor what is right for you.

- Cold turkey: Quitting on your own because you are motivated to have a successful surgery.

- Smoking cessation counseling with your doctor/professional.

- Telephone counseling: Call the Quit Line at 1-800-QUIT-NOW (1-800-784-8669). Help is free and all information is confidential.

- Behavior therapy: Training to help you cope when you want a smoke.

- Medications, including:
  - Varenicline (Chantix) and bupropion SR (Zyban) both require a prescription and are started 1 to 2 weeks before quitting.

- Nicotine replacement therapy (NRT) delivers a safer source of nicotine than cigarettes, may decrease the withdrawal effect, and may help prevent overeating.

- The health effects of electronic cigarettes (e-cigarettes) as a quit method and the vapors they give off are unknown. Initial lab tests conducted by the FDA found levels of toxic cancer-causing chemicals.

Table 14.1. Medicines for Smoking Cessation

Medication	How Do I Take This?	When Do I Begin?
Varenicline*	Orally with a meal and water	1 to 2 weeks before quitting
Bupropion*	Orally; dose is decreased day by day	1 to 2 weeks before quitting
Nicotine patch	Apply patch to the skin	Do not smoke; use as directed
Nicotine gum	Chew	Do not smoke; use as directed
Nicotine lozenge	Dissolve in the mouth	Do not smoke; use as directed
Nicotine inhaler*	Spray in the back of the throat	Do not smoke; use as directed
Nicotine nasal spray*	Spray in the nose	Do not smoke; use as directed

Available only with a prescription

Chapter 15

Blood Donation

Chapter Contents

Section 15.1

Donating Blood for Surgery

This section includes text excerpted from "Have You
Given Blood Lately?" U.S. Food and Drug
Administration (FDA), December 21, 2016.

Every day, hospitals throughout the United States transfuse blood
or blood components, such as platelets, to save the lives of people
who are in motor vehicle accidents, and victims of fires and other
emergencies.

Blood is also required for many people with life-threatening illnesses and others undergoing routine surgeries. According to the Centers for Disease Control and Prevention (CDC), an estimated 5 million
patients receive blood annually.

In fact, every two seconds, someone in America needs blood, according to the American Red Cross (ARC). This may include:

- cancer patients undergoing chemotherapy

- people with sickle cell disease or other types of inherited anemia

- organ transplant recipients

- people undergoing elective surgery

- women during and following labor and delivery

- premature babies

- trauma victims

Blood products from healthy donors are often lifesaving or life
enhancing.

U.S. Food and Drug Administration (FDA) Oversight

U.S. Food and Drug Administration (FDA), through the Center for
Biologics and Research (CBER), is responsible for ensuring the safety
of the more than the approximately 19 million units of whole blood
donated each year in the United States. These donations can be further

processed into blood components such as Red Blood Cells (RBCs), platelets, and plasma. FDA's standards and regulations regarding blood donor selection, blood donation, and processing help protect the health of both the donor and the recipient.

FDA's oversight of the blood industry includes:

- approving licenses for blood products
- approving devices used for blood collection, infectious disease testing and pathogen reduction technologies
- developing and enforcing quality standards
- providing guidance on emerging infectious diseases
- inspecting all blood facilities at least every two years
- inspecting "problem" facilities more often
- monitoring reports of errors and adverse events associated with blood donation or transfusion
- taking regulatory or legal actions if problems are found

Five Layers of Safety

FDA's blood safety efforts focus on minimizing the risk of transmitting infectious diseases, while maintaining an adequate supply of blood for the nation.

Blood safety is based on five layers of overlapping safeguards:

1. **Donor screening.** Donors are provided with educational material and asked to self-defer if they have risk factors that may affect blood safety. Donors are then asked specific questions about their medical history and other risk factors that may affect the safety of their donation. This "up-front" screening identifies ineligible donors.

2. **Donor deferral lists.** Blood establishments must keep current a list of deferred donors. They must also check all potential donors against that list to prevent the collection or use of blood from deferred donors.

3. **Blood testing.** After donation, blood establishments are required to test each unit of donated blood for the following transfusion-transmitted infections:

   - Hepatitis B

137

- Hepatitis C
- Human immunodeficiency viruses (HIV) 1 and 2
- Human T-cell lymphotropic viruses (HTLV) I and II
- Treponema pallidum, which causes syphilis
- West Nile Virus
- Trypanosoma cruzi (Chagas disease)
- Zika virus

4. **Quarantine.** Donated blood must be quarantined until it is tested and shown to be free of infectious agents.

5. **Problems and deficiencies.** Blood establishments must investigate manufacturing problems, correct all deficiencies, and notify U.S. Food and Drug Administration (FDA) when product deviations occur in distributed products.

If a violation of any one of these safeguards occurs, the blood product is considered unsuitable for transfusion and may be subject to recall.

Ongoing Safety Efforts

Emerging threats to the blood supply and other potential risks mean FDA's Blood Safety Team never stops looking for ways to ensure and preserve the safety of blood and blood products.

FDA scientists are working to develop sensitive donor screening tests to detect emerging diseases and potential bioterrorism agents in blood donations. They are also working to improve blood donor screening tests to detect variant strains of HIV, West Nile virus and hepatitis viruses. In addition, FDA's Office of Blood Research and Review (OBRR) addresses donor deferral issues and updates eligibility requirements when appropriate.

Also, FDA is a member of the AABB Inter-organizational Task Force on Domestic Disasters and Acts of Terrorism that includes other blood organizations, government agencies, and device manufacturers. As such, it works with others to help assure that blood facilities maintain adequate blood inventories at all times in case of a disaster.

The Process of Donating Blood

Blood is critically needed every day, yet only a small percentage of the eligible United States population donates blood in any given year.

The entire procedure takes about an hour and includes:

- registering at the donation site
- answering questions about your health and travel history
- getting a limited physical assessment that includes measuring vital signs and hemoglobin levels
- donating the blood (This takes about 15 to 20 minutes.)
- having a light refreshment to boost your energy level before leaving the facility.

Am I Eligible to Donate Blood?

To meet the basic requirements for donating blood, you must be in good health and,

- have a pulse and blood pressure within normal limits
- have a normal temperature
- meet the minimum age requirement per applicable state law
- have a normal blood hemoglobin level
- be free of infections that can be transmitted through blood transfusion, or risk factors closely associated with exposure to these infections
- not have donated blood in the last 56 days

There are a number of potential reasons which may cause you to be temporarily or permanently deferred from donating blood. These include but are not limited to:

- not feeling well on the day of donation
- past use of needles to take drugs that were not prescribed by a healthcare professional
- being a male who has had sexual contact with another male in the past 12 months
- getting tattooed in the last year (unless done under sterile conditions and at a state-licensed facility)
- having certain medical conditions or receiving certain medical treatments or medications

- living in or travelling to certain areas for a designated period of time; for example, travelling to an area where malaria is endemic

Section 15.2

Blood Donation Types

This section contains text excerpted from the following sources:
Text under the heading "Blood Donor Types" is excerpted from "BER Instructions for Completing the Electronic Blood Establishment Registration and Product Listing Form," U.S. Food and Drug Administration (FDA), August 6, 2014; Text beginning with heading "Blood Types" is excerpted from "What Is a Blood Transfusion?" National Heart, Lung, and Blood Institute (NHLBI), January 30, 2012. Reviewed June 2017.

Blood Donor Types

Donor types include: Allogeneic, Autologous, or Directed. Allogeneic donors donate blood intended for transfusion to other than the donor or a known recipient. Autologous donors donate blood intended for transfusion at a later time to the donor. Directed donors donate blood intended for transfusion to a known recipient.

Blood Types

Every person has one of the following blood types: A, B, AB, or O. Also, every person's blood is either Rh-positive or Rh-negative. So, if you have type A blood, it's either A positive or A negative. The blood used in a transfusion must work with your blood type. If it doesn't, antibodies (proteins) in your blood attack the new blood and make you sick.

Type O blood is safe for almost everyone. About 40 percent of the population has type O blood. People who have this blood type are called universal donors. Type O blood is used for emergencies when there's no time to test a person's blood type. People who have type AB blood are called universal recipients. This means they can get any type of blood.

If you have Rh-positive blood, you can get Rh-positive or Rh-negative blood. But if you have Rh-negative blood, you should only get Rh-negative blood. Rh-negative blood is used for emergencies when there's no time to test a person's Rh type.

Blood Banks

Blood banks collect, test, and store blood. They carefully screen all donated blood for possible infectious agents, such as viruses, that could make you sick.

Blood bank staff also screen each blood donation to find out whether it's type A, B, AB, or O and whether it's Rh-positive or Rh-negative. Getting a blood type that doesn't work with your own blood type will make you very sick. That's why blood banks are very careful when they test the blood.

To prepare blood for a transfusion, some blood banks remove white blood cells. This process is called white cell or leukocyte reduction. Although rare, some people are allergic to white blood cells in donated blood. Removing these cells makes allergic reactions less likely. Not all transfusions use blood donated from a stranger. If you're going to have surgery, you may need a blood transfusion because of blood loss during the operation. If it's surgery that you're able to schedule months in advance, your doctor may ask whether you would like to use your own blood, rather than donated blood.

If you choose to use your own blood, you will need to have blood drawn one or more times prior to the surgery. A blood bank will store your blood for your use.

Chapter 16

Reducing Anxiety before Surgery

It is natural to feel anxious before surgery no matter how major or minor the procedure is. Even though most of the surgeries occur with relatively few complications, patients tend to feel anxious beforehand. Sometimes, the fear becomes significant, with the patient experiencing physical symptoms including chest pain, racing heart, and nausea.

The source of this anxiety could be an unknown fear, a previous bad experience with surgery, or fear about the outcome of surgery. It is important not to become overwhelmed by anxiety before surgery. While a magic cure for anxiety does not exist, but things such as relaxation techniques and support from family, friends, and hospital staff go a long way in reducing presurgery stress.

What Are the Effects of Anxiety before Surgery?

For many patients, it is hard not to have anxious feeling about the inherent risks of surgery. Anxiety leads to stress and other related symptoms such as a fast pulse, racing heart, nervous stomach, sleeplessness, and shortness of breath. These symptoms might make it difficult for the patient to properly prepare for surgery or to remember postsurgery instructions.

"Reducing Anxiety before Surgery," © 2017 Omnigraphics. Reviewed June 2017.

What Can Be Done to Relieve Anxiety before Surgery?

Anxiety is a normal human response. The body is conditioned to protect itself by going into a defensive stance or escaping from danger. This is known as the "fight-or-flight response" And it is responsible for causing the physiological responses in the body when you are anxious. Unfortunately, they are not of much use when no inherent danger exists Most people learn to adapt to frightening situations over time, but surgery can often be a new and anxiety-inducing event.

Taking the following steps may help ease your anxiety.

Share Your Fears

Talking about your fears is the first step in controlling it. Sharing your thoughts lifts the burden from your mind and results in relief. Also, seek information and determine if there is any basis to your fears or if they are simply unfounded. Talk to the hospital clinical counselor or physician assistant or nurse about your fears. They will be able to understand your anxiety and help alleviate it.

Understand the Surgical Procedure

Fear of the unknown is a primary cause of anxiety and the best way to handle it is to understand what you are getting into. Talk to the surgeon and get to know the surgical procedure and what to expect when it is over. If you are searching the Internet for information, be sure you are sourcing it from credible websites. It is the unanswered questions that cause anxiety. Understanding what you will undergo will calm your nerves. Though it may be clear that surgery is essential for you, it is easy to be confused by medical jargon. Make sure you understand why you need surgery and do not be afraid to get a second opinion.

Learn about Anesthesia

Educate yourself about anesthesia. You may not get a chance to meet the anesthesiologist the day before surgery. So, make an appointment with him or her beforehand. Understand what choices will be available to you. Research the kind of anesthesia you will be given using authoritative websites. You may not have much choice in anesthesia because, after an evaluation of all factors involved, the specific kind of anesthesia to be used is decided only shortly before surgery.

Keep Yourself Busy

Prepare yourself to avoid stress. Take care of chores at home before surgery. Clean your house or if possible make a thorough clean up. Take care of your work and apply for leave if needed. If you have kids, make arrangements for their care while you are in recovery. Tell your partner about things to take care at home, such as cooking meals, so that your absence will not be felt.

Distract Yourself

It is easy to dwell on negative thoughts and brood over them. Don't let your imagination get the better of you. Use common distraction techniques such as reading a book, watching a TV show or movie, or listening to your favorite music. This should keep your mind relaxed and delay your thoughts about surgery until much later.

Use Relaxation Techniques

If you are prone to anxiety, then find out about specific techniques to reduce it. Breathing exercises, meditation, and mindfulness help reduce anxiety, stress, and lowers blood pressure. Such techniques have been scientifically proven to reduce stress and anxiety.

Allow Hospital Staff to Help You

Doctors and nurses at the hospital are well aware of patients' potential anxiety. Most staff try to make wait times minimal and your stay as pleasant as possible. Hospitals have counselors and volunteers on call to offer support and assistance. Make use of their services. Personal coping strategies serve the purpose best, but they tend to be different for each individual.

Do Not Smoke before Surgery

Smoking before surgery is linked to complications and is best avoided even though you think it will help relax you. Smoking adversely affects healing of wounds and you should begin nicotine replacement therapy a few months before surgery if possible in order to reduce risk of complications.

Use of Sedatives

If you are admitted to the hospital the night before surgery you might be given a sedative, usually a benzodiazepine, to make you sleep better and to control anxiety. Sedatives make you drowsy and can cause nausea but they also make you relax and reduce anxiety. You may also be given a sedative an hour or two before anesthesia is administered.

Helping Your Child Who Is Anxious about Surgery

It is very important to address concerns about surgery in children because this usually translates to better outcomes after surgery. Children tend to emulate the attitude of parents when it comes to surgery, be it good or bad. If a parent is fearful or anxious, chances are the child becoming fearful too. Children should be told about the surgery in advance and allowed to ask questions. Any anxiety or fearfulness about surgery should be put to rest. It is best not to surprise a child because it could result in a lasting fear of healthcare. Also, it is better to sound positive and upbeat about surgery with your child. He or she should know what the advantages are that will come after surgery.

The approach adopted with children varies with age. Very young children need to be informed just a few days before surgery. Slightly older children may already know what surgery entails and should be given enough opportunities to voice their doubts and fears with doctors and parents. Older children may know the surgical procedure in detail from books, TV, or the Internet. They should meet the surgeon with their parent for a 'reality check' so they understand what the procedure actual entails. Most hospitals offer a presurgery tour and information presentations to relieve anxiety before surgery.

References

1. "What Can Help Relieve Anxiety Before Surgery?" PubMed Health, IQWiG (Institute for Quality and Efficiency in Health Care), May 21, 2014.

2. "5 Ways to Calm Your Nerves Before Surgery," The Healthcare Management Trust, July 26, 2016.

3. TahoeDoc. "How to Calm Yourself Down Before a Day Surgery Procedure," HealDove, April 28, 2017.

4. Whitlock, Jennifer., RN, MSN, FNP-C. "Understanding and Dealing with a Fear of Surgery," VeryWell, April 21, 2016.

Chapter 17

Understanding Informed Consent

The right to make informed decisions means that the patient or patient's representative is given the information needed in order to make "informed" decisions regarding his/her care.

A patient may wish to delegate his/her right to make informed decisions to another person. To the degree permitted by state law, and to the maximum extent practicable, the hospital must respect the patient's wishes and follow that process. In some cases, the patient may be unconscious or otherwise incapacitated. If the patient is unable to make a decision, the hospital must consult the patient's advance directives, medical power of attorney or patient representative, if any of these are available. In the advance directive or the medical power of attorney, the patient may provide guidance as to his/her wishes in certain situations, or may delegate decisionmaking to another individual as permitted by state law. If such an individual has been selected by the patient, or if a person willing and able under applicable state law is available to make treatment decisions, relevant information should be provided to the representative so that informed healthcare decisions can be made for the patient. However, as soon as the patient is able to be informed of his/her rights, the hospital should provide that information to the patient.

This chapter includes text excerpted from "Revisions to the Hospital Interpretive Guidelines for Informed Consent," Centers for Medicare and Medicaid Services (CMS), April 13, 2007. Reviewed June 2017.

Information about Health Status

The right to make informed decisions regarding care presumes that the patient has been provided information about his/her health status, diagnosis, and prognosis. Furthermore, it includes the patient's participation in the development of the plan of care, including providing consent to, or refusal of, medical or surgical interventions, and in planning for care after discharge from the hospital. The patient or the patient's representative should receive adequate information, provided in a manner that the patient or the patient's representative can understand, to assure that the patient can effectively exercise the right to make informed decisions.

Hospitals must establish processes to assure that each patient or the patient's representative is given information on the patient's health status, diagnosis, and prognosis.

Informed Consent

Giving informed consent to a treatment or a surgical procedure is one type of informed decision that a patient or patient's representative may need to make regarding the patient's plan of care. Hospitals must utilize an informed consent process that assures patients or their representatives are given the information and disclosures needed to make an informed decision about whether to consent to a procedure, intervention, or type of care that requires consent. See the guidelines for 482.51(b)(2) pertaining to surgical services informed consent and the guidelines for 482.24(c)(2)(v) pertaining to medical records.

Informed decisions related to care planning also extend to discharge planning for the patient's postacute care. See the guidelines for 482.43(c) pertaining to discharge planning for discussion of pertinent requirements.

Hospitals must also establish policies and procedures that assure a patient's right to request or refuse treatment. Such policies should indicate how the patient's request will be addressed. However, hospitals are under no obligation to fulfill a patient's request for a treatment or service that the responsible practitioner has deemed medically unnecessary or even inappropriate.

Informed Consent for Surgical Services

The primary purpose of the informed consent process for surgical services is to ensure that the patient, or the patient's representative, is provided information necessary to enable him/her to evaluate a proposed surgery before agreeing to the surgery. Typically, this information would include potential short- and longer-term risks and benefits to the patient of the proposed intervention, including the likelihood of each, based on the available clinical evidence, as informed by the responsible practitioner's professional judgment. Informed consent must be obtained, and the informed consent form must be placed in the patient's medical record, prior to surgery, except in the case of emergency surgery.

"Surgery" includes any procedure that is listed as a surgical procedure in any of the various billing coding systems used by CMS or the hospital, regardless of whether Medicare pays for that surgical procedure. Hospitals must assure that the practitioner(s) responsible for the surgery obtain informed consent from patients in a manner consistent with the hospital's policies governing the informed consent process. It should be noted that there is no specific requirement for informed consent within the regulation at §482.52 governing anesthesia services. However, given that surgical procedures generally entail use of anesthesia, hospitals may wish to consider specifically extending their informed consent policies to include obtaining informed consent for the anesthesia component of the surgical procedure.

Surgical Informed Consent Policy

The hospital's surgical informed consent policy should describe the following:

- Who may obtain the patient's informed consent;

- Which procedures require informed consent;

- The circumstances under which surgery is considered an emergency, and may be undertaken without an informed consent;

- The circumstances when a patient's representative, rather than the patient, may give informed consent for a surgery;

- The content of the informed consent form and instructions for completing it;

- The process used to obtain informed consent, including how informed consent is to be documented in the medical record;

- Mechanisms that ensure that the informed consent form is properly executed and is in the patient's medical record prior to the surgery (except in the case of emergency surgery); and

149

- If the informed consent process and informed consent form are obtained outside the hospital, how the properly executed informed consent form is incorporated into the patient's medical record prior to the surgery.

If there are additional requirements under state law for informed consent, the hospital must comply with those requirements.

Example of a Well-Designed Informed Consent Process

A well-designed informed consent process would include discussion of the following elements:

- A description of the proposed surgery, including the anesthesia to be used;

- The indications for the proposed surgery;

- Material risks and benefits for the patient related to the surgery and anesthesia, including the likelihood of each, based on the available clinical evidence, as informed by the responsible practitioner's clinical judgment. Material risks could include risks with a high degree of likelihood but a low degree of severity, as well as those with a very low degree of likelihood but high degree of severity;

- Treatment alternatives, including the attendant material risks and benefits;

- The probable consequences of declining recommended or alternative therapies;

- Who will conduct the surgical intervention and administer the anesthesia;

- Whether physicians other than the operating practitioner, including but not limited to residents, will be performing important tasks related to the surgery, in accordance with the hospital's policies. Important surgical tasks include: opening and closing, dissecting tissue, removing tissue, harvesting grafts, transplanting tissue, administering anesthesia, implanting devices, and placing invasive lines;

  - For surgeries in which residents will perform important parts of the surgery, discussion is encouraged to include the following:

- That it is anticipated that physicians who are in approved postgraduate residency training programs will perform portions of the surgery, based on their availability and level of competence;

- That it will be decided at the time of the surgery which residents will participate and their manner or participation, and that this will depend on the availability of residents with the necessary competence; the knowledge the operating practitioner/teaching surgeon has of the resident's skill set; and the patient's condition; and

- That residents performing surgical tasks will be under the supervision of the operating practitioner/teaching surgeon.

- Whether, based on the resident's level of competence, the operating practitioner/teaching surgeon will not be physically present in the same operating room for some or all of the surgical tasks performed by residents.

Note: a "moonlighting" resident or fellow is a postgraduate medical trainee who is practicing independently, outside the scope of his/her residency training program and would be treated as a physician within the scope of the privileges granted by the hospital.

- Whether, as permitted by state law, qualified medical practitioners who are not physicians will perform important parts of the surgery or administer the anesthesia, and if so, the types of tasks each type of practitioner will carry out; and that such practitioners will be performing only tasks within their scope of practice for which they have been granted privileges by the hospital.

Chapter 18

Ensuring Patient Safety

Chapter Contents

Section 18.1

Twenty Tips to Prevent Medical Errors

This section includes text excerpted from "20 Tips to Help Prevent
Medical Errors: Patient Fact Sheet," Agency for Healthcare Research
and Quality (AHRQ), U.S. Department of Health and Human
Services (HHS), December 2014.

Medical errors can occur anywhere in the healthcare system: In hospitals, clinics, surgery centers, doctors' offices, nursing homes, pharmacies, and patients' homes. Errors can involve medicines, surgery, diagnosis, equipment, or lab reports. These tips tell what you can do to get safer care.

One in seven Medicare patients in hospitals experience a medical error. But medical errors can occur anywhere in the healthcare system: In hospitals, clinics, surgery centers, doctors' offices, nursing homes, pharmacies, and patients' homes. Errors can involve medicines, surgery, diagnosis, equipment, or lab reports. They can happen during even the most routine tasks, such as when a hospital patient on a salt-free diet is given a high-salt meal.

Most errors result from problems created by complex healthcare system. But errors also happen when doctors and patients have problems communicating. These tips tell what you can do to get safer care.

What You Can Do to Stay Safe

The best way you can help to prevent errors is to be an active member of your healthcare team. That means taking part in every decision about your healthcare. Research shows that patients who are more involved with their care tend to get better results.

Medicines

1. **Make sure that all of your doctors know about every medicine you are taking.** This includes prescription and over-the-counter medicines and dietary supplements, such as vitamins and herbs.

2. **Bring all of your medicines and supplements to your doctor visits.** "Brown bagging" your medicines can help you and your doctor talk about them and find out if there are any problems. It can also help your doctor keep your records up to date and help you get better quality care.

3. **Make sure your doctor knows about any allergies and adverse reactions you have had to medicines.** This can help you to avoid getting a medicine that could harm you.

4. **When your doctor writes a prescription for you, make sure you can read it.** If you cannot read your doctor's handwriting, your pharmacist might not be able to either.

5. **Ask for information about your medicines in terms you can understand—both when your medicines are prescribed and when you get them:**

   - What is the medicine for?
   - How am I supposed to take it and for how long?
   - What side effects are likely? What do I do if they occur?
   - Is this medicine safe to take with other medicines or dietary supplements I am taking?
   - What food, drink, or activities should I avoid while taking this medicine?

6. **When you pick up your medicine from the pharmacy, ask: Is this the medicine that my doctor prescribed?**

7. **If you have any questions about the directions on your medicine labels, ask.** Medicine labels can be hard to understand. For example, ask if "four times daily" means taking a dose every 6 hours around the clock or just during regular waking hours.

8. **Ask your pharmacist for the best device to measure your liquid medicine.** For example, many people use household teaspoons, which often do not hold a true teaspoon of liquid. Special devices, like marked syringes, help people measure the right dose.

9. **Ask for written information about the side effects your medicine could cause.** If you know what might happen, you will be better prepared if it does or if something unexpected happens.

155

Hospital Stays

10. **If you are in a hospital, consider asking all healthcare workers who will touch you whether they have washed their hands.** Hand washing can prevent the spread of infections in hospitals.

11. **When you are being discharged from the hospital, ask your doctor to explain the treatment plan you will follow at home.** This includes learning about your new medicines, making sure you know when to schedule follow-up appointments, and finding out when you can get back to your regular activities.

It is important to know whether or not you should keep taking the medicines you were taking before your hospital stay. Getting clear instructions may help prevent an unexpected return trip to the hospital.

Surgery

12. **If you are having surgery, make sure that you, your doctor, and your surgeon all agree on exactly what will be done.** Having surgery at the wrong site (for example, operating on the left knee instead of the right) is rare. But even once is too often. The good news is that wrong-site surgery is 100 percent preventable. Surgeons are expected to sign their initials directly on the site to be operated on before the surgery.

13. **If you have a choice, choose a hospital where many patients have had the procedure or surgery you need.** Research shows that patients tend to have better results when they are treated in hospitals that have a great deal of experience with their condition.

Other Steps

14. **Speak up if you have questions or concerns.** You have a right to question anyone who is involved with your care.

15. **Make sure that someone, such as your primary care doctor, coordinates your care.** This is especially important if you have many health problems or are in the hospital.

16. **Make sure that all your doctors have your important health information.** Do not assume that everyone has all the information they need.

17. **Ask a family member or friend to go to appointments with you.** Even if you do not need help now, you might need it later.

18. **Know that "more" is not always better.** It is a good idea to find out why a test or treatment is needed and how it can help you. You could be better off without it.

19. **If you have a test, do not assume that no news is good news.** Ask how and when you will get the results.

20. **Learn about your condition and treatments by asking your doctor and nurse and by using other reliable sources.** Ask your doctor if your treatment is based on the latest evidence.

Section 18.2

Strategies to Reduce Medication Errors

This section includes text excerpted from "Strategies to Reduce Medication Errors: Working to Improve Medication Safety," U.S. Food and Drug Administration (FDA), October 23, 2015.

Since 1992, the U.S. Food and Drug Administration (FDA) has received nearly 30,000 reports of medication errors. These are voluntary reports, so the number of medication errors that actually occur is thought to be much higher. There is no "typical" medication error, and health professionals, patients, and their families are all involved. Some examples:

- A physician ordered a 260-milligram preparation of Taxol for a patient, but the pharmacist prepared 260 milligrams of Taxotere instead. Both are chemotherapy drugs used for different types of cancer and with different recommended doses. The patient died several days later, though the death couldn't be linked to the error because the patient was already severely ill.

- An older patient with rheumatoid arthritis died after receiving an overdose of methotrexate—a 10-milligram daily dose of the drug rather than the intended 10-milligram weekly dose. Some dosing mix-ups have occurred because daily dosing of methotrexate is typically used to treat people with cancer, while low weekly doses of the drug have been prescribed for other conditions, such as arthritis, asthma, and inflammatory bowel disease.

- One patient died because 20 units of insulin was abbreviated as "20 U," but the "U" was mistaken for a "zero." As a result, a dose of 200 units of insulin was accidentally injected.

- A man died after his wife mistakenly applied six transdermal patches to his skin at one time. The multiple patches delivered an overdose of the narcotic pain medicine fentanyl through his skin.

- A patient developed a fatal hemorrhage when given another patient's prescription for the blood thinner warfarin.

These and other medication errors reported to the FDA may stem from poor communication; misinterpreted handwriting; drug name confusion; confusing drug labels, labeling, and packaging; lack of employee knowledge; and lack of patient understanding about a drug's directions. "But it's important to recognize that such errors are due to multiple factors in a complex medical system," says Paul Seligman, M.D., director of the FDA's Office of Pharmacoepidemiology and Statistical Science (OPaSS). "In most cases, medication errors can't be blamed on a single person."

A medication error is "any preventable event that may cause or lead to inappropriate medication use or patient harm while the medication is in the control of the healthcare professional, patient, or consumer," according to the National Coordinating Council for Medication Error Reporting and Prevention (NCC MERP). The council, a group of more than 25 national and international organizations, including the FDA, examines and evaluates medication errors and recommends strategies for error prevention.

A Regulatory Approach

The public took notice in 1999 when the Institute of Medicine (IOM) released a report, "To Err is Human: Building a Safer Health System." According to the report, between 44,000 and 98,000 deaths may result each year from medical errors in hospitals alone. And more than 7,000 deaths each year are related to medications. In response to the IOM's report, all parts of the U.S. health system put error reduction strategies into high gear by re-evaluating and strengthening checks and balances to prevent errors.

In addition, the U.S. Department of Health and Human Services (HHS) and other federal agencies formed the Quality Interagency Coordination Task Force (QuIC) in 2000 and issued an action plan for reducing medical errors. In 2001, former HHS Secretary Tommy G. Thompson announced a Patient Safety Task Force to coordinate a joint effort to improve data collection on patient safety. The lead agencies are the FDA, the Centers for Disease Control and Prevention (CDC), the Centers for Medicare and Medicaid Services (CMS), and the Agency for Healthcare Research and Quality (AHRQ).

The FDA enhanced its efforts to reduce medication errors by dedicating more resources to drug safety, which included forming a new division on medication errors at the agency in 2002. "FDA works to prevent medication errors before a drug reaches the market and monitors any errors that may occur after that," says Jerry Phillips, R.Ph., former director of the FDA's Division of Medication Errors and Technical Support.

Here's a look at key areas in which the FDA is working to reduce medication errors.

Bar code label rule. After a public meeting in July 2002, the FDA decided to propose a new rule requiring bar codes on certain drug and biological product labels. Healthcare professionals would use bar code scanning equipment, similar to that used in supermarkets, to make sure that the right drug in the right dose and route of administration is given to the right patient at the right time.

"It's a promising way to automate aspects of medication administration," says Robert Krawisz, former executive director of the National Patient Safety Foundation. "The technology's impact at VA hospitals so far has been amazing." The Department of Veterans Affairs (VA) already uses bar codes nationwide in its hospitals, and the result has been a drastic reduction in medication errors. For example, the VA medical center in Topeka, Kan., has reported that bar coding reduced its medication error rate by 86 percent over a nine-year period.

How it works. When patients enter the hospital, they get a bar-coded identification wristband that can transmit information to the hospital's computer, says Lottie Lockett, R.N., a nursing administrator at the Houston VA Medical Center. Nurses have laptop computers and scanners on top of medication carts that they bring to patients' rooms. Nurses use the scanners to scan the patient's wristband and the medications to be given. The bar codes provide unique, identifying information about drugs given at the patient's bedside. "Before giving medications, nurses use the scanner to pull up a patient's full name and social security number on the laptops, along with the medications," Lockett says. "If there is not a match between the patient and the medication or some other problem, a warning box pops up on the screen."

The FDA's final rule on bar code labeling was published on Feb. 26, 2004. The rule, which took effect on April 26, 2004, applies to prescription drugs, biological products (other than blood, blood components, and devices regulated by the Center for Biologics Evaluation and Research (CBER)), and over-the-counter (OTC) drugs that are commonly used in hospitals. Manufacturers, repackers, relabelers, and private label distributors of prescription and OTC drugs would be subject to the bar code requirements. The agency continues to study whether it also should develop a rule requiring bar code labeling on medical devices.

Drug name confusion. To minimize confusion between drug names that look or sound alike, the FDA reviews about 300 drug names a year before they are marketed. "About one-third of the names that drug companies propose are rejected," says Phillips. The agency tests drug names with the help of about 120 FDA health professionals who volunteer to simulate real-life drug order situations. "FDA also created a computerized program that assists in detecting similar names and that will help take a more scientific approach to comparing names," Phillips says.

After drugs are approved, the FDA tracks reports of errors due to drug name confusion and spreads the word to health professionals, along with recommendations for avoiding future problems. For example, the FDA has reported errors involving the inadvertent administration of methadone, a drug used to treat opiate dependence, rather than the intended Metadate ER (methylphenidate) for the treatment of attention deficit hyperactivity disorder (ADHD). One report involved the death of an 8-year-old boy after a possible medication error at the dispensing pharmacy. The child, who was being treated for ADHD, was found dead at home. Methadone substitution was the suspected cause of death. Some FDA recommendations regarding drug name confusion have encouraged pharmacists to separate similar drug products on pharmacy shelves and have encouraged physicians to indicate both brand and generic drug names on prescription orders, as well as what the drug is intended to treat.

The last time the FDA changed a drug name after it was approved was in 2004 when the cholesterol-lowering medicine Altocor was being confused with the cholesterol-lowering medicine Advicor. Now Altocor is called Altoprev, and the agency hasn't received reports of errors since the name change. Other examples of drug name confusion reported to the FDA include:

- Serzone (nefazodone) for depression and Seroquel (quetiapine) for schizophrenia

- Lamictal (lamotrigine) for epilepsy, Lamisil (terbinafine) for nail infections, Ludiomil (maprotiline) for depression, and Lomotil (diphenoxylate) for diarrhea

- Taxotere (docetaxel) and Taxol (paclitaxel), both for chemotherapy

- Zantac (ranitidine) for heartburn, Zyrtec (cetirizine) for allergies, and Zyprexa (olanzapine) for mental conditions

- Celebrex (celecoxib) for arthritis and Celexa (citalopram) for depression.

Drug labeling. Consumers tend to overlook important label information on OTC drugs, according to a Harris Interactive Market Research Poll conducted for the National Council on Patient Information and Education (NCPIE) and released in January 2002. In May 2002, an FDA regulation went into effect that aims to help consumers use OTC drugs more wisely.

The regulation requires a standardized "Drug Facts" label on more than 100,000 OTC drug products. Modeled after the Nutrition Facts label on foods, the label helps consumers compare and select OTC medicines and follow instructions. The label clearly lists active ingredients, uses, warnings, dosage, directions, other information, such as how to store the medicine, and inactive ingredients.

As for health professionals, the FDA proposed a new format in 2000 to improve prescription drug labeling for physicians, also known as the package insert. One FDA study showed that practitioners found the labeling to be lengthy, complex, and hard to use. The proposed redesign would feature a user-friendly format and would highlight critical information more clearly. The FDA is still reviewing public comments on this proposed rule. The agency also has been working on a project called DailyMed, a computer system that will be available without cost from the National Library of Medicine (NLM) next year. DailyMed will have new information added daily, and will allow health professionals to pull up drug warnings and label changes electronically.

Error tracking and public education. The FDA reviews medication error reports that come from drug manufacturers and through MedWatch, the agency's safety information and adverse event reporting program. The agency also receives reports from the Institute for Safe Medication Practices (ISMP) and the U.S. Pharmacopeia or USP.

An ISMP survey on medication error reporting practices showed that health professionals submit reports more often to internal reporting programs such as hospitals than to external programs such as the FDA. According to the ISMP, one reason may be health professionals' limited knowledge about external reporting programs.

The FDA receives and reviews about 300 medication error reports each month and classifies them to determine the cause and type of error. Depending on the findings, the FDA can change the way it labels, names, or packages a drug product. In addition, once a problem is discovered, the FDA educates the public on an ongoing basis to prevent repeat errors.

In 2001, the agency released a public health advisory to hospitals, nursing homes, and other healthcare facilities about the hazards of mix-ups between medical gases, which are prescription drugs. In one case, a nursing home in Ohio reported four deaths after an employee mistakenly connected nitrogen to the oxygen system.

The ISMP reports medication errors through various newsletters that target health professionals in acute care, nursing, and community/ambulatory care. The ISMP also has launched a newsletter for consumers called Safe Medicine.

In December 2003, the USP released an analysis of medication errors captured in 2002 by its anonymous national reporting database, MedMARX. Of the errors reported to MedMARX, slightly more than one-third reached the patient and involved a geriatric patient. Many of these medication errors were found to be harmful.

What Consumers Can Do

In one case reported to the ISMP, a doctor called in a prescription for the antibiotic Noroxin (norfloxacin) for a patient with a bladder infection. But the pharmacist thought the order was for Neurontin (gabapentin), a medication used to treat seizures. The good news is that the patient read the medication leaflet stapled to his medication bag, noticed the drug he received is used to treat seizures, and then asked about it. ISMP president Michael Cohen, R.Ph., Sc.D., says, "You should expect to count on the health system to keep you safe, but there are also steps you can take to look out for yourself and your family."

- **Know what kind of errors occur.** The FDA evaluated reports of fatal medication errors that it received from 1993 to 1998 and found that the most common types of errors involved administering an improper dose (41%), giving the wrong drug (16%), and using the wrong route of administration (16%). The most common causes of the medication errors were performance and knowledge deficits (44%) and communication errors (16%). Almost half of the fatal medication errors occurred in people over 60. Older people are especially at risk for errors because they often take multiple medications. Children are also a vulnerable population because drugs are often dosed based on their weight, and accurate calculations are critical.

- **Find out what drug you're taking and what it's for.** Rather than simply letting the doctor write you a prescription and send you on your way, be sure to ask the name of the drug. Cohen says, "I would also ask the doctor to put the purpose of the prescription on the order." This serves as a check in case there is some confusion about the drug name. If you're in the hospital, ask (or have a friend or family member ask) what drugs you are being given and why.

- **Find out how to take the drug and make sure you understand the directions.** If you are told to take a medicine three times a day, does that mean eight hours apart exactly or at mealtimes? Should the medicine be stored at room temperature or in the refrigerator? Are there any medications, beverages, or foods you should avoid? Also, ask about what medication side effects you might expect and what you should do about them. And read the bottle's label every time you take a drug to avoid mistakes. In the middle of the night, you could mistake ear drops for eye drops, or accidentally give your older child's medication to the baby if you're not careful. Use the measuring device that comes with the medicine, not spoons from the kitchen drawer. If you take multiple medications and have trouble keeping them straight, ask your doctor or pharmacist about compliance aids, such as containers with sections for daily doses. Family members can help by reminding you to take your medicine.

- **Keep a list of all medications,** including OTC drugs, as well as dietary supplements, medicinal herbs, and other substances you take for health reasons, and report it to your healthcare providers. The often-forgotten things that you should tell your doctor about include vitamins, laxatives, sleeping aids, and birth control pills. One National Institutes of Health (NIH) study showed a significant drug interaction between the herbal product St. John's wort and indinavir, a protease inhibitor used to treat human immunodeficiency virus (HIV) infection. Some antibiotics can lower the effectiveness of birth control pills. If you see different doctors, it's important that they all know what you are taking. If possible, get all your prescriptions filled at the same pharmacy so that all of your records are in one place. Also, make sure your doctors and pharmacy know about your medication allergies or other unpleasant drug reactions you may have experienced.

- **If in doubt, ask, ask, ask.** Be on the lookout for clues of a problem, such as if your pills look different than normal or if you notice a different drug name or different directions than what you thought. Krawisz says it's best to be cautious and ask questions if you're unsure about anything. "If you forget, don't hesitate to call your doctor or pharmacist when you get home," he says. "It can't hurt to ask."

Hospital Strategies

Hospitals and other healthcare organizations work to reduce medication errors by using technology, improving processes, zeroing in on errors that cause harm, and building a culture of safety. Here are a couple of examples.

Pharmacy intervention. It was a challenge for healthcare providers, especially surgeons, at Fairview Southdale Hospital in Edina, Minn., to ensure that patients continued taking their regularly prescribed medicines when they entered the hospital, says Steven Meisel, Pharm.D., director of medication safety at Fairview Health Services. "Surgeons are not typically the original prescribers," he says. The solution was to have pharmacy technicians record complete medication histories on a form. In a pilot program, the technicians called most patients on the phone a couple of days before surgery. A pharmacist reviewed the information, and then the surgeon decided which medications should be continued. After three months, the number of order errors per patient dropped by 84 percent, and the pilot program became permanent.

Computerized Physician Order Entry (CPOE). Studies have shown that CPOE is effective in reducing medication errors. It involves entering medication orders directly into a computer system rather than on paper or verbally. The Institute for Safe Medication Practices conducted a survey of 1,500 hospitals in 2001 and found that about 3 percent of hospitals were using CPOE, and the number is rising. Eugene Wiener, M.D., medical director at the Children's Hospital of Pittsburgh, says, "There is no misinterpretation of handwriting, decimal points, or abbreviations. This puts everything in a digital world."

The Pittsburgh hospital unveiled its CPOE system in October 2002. Developed by the hospital and the Cerner Corp. in Kansas City, Mo., Children'sNet has replaced most paper forms and prescription pads. Wiener says that, unlike with adults, most drug orders for children are generally based on weight. "The computer won't let you put an order in if the child's weight isn't in the system," he says, "and if the weight changes, the computer notices." The system also provides all kinds of information about potential drug complications that the doctor might not have thought about. "Doctors always have a choice in dealing with the alerts," Wiener says. "They can choose to move past an alert, but the alert makes them stop and think based on the specific patient indications."

Patient Safety Proposals

In March 2003, the U.S. Department of Health and Human Services (HHS) announced two new FDA strategies that will use state-of-the-art technology to improve patient safety.

- **Bar codes.** Just as the technology is used in retail and other industries, required bar codes would contain unique identifying information about drugs. When used with bar code scanners and computerized patient information systems, bar code technology can prevent many medication errors, including administering the wrong drug or dose, or administering a drug to a patient with a known allergy. The requirement took effect in April 2004.

- **Safety reporting.** A proposed revamping of safety reporting requirements aims to enhance the FDA's ability to monitor and improve the safe use of drugs and biologics. In 2003, the FDA published a proposed rule. The rule, if enacted, would improve the quality and consistency of safety reports, require the submission of all suspected serious reactions for blood and blood products, and require reports on important potential medication errors.

Section 18.3

Things You Can Do to Be a Safe Patient

This section includes text excerpted from "Getting Medical Care? How to Avoid Getting an Infection," Centers for Disease Control and Prevention (CDC), March 13, 2017.

People receiving medical care sometimes develop infections so serious they may lead to sepsis or death. It can happen in any medical facility such as a hospital, outpatient clinic, dialysis center, or long-term care facility.

These are called healthcare-associated infections—and are often associated with devices used in medical procedures, such as catheters or ventilators.

Healthcare-associated infections (HAIs) can be caused by bacteria that are resistant to antibiotics, making them difficult to treat. Although national progress is being made to prevent these infections, there's more to do, especially in fighting antibiotic-resistant bacteria. As a patient, you can help prevent the spread of infections and improve antibiotic use.

Be informed. Be empowered. Be prepared.

Here are ten things you can do to protect yourself and your loved ones:

1. **Speak up**. Talk to your doctor about any questions or worries. Ask what they're doing to protect you.

2. **Keep hands clean**. Make sure everyone, including friends and family, clean their hands before touching you. If you don't see your healthcare providers clean their hands, ask them to do so.

3. **Ask each day if your central line catheter or urinary catheter is necessary**. Leaving a catheter in place too long increases the chances you'll get an infection. Let your doctor or nurse know immediately if the area around the central line becomes sore or red, or if the bandage falls off or looks wet or dirty.

4. **Prepare for surgery**. Let your doctor know about any medical problems you have. Ask your doctor how he/she prevents surgical site infections.

5. **Ask your healthcare provider**, "Will there be a new needle, new syringe, and a new vial for this procedure or injection?" Insist that your healthcare providers never reuse a needle or syringe on more than one patient.

6. **Get Smart about antibiotics**. Antibiotics only treat bacterial infections—they don't work for viruses like the ones that cause colds and flu. Ask your healthcare provider if there are steps you can take to feel better without using antibiotics. If you're prescribed an antibiotic, make sure to take the prescribed antibiotic exactly as your healthcare provider tells you and do not skip doses.

7. **Watch out for deadly diarrhea** (*Clostridium difficile*). Tell your doctor if you have 3 or more diarrhea episodes in 24 hours, especially if you've been taking an antibiotic.

8. **Know the signs and symptoms of infection**. Some skin infections, such as Methicillin-resistant *Staphylococcus aureus* (MRSA), appear as redness, pain, or drainage at an IV catheter site or surgery site and come with a fever. Infections can also lead to sepsis, a complication caused by the body's overwhelming and life-threatening response to an infection.

9. **Get Vaccinated**. Getting yourself, family, friends, and caregivers vaccinated against the flu and other infections prevents spread of disease.

10. **Cover your mouth and nose**. When you sneeze or cough, germs can travel 3 feet or more. Use a tissue to avoid spreading germs with your hands.

Healthcare-associated Infections are not only a problem for healthcare facilities–they represent a public health issue. Many people and organizations are working together to attack these largely preventable infections. Centers for Disease Control and Prevention (CDC) is committed to preventing healthcare-associated infections and making healthcare safer for everyone.

Visit the United for Patient Safety website (www.unitedforpatientsafety.org) to see how you can make healthcare safer.

Section 18.4

Wrong-Site Surgery: Help Avoid Mistakes in Your Surgery

This section includes text excerpted from "Wrong-Site, Wrong-Procedure, and Wrong-Patient Surgery," Agency for Healthcare Research and Quality (AHRQ), U.S. Department of Health and Human Services (HHS), July 2016.

Few medical errors are as vivid and terrifying as those that involve patients who have undergone surgery on the wrong body part, undergone the incorrect procedure, or had a procedure intended for another patient. These "wrong-site, wrong-procedure, wrong-patient errors" (WSPEs) are rightly termed never events—errors that should never occur and indicate serious underlying safety problems.

Wrong-site surgery may involve operating on the wrong side, as in the case of a patient who had the right side of her vulva removed when the cancerous lesion was on the left, or the incorrect body site. One example of surgery on the incorrect site is operating on the wrong level of the spine, a surprisingly common issue for neurosurgeons. A classic case of wrong-patient surgery involved a patient who underwent a cardiac procedure intended for another patient with a similar last name.

While much publicity has been given to these high-profile cases of WSPEs, these errors are in fact relatively rare. A seminal study estimated that such errors occur in approximately 1 of 112,000 surgical procedures, infrequent enough that an individual hospital would only experience one such error every 5–10 years. However, this estimate only included procedures performed in the operating room; if procedures performed in other settings (for example, ambulatory surgery or interventional radiology) are included, the rate of such errors may be significantly higher. One study using Veterans Affairs data found that fully half of WSPEs occurred during procedures outside of the operating room.

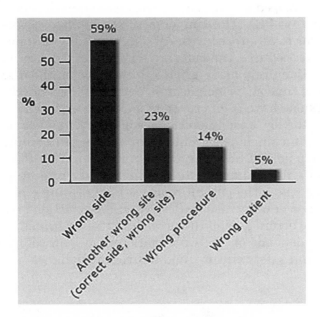

Figure 18.1. *Types of Wrong-Site Surgery Observed*

Preventing Wrong-Site, Wrong-Procedure, and Wrong-Patient Surgery

Early efforts to prevent WSPEs focused on developing redundant mechanisms for identifying the correct site, procedure, and patient, such as "sign your site" initiatives, that instructed surgeons to mark the operative site in an unambiguous fashion. However, it soon became clear that even this seemingly simple intervention was problematic. An analysis of the United Kingdom's efforts to prevent WSPEs found that, although dissemination of a site-marking protocol did increase use of preoperative site marking, implementation and adherence to the protocol differed significantly across surgical specialties and hospitals, and many clinicians voiced concerns about unintended consequences of the protocol. In some cases, there was even confusion over whether the marked site indicates the area to be operated on, or the area to be avoided. Site marking remains a core component of The Joint Commission's Universal Protocol to prevent WSPEs.

169

Root cause analyses of WSPEs consistently reveal communication issues as a prominent underlying factor. The concept of the surgical timeout—a planned pause before beginning the procedure in order to review important aspects of the procedure with all involved personnel—was developed to improve communication in the operating room and prevent WSPEs. The Universal Protocol also specifies use of a timeout prior to all procedures. Although initially designed for operating room procedures, timeouts are now required before any invasive procedure. Comprehensive efforts to improve surgical safety have incorporated timeout principles into surgical safety checklists; while these checklists have been proven to improve surgical and postoperative safety, the low baseline incidence of WSPEs makes it difficult to establish that a single intervention can reduce or eliminate WSPEs.

It is worth noting, however, that many cases of WSPEs would still occur despite full adherence to the Universal Protocol. Errors may happen well before the patient reaches the operating room, a timeout may be rushed or otherwise ineffective, and production pressures may contribute to errors during the procedure itself. Ultimately, preventing WSPEs depends on the combination of system solutions, strong teamwork and safety culture, and individual vigilance.

Chapter 19

What Medicare Covers If You Are Having Surgery

If you're enrolled in Original Medicare, finding out if Medicare will cover a service or supply that you need isn't always easy. Generally, Medicare covers services (like lab tests, surgeries, and doctor visits) and supplies (like wheelchairs and walkers) that Medicare considers "medically necessary" to treat a disease or condition.

What Medicare covers may be based on several factors, like:

- Federal laws describing Medicare benefits or state laws that tell what services a particular type of practitioner is licensed to provide.

- National coverage decisions made by Medicare about whether a particular item or service is covered nationally under Medicare's rules.

- Local coverage decisions made by local companies in each state that process claims for Medicare. These companies decide whether an item or service is medically necessary and should be covered in that area under Medicare's rules.

There may be other coverage rules and policies that also apply. Some services may only be covered when provided in certain settings or covered for patients with certain conditions. For example, some surgeries, like organ transplants, can only be done in certain approved hospitals.

This chapter includes text excerpted from "Learning What Medicare Covers and How Much You Pay," Centers for Medicare and Medicaid Services (CMS), December 2016.

If you're in a Medicare Advantage Plan or other Medicare health plan, you may have different rules, but your plan must give you at least the same coverage as Original Medicare.

Learning More about Medicare Coverage

1. Talk to your doctor or other healthcare provider about why you need the service or supply and ask whether he or she thinks Medicare will cover it. Your doctor or provider knows more than anyone about your individual medical needs.

2. Check your "Medicare and You" handbook mailed to you each fall. Your handbook has this information:

    *   You can call 1-800-MEDICARE (1-800-633-4227). TTY users can call 1-877-486-2048.

    *   A general list of services covered by Medicare Part A (Hospital Insurance), like inpatient hospital stays, home health services, hospice care, and care in a skilled nursing facility.

    *   A general list of services covered by Medicare Part B (Medical Insurance), including preventive services, lab tests, X-rays, doctor services, and more.

    *   Information on getting Medicare benefits through private health plans (Part C) and Medicare prescription drug coverage (Part D).

    *   General information on coinsurance and copayment amounts.

    *   Yearly deductibles for Part A and Part B services, and other costs under Part C and Part D.

3. Call 1-800-MEDICARE (1-800-633-4227) to see if they have information on any related local or national coverage policies.

If there's a service or supply that Medicare usually covers that your doctor, healthcare provider, or supplier thinks Medicare won't cover in your specific case, he or she must give you a Medicare notice, like an "Advance Beneficiary Notice of Noncoverage," and ask you to sign it. Read this notice carefully to understand your options and payment responsibilities. You'll be asked if you want to get the items or services listed on the notice and you will have to pay for them if Medicare doesn't.

The type of notice you get depends on the healthcare setting and services you're getting.

How Much to Pay for Surgery

For surgeries or procedures, it may be difficult to know the exact costs in advance because no one knows exactly the amount or type of services you'll need. For example, if you experience complications during surgery, your costs could be higher.

If you're having surgery or a procedure, there are some things you can do in advance to determine approximately what your share of the cost may be:

- Ask the doctor or healthcare provider if they can tell you how much the surgery or procedure will cost and how much you'll have to pay. Learn how Medicare covers inpatient versus outpatient hospital services.

- Look at your last "Medicare Summary Notice" to see if you met the deductible for Part A (Hospital Insurance) if you expect to be admitted to the hospital, or the deductible for Part B (Medical Insurance) for a doctor's visit and other outpatient care. You'll need to pay the deductible amounts before Medicare will start to pay. After Medicare starts to pay, you may have copayments for the care you get.

- Check with any other insurance you may have like Medigap (Medicare Supplement Insurance), Medicaid, or an employer retiree insurance plan, to see what they'll pay. If you belong to a Medicare health plan, contact the plan for more information.

- Call the hospital or facility and ask them to tell you the copayment for the specific surgery or procedure the doctor is planning. It's important to remember that if you need other unexpected services, your costs may be higher.

- Ask your doctor, surgeon, or other healthcare provider, or their staff what kind of care or services you may need after your surgery or procedure and how much you'll have to pay.

Keeping Surgery Costs Down

- Make sure that your Medicare card is valid and that you've paid your Medicare Part B premium.

- Ask your doctor, other healthcare provider, or supplier if they accept assignment. Assignment means your doctor, provider, or supplier has signed an agreement with Medicare (or is required by law) to accept the Medicare-approved amount as full payment for covered services. This can help keep your costs down.

- If you have limited income and resources, you might qualify for extra help to pay for some of your healthcare and prescription drug costs. Check your "Medicare and You" handbook, or visit www.medicare.gov.

Ask Questions!

Your doctor or other healthcare provider is a great resource. Ask them to explain why you're getting certain services or supplies and if they think Medicare will cover them.

Chapter 20

Advanced Care Planning

Because of advances in medicine, each of us, as well as our families and friends, may face many decisions about the dying process. As hard as it might be to face the idea of your own death, you might take time to consider how your individual values relate to your wishes for end-of-life care.

By deciding what end-of-life care best suits your needs when you are healthy, you can help those close to you make the right choices when the time comes. This not only respects your values, but also may give your loved ones, comfort.

There are several ways to make sure others know the kind of care you want when dying.

Talk about End-of-Life Wishes

The simplest, but not always the easiest, way is to talk about end-of-life care before an illness. Discussing your thoughts, values, and desires about end-of-life care before you become sick will help people who are close to you to know what care you want. You could discuss how you feel about using life-prolonging measures, for example cardiopulmonary resuscitation (CPR) or a ventilator, or where you would like to be cared for (for example, home or nursing home). Doctors should be told about these wishes as well.

This chapter includes text excerpted from "Planning for End-of-Life Care Decisions," National Institute on Aging (NIA), National Institutes of Health (NIH), July 2016.

For some people, it makes sense to bring this up at a small family gathering. Some may find that telling their family they have made a will (or updated an existing one) provides an opportunity to bring up this subject with other family members. As hard as it might be to talk about your end-of-life wishes, knowing your preferences ahead of time can make decision-making easier for your family. You may also have some comfort knowing that your family can choose what you want.

On the other hand, if your parents (or another close relative or friend) are aging and you are unsure about what they want, you might introduce the subject. You can try to explain that having this conversation will help you care for them and do what they want. You might start by talking about what you think their values are, instead of talking about specific treatments. Try saying something like, "When Uncle Isaiah had a stroke, I thought you seemed upset that his kids wanted to put him on a respirator." Or, "I've always wondered why Grandpa didn't die at home. Do you know?"

Encourage your parents to share the type of care they would choose to have at the end of life, rather than what they don't want. There is no right or wrong plan, only what they would like. If they are reluctant to have this conversation, don't force it, but try to bring it up again at a later time.

Prepare Advance Directives and Other Documents

Written instructions letting others know the type of care you want if you are seriously ill or dying are called advance directives. These include a living will and healthcare power of attorney. A living will records your end-of-life care wishes in case you are no longer able to speak or make decisions for yourself.

You might want to talk with your doctor or other healthcare provider before preparing a living will. This will help you have a better understanding of what types of decisions might need to be made. Make sure your doctor and family have seen your living will and understand your instructions.

Because a living will cannot give guidance for every possible situation, you probably want to name someone to make care decisions for you if you are unable to do so for yourself. You might choose a family member, friend, lawyer, or someone in your religious community. Of course, you should make sure the person you have named (and alternates) understand your views about end-of-life care and are willing to make those decisions on your behalf. You can do this either in the advance directives or through a durable power of attorney for healthcare that names a healthcare proxy, who is also called a representative, surrogate, agent, or attorney-in-fact.

Durable means it remains in effect even if you are unable to make decisions. A durable power of attorney for healthcare is a useful document if you don't want to be specific—if you'd rather let a proxy evaluate each situation or treatment option independently. This document is particularly important if your healthcare proxy—the person you want to make choices for you—is not a legal member of your family.

If you don't name someone, the State you live in probably has an order of priority based on family relationships to determine who decides for you.

Don't confuse a durable power of attorney for healthcare with a durable power of attorney. The first is limited to decisions related to healthcare, while the latter covers decisions regarding property or financial matters.

A lawyer can prepare these papers, or you can do them yourself. Forms are available from your local or State government, from private groups, or on the Internet. Often, these forms need to be witnessed. That means that people who are not related to you watch as you sign and date the paperwork and then sign and date it themselves as proof that the signature is indeed yours.

Make sure you give copies to your primary doctor and your healthcare proxy. Have copies in your files as well. Hospitals might ask for a copy when you are admitted, even if you are not seriously ill.

You should also give permission to your doctors and insurance companies to share your personal information with your healthcare proxy. This lets your proxy discuss your case with the doctor and handle insurance issues that may come up.

Sometimes, people change their minds as they get older or after they become ill. Review the decisions in your advance directives from time to time, and make changes if your views or your health needs have changed. Be sure to discuss these changes with your healthcare proxy and your doctor. Replace all copies of the older version with the updated ones, witnessed and signed if appropriate.

Do you live in one State, but spend a lot of time in another? Maybe you live in the north and spend winter months in a southern State. Or, perhaps your children and grandchildren live in a different State and you visit them often. Because States' rules and regulations may differ, make sure your forms are legal in both your home State and the State you travel to often. If not, make an advance directive with copies for that State, too, and be sure your family there has a copy.

177

Physician Orders for Life-Sustaining Treatment (POLST) or Medical Orders for Life-Sustaining Treatment (MOLST)

A number of States use an advance care planning form known as POLST (Physician Orders for Life-Sustaining Treatment) or MOLST (Medical Orders for Life-Sustaining Treatment). This form provides more detailed guidance about your medical care preferences.

The form is filled out by your doctor, or sometimes a nurse practitioner or physician's assistant, after discussing your wishes with you and your family. Once signed by your doctor, this form has the same authority as any other medical order.

Chapter 21

Medical Tourism

Medical Tourism: Going Abroad for Medical Care

"Medical tourism" refers to traveling to another country for medical care. It's estimated that thousands of U.S. residents travel abroad for care each year. Many factors influence the decision to seek medical care overseas. Some people travel for care because treatment is cheaper in another country. Other medical tourists may be immigrants to the United States who prefer to return to their home country for healthcare. Still others may travel to receive a procedure or therapy not available in the United States. The most common procedures that people undergo on medical tourism trips include cosmetic surgery, dentistry, and heart surgery.

Risks of Medical Tourism

The specific risks of medical tourism depend on the area being visited and the procedures performed, but some general issues have been identified:

- Communication may be a problem. Receiving care at a facility where you do not speak the language fluently might increase the chance that misunderstandings will arise about your care.

This chapter includes text excerpted from "Medical Tourism," Centers for Disease Control and Prevention (CDC), December 5, 2016.

- Medication may be counterfeit or of poor quality in some countries.

- Antibiotic resistance is a global problem, and resistant bacteria may be more common in other countries than in the United States.

- Flying after surgery can increase the risk for blood clots.

What You Can Do

- If you are planning to travel to another country for medical care, see a travel medicine practitioner at least 4–6 weeks before the trip to discuss general information for healthy travel and specific risks related to the procedure and travel before and after the procedure.

- Make sure that any current medical conditions you have are well controlled, and that your regular healthcare provider knows about your plans for travel and medical care overseas.

- Check the qualifications of the healthcare providers who will be doing the procedure and the credentials of the facility where the procedure will be done. Remember that foreign standards for healthcare providers and facilities may be different from those of the United States. Accrediting groups, including Joint Commission International (JCI), DNV International Accreditation for Hospitals, and the International Society for Quality in Healthcare (ISQua), have lists of standards that facilities need to meet to be accredited.

- Make sure that you have a written agreement with the healthcare facility or the group arranging the trip, defining what treatments, supplies, and care are covered by the costs of the trip.

- If you go to a country where you do not speak the language, determine ahead of time how you will communicate with your doctor and other people who are caring for you.

- Take with you copies of your medical records that include the lab and other studies done related to the condition for which you are obtaining care and any allergies you may have.

- Bring copies of all your prescriptions and a list of all the medicines you take, including their brand names, generic names, manufacturers, and dosages.

- Arrange for follow-up care with your local healthcare provider before you leave.

- Before planning vacation activities, such as sunbathing, drinking alcohol, swimming, or taking long tours, find out if those activities are permitted after surgery.

- Get copies of all your medical records before you return home.

Part Three

Common Types of Surgery and Surgical Procedures

Chapter 22

Head and Neck Surgery

Chapter Contents

185

Section 22.1

Treating Head and Neck Cancers

This section includes text excerpted from "Head and Neck Cancers,"
National Cancer Institute (NCI), March 29, 2017.

Cancers that are known collectively as head and neck cancers usually begin in the squamous cells that line the moist, mucosal surfaces
inside the head and neck (for example, inside the mouth, the nose,
and the throat). These squamous cell cancers are often referred to as
squamous cell carcinomas of the head and neck. Head and neck cancers
can also begin in the salivary glands, but salivary gland cancers are
relatively uncommon. Salivary glands contain many different types
of cells that can become cancerous, so there are many different types
of salivary gland cancer.

Cancers of the head and neck are further categorized by the area of
the head or neck in which they begin. These areas are described below
and labeled in the image of head and neck cancer regions.

Treatment for Cancer

The treatment plan for an individual patient depends on a number
of factors, including the exact location of the tumor, the stage of the
cancer, and the person's age and general health. Treatment for head
and neck cancer can include surgery, radiation therapy, chemotherapy,
targeted therapy, or a combination of treatments.

People who are diagnosed with human papillomavirus (HPV)-posi-
tive oropharyngeal cancer may be treated differently than people with
oropharyngeal cancers that are HPV-negative. Research has shown
that patients with HPV-positive oropharyngeal tumors have a better
prognosis and may do just as well on less intense treatment. An ongoing clinical trial is investigating this question.

The patient and the doctor should consider treatment options carefully. They should discuss each type of treatment and how it might
change the way the patient looks, talks, eats, or breathes.

Side Effect of Treatment

Surgery for head and neck cancers often changes the patient's ability to chew, swallow, or talk. The patient may look different after surgery, and the face and neck may be swollen. The swelling usually goes away within a few weeks. However, if lymph nodes are removed, the flow of lymph in the area where they were removed may be slower and lymph could collect in the tissues, causing additional swelling; this swelling may last for a long time.

After a laryngectomy (surgery to remove the larynx) or other surgery in the neck, parts of the neck, and throat may feel numb because nerves have been cut. If lymph nodes in the neck were removed, the shoulder and neck may become weak and stiff.

Patients who receive radiation to the head and neck may experience redness, irritation, and sores in the mouth; a dry mouth or thickened saliva; difficulty in swallowing; changes in taste; or nausea. Other problems that may occur during treatment are loss of taste, which may decrease appetite and affect nutrition, and earaches (caused by the hardening of ear wax). Patients may also notice some swelling or drooping of the skin under the chin and changes in the texture of the skin. The jaw may feel stiff, and patients may not be able to open their mouth as wide as before treatment.

Patients should report any side effects to their doctor or nurse, and discuss how to deal with them.

Rehabilitation and Support Options

The goal of treatment for head and neck cancers is to control the disease, but doctors are also concerned about preserving the function of the affected areas as much as they can and helping the patient return to normal activities as soon as possible after treatment. Rehabilitation is a very important part of this process. The goals of rehabilitation depend on the extent of the disease and the treatment that a patient has received.

Depending on the location of the cancer and the type of treatment, rehabilitation may include physical therapy, dietary counseling, speech therapy, and/or learning how to care for a stoma. A stoma is an opening into the windpipe through which a patient breathes after a laryngectomy, which is surgery to remove the larynx.

Sometimes, especially with cancer of the oral cavity, a patient may need reconstructive and plastic surgery to rebuild bones or tissues.

However, reconstructive surgery may not always be possible because of damage to the remaining tissue from the original surgery or from radiation therapy. If reconstructive surgery is not possible, a prosthodontist may be able to make a prosthesis (an artificial dental and/or facial part) to restore satisfactory swallowing, speech, and appearance. Patients will receive special training on how to use the device.

Patients who have trouble speaking after treatment may need speech therapy. Often, a speech-language pathologist will visit the patient in the hospital to plan therapy and teach speech exercises or alternative methods of speaking. Speech therapy usually continues after the patient returns home.

Eating may be difficult after treatment for head and neck cancer. Some patients receive nutrients directly into a vein after surgery or need a feeding tube until they can eat on their own. A feeding tube is a flexible plastic tube that is passed into the stomach through the nose or an incision in the abdomen. A nurse or speech-language pathologist can help patients learn how to swallow again after surgery.

Section 22.2

Brain Tumor Surgery

This section includes text excerpted from "What You Need to Know about Brain Tumors," National Cancer Institute (NCI), February 2009. Reviewed June 2017.

Brain Tumor and Its Types

When most normal cells grow old or get damaged, they die, and new cells take their place. Sometimes, this process goes wrong. New cells form when the body doesn't need them, and old or damaged cells don't die as they should. The buildup of extra cells often forms a mass of tissue called a growth or tumor.

Primary brain tumors can be benign or malignant:

- Benign brain tumors do not contain cancer cells:

    - Usually, benign tumors can be removed, and they seldom grow back.

- Benign brain tumors usually have an obvious border or edge. Cells from benign tumors rarely invade tissues around them. They don't spread to other parts of the body. However, benign tumors can press on sensitive areas of the brain and cause serious health problems.

- Unlike benign tumors in most other parts of the body, benign brain tumors are sometimes life threatening.

- Benign brain tumors may become malignant.

- Malignant brain tumors (also called brain cancer) contain cancer cells:

  - Malignant brain tumors are generally more serious and often are a threat to life.

  - They are likely to grow rapidly and crowd or invade the nearby healthy brain tissue.

  - Cancer cells may break away from malignant brain tumors and spread to other parts of the brain or to the spinal cord. They rarely spread to other parts of the body.

Surgery for Brain Tumor

Surgery is the usual first treatment for most brain tumors. Before surgery begins, you may be given general anesthesia, and your scalp is shaved. You probably won't need your entire head shaved.

Craniotomy

Surgery to open the skull is called a craniotomy. The surgeon makes an incision in your scalp and uses a special type of saw to remove a piece of bone from the skull. You may be awake when the surgeon removes part or all of the brain tumor. The surgeon removes as much tumor as possible. You may be asked to move a leg, count, say the alphabet, or tell a story. Your ability to follow these commands helps the surgeon protect important parts of the brain.

After the tumor is removed, the surgeon covers the opening in the skull with the piece of bone or with a piece of metal or fabric. The surgeon then closes the incision in the scalp.

Sometimes surgery isn't possible. If the tumor is in the brain stem or certain other areas, the surgeon may not be able to remove the tumor without harming normal brain tissue. People who can't have surgery may receive radiation therapy or other treatment.

Recovering from Surgery

You may have a headache or be uncomfortable for the first few days after surgery. However, medicine can usually control pain. Before surgery, you should discuss the plan for pain relief with your healthcare team. After surgery, your team can adjust the plan if you need more relief.

You may also feel tired or weak. The time it takes to heal after surgery is different for everyone. You will probably spend a few days in the hospital.

Problems after Surgery

Other, less common problems may occur after surgery for a brain tumor. The brain may swell or fluid may buildup within the skull. The healthcare team will monitor you for signs of swelling or fluid buildup. You may receive steroids to help relieve swelling. A second surgery may be needed to drain the fluid. The surgeon may place a long, thin tube (shunt) in a ventricle of the brain. (For some people, the shunt is placed before performing surgery on the brain tumor.) The tube is threaded under the skin to another part of the body, usually the abdomen. Excess fluid is carried from the brain and drained into the abdomen. Sometimes the fluid is drained into the heart instead.

Infection is another problem that may develop after surgery. If this happens, the healthcare team will give you an antibiotic.

Brain surgery may harm normal tissue. Brain damage can be a serious problem. It can cause problems with thinking, seeing, or speaking. It can also cause personality changes or seizures. Most of these problems lessen or disappear with time. But sometimes damage to the brain is permanent. You may need physical therapy, speech therapy, or occupational therapy.

Section 22.3

Ear Tube Surgery for Ear Infections

This section contains text excerpted from the following sources:
Text beginning with the heading "Ear Infection" is excerpted from
"Ear Infections in Children," National Institute on Deafness and
Other Communication Disorders (NIDCD), February 13, 2017; Text
under the heading "Myringotomy" is excerpted from "Myringotomy,"
U.S. Department of Veterans Affairs (VA), 2005.
Reviewed June 2017.

Ear Infection

An ear infection is an inflammation of the middle ear, usually caused by bacteria, that occurs when fluid builds up behind the eardrum. Anyone can get an ear infection, but children get them more often than adults. Five out of six children will have at least one ear infection by their third birthday. The scientific name for an ear infection is otitis media (OM).

Diagnosing a Middle Ear Infection

The first thing a doctor will do is ask you about your child's health. Has your child had a head cold or sore throat recently? Is he having trouble sleeping? Is she pulling at her ears? If an ear infection seems likely, the simplest way for a doctor to tell is to use a lighted instrument, called an otoscope, to look at the eardrum. A red, bulging eardrum indicates an infection.

A doctor also may use a pneumatic otoscope, which blows a puff of air into the ear canal, to check for fluid behind the eardrum. A normal eardrum will move back and forth more easily than an eardrum with fluid behind it.

Tympanometry, which uses sound tones and air pressure, is a diagnostic test a doctor might use if the diagnosis still isn't clear. A tympanometer is a small, soft plug that contains a tiny microphone and speaker as well as a device that varies air pressure in the ear. It measures how flexible the eardrum is at different pressures.

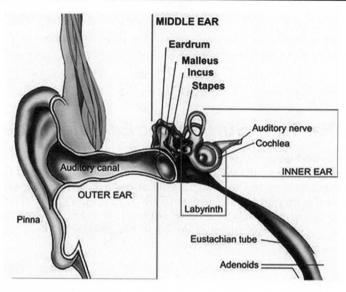

Figure 22.1. *Parts of the Ear*

Treating Acute Middle Ear Infection

Many doctors will prescribe an antibiotic, such as amoxicillin, to be taken over seven to 10 days. Your doctor also may recommend over-the-counter pain relievers such as acetaminophen or ibuprofen, or eardrops, to help with fever and pain. (Because aspirin is considered a major preventable risk factor for Reye syndrome, a child who has a fever or other flu-like symptoms should not be given aspirin unless instructed to by your doctor.)

If your doctor isn't able to make a definite diagnosis of OM and your child doesn't have severe ear pain or a fever, your doctor might ask you to wait a day or two to see if the earache goes away. The American Academy of Pediatrics (AAP) issued guidelines that encourage doctors to observe and closely follow these children with ear infections that can't be definitively diagnosed, especially those between the ages of 6 months to 2 years. If there's no improvement within 48 to 72 hours from when symptoms began, the guidelines recommend doctors start antibiotic therapy. Sometimes ear pain isn't caused by infection, and some ear infections may get better without antibiotics. Using antibiotics cautiously and with good reason helps prevent the development of bacteria that become resistant to antibiotics.

If your doctor prescribes an antibiotic, it's important to make sure your child takes it exactly as prescribed and for the full amount of time.

Even though your child may seem better in a few days, the infection still hasn't completely cleared from the ear. Stopping the medicine too soon could allow the infection to come back. It's also important to return for your child's follow-up visit, so that the doctor can check if the infection is gone.

Myringotomy

A myringotomy is a tiny opening made in the eardrum so fluid can drain from the middle ear.

Why Is It Done?

The eustachian tube is the narrow passage between the middle ear and the space behind the nose. Repeated infections can block the eustachian tube. Prolonged blockage may cause some discomfort, decreased hearing, and fluid formation in the middle ear space.

How Is It Done?

The doctor makes a very small opening in your eardrum and suctions (vacuums) out the fluid. This relieves pressure and lets air flow through the middle ear. A small tube may be placed in this opening to help drainage and airflow.

Care after Tube Placement

If you are given a prescription for ear drops, use them as prescribed. Follow these steps to put the drops in your ear:

1. Lie down on your side.

2. Gently pull the ear up, back, and out to straighten the ear canal.

3. Use the dropper to put the prescribed number of drops into your ear.

4. Remain on your side for about five minutes to let the drops work their way into the ear canal.

The tube falls out as the eardrum heals, this is normal. Do not swim until you are given permission.

Section 22.4

Cochlear Implant Surgery

This section contains text excerpted from the following sources:
Text in this section begins with excerpts from "Cochlear Implant,"
National Institute on Deafness and Other Communication Disorders
(NIDCD), March 6, 2017; Text beginning with the heading "Before
Surgery" is excerpted from "Cochlear Implants—Before, during, and
after Implant Surgery," U.S. Food and Drug Administration (FDA),
June 6, 2014.

A cochlear implant is a small, complex electronic device that can
help to provide a sense of sound to a person who is profoundly deaf or
severely hard-of-hearing. The implant consists of an external portion
that sits behind the ear and a second portion that is surgically placed
under the skin (see Figure 22.2). An implant has the following parts:

- A microphone, which picks up sound from the environment.

- A speech processor, which selects and arranges sounds picked
  up by the microphone.

- A transmitter and receiver/stimulator, which receive signals from the speech processor and convert them into electric
  impulses.

- An electrode array, which is a group of electrodes that collects
  the impulses from the stimulator and sends them to different
  regions of the auditory nerve.

An implant does not restore normal hearing. Instead, it can give a
deaf person a useful representation of sounds in the environment and
help him or her to understand speech.

How It Works

A cochlear implant is very different from a hearing aid. Hearing aids
amplify sounds so they may be detected by damaged ears. Cochlear
implants bypass damaged portions of the ear and directly stimulate
the auditory nerve. Signals generated by the implant are sent by way

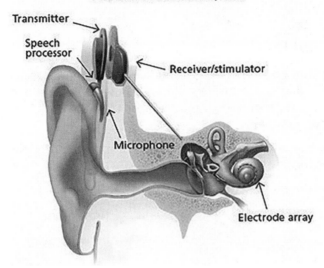

Figure 22.2. *Cochlear Implant*

of the auditory nerve to the brain, which recognizes the signals as sound. Hearing through a cochlear implant is different from normal hearing and takes time to learn or relearn. However, it allows many people to recognize warning signals, understand other sounds in the environment, and understand speech in person or over the telephone.

Getting a Cochlear Implant

Use of a cochlear implant requires both a surgical procedure and significant therapy to learn or relearn the sense of hearing. Not everyone performs at the same level with this device. The decision to receive an implant should involve discussions with medical specialists, including an experienced cochlear-implant surgeon. The process can be expensive. For example, a person's health insurance may cover the expense, but not always.

Some individuals may choose not to have a cochlear implant for a variety of personal reasons. Surgical implantations are almost always safe, although complications are a risk factor, just as with any kind of surgery. An additional consideration is learning to interpret the sounds created by an implant. This process takes time and practice. Speech-language pathologists and audiologists are frequently involved in this learning process. Prior to implantation, all of these factors need to be considered.

Before Surgery

Primary care doctors usually refer patients to ear, nose, and throat doctors (ENT doctors or otolaryngologists) to test them to see if they are candidates for cochlear implants.

Tests often done are:

- examination of external, middle, and inner ear for signs of infection or abnormality

- various tests of hearing, such as an audiogram

- a trial of hearing aid use to assess its potential benefit

- exams to evaluate middle and inner ear structures:

  - CT (computerized tomography) scan. This type of X-ray helps the doctor see if the cochlea has a normal shape. This scan is especially important if the patient has a history of meningitis because it helps see if there is new bone growth in the cochlea that could interfere with the insertion of the implant. This scan also may indicate which ear should be implanted.

  - MRI (magnetic resonance imaging) scan

- psychological examination to see if the patient can cope with the implant

- physical exam to prepare for general anesthesia

During Surgery

The doctor or other hospital staff may:

- insert some intravenous (I.V.) lines

- shave or clean the scalp around the site of the implant

- attach cables, monitors and patches to the patient's skin to monitor vital signs

- put a mask on the patient's face to provide oxygen and anesthetic gas

- administer drugs through the I.V. and the face mask to cause sleep and general anesthesia

- awaken the patient in the operating room and take him or her to a recovery room until all the anesthesia is gone

After Surgery

Immediately after waking, a patient may feel:

- pressure or discomfort over his (or her) implanted ear
- dizziness
- sick to the stomach (have nausea)
- disoriented or confused for a while
- a sore throat for a while from the breathing tube used during general anesthesia

Then, a patient can expect to:

- keep the bandages on for a while
- have the bandages be stained with some blood or fluid
- go home in about a day after surgery
- have stitches for a while
- get instructions about caring for the stitches, washing the head, showering, and general care and diet
- have an appointment in about a week to the stitches removed and have the implant site examined
- have the implant "turned on" (activated) about 3–6 weeks later

Frequently Asked Questions on Cochlear Implant

Can a Patient Hear Immediately after the Operation?

No. Without the external transmitter part of the implant a patient cannot hear. The clinic will give the patient the external components about a month after the implant surgery in the first programming session.

Why Is It Necessary to Wait 3 to 6 weeks after the Operation before Receiving the External Transmitter and Sound Processor?

The waiting period provides time for the operative incision to heal completely. This usually takes 3 to 6 weeks. After the swelling is gone, your clinician can do the first fitting and programming.

What Happens during the Initial Programming Session?

An audiologist adjusts the sound processor to fit the implanted patient, tests the patient to ensure that the adjustments are correct, determines what sounds the patient hears, and gives information on the proper care and use of the device.

Is It Beneficial If a Family Member Participates in the Training Program?

Yes! A family member should be included in the training program whenever possible to provide assistance. The family member should know how to manage the operations of the sound processor.

Do Patients Have More than One Implant?

Usually, patients have only one ear implanted, though a few patients have implants in both ears.

How can I help my child receive the most benefit from their cochlear implant?

- try to make hearing and listening as interesting and fun as possible

- encourage your child to make noises

- talk about things you do as you do them

- Show your child that he or she can consciously use and evaluate the sounds he or she receives from his or her cochlear implant

- realize that the more committed you, your child's teachers, and your health professionals are to helping your child, the more successful he or she will be

Section 22.5

Sinus Surgery

This section includes text excerpted from "Endoscopic Sinus Surgery," U.S. Department of Veterans Affairs (VA), July 2013. Reviewed June 2017.

Sinuses

Your sinuses are air-filled spaces in the bones of the face and head. The sinuses drain mucous through small openings that are linked to the inside of the nose. They play a big role in how we breathe and make mucous. Mucous does not drain well when you have swelling of the lining of the nose and sinuses. An acute or chronic infection can result. When medical therapies and sinus rinses do not clear up the swelling, surgery may be needed to open up the sinuses and allow them to drain. Some people grow polyps (small growth sticking out from the mucous lining). Surgery may be needed to remove the polyps.

Endoscopic Sinus Surgery

You will be given medicine to keep you asleep and free from pain during surgery. There will be no incisions (cuts) made on the outside of your nose. All surgery is done through your nostrils, using scopes. Your doctor can see the images on a monitor. The opening to each sinus that is blocked will be opened. Any polyps are removed. This is a detailed surgery and must be done carefully. The surgery may take 3–4 hours. If the divider between the two sides of your nose (the nasal septum) is too crooked it may have to be straightened. This will allow drainage of all the sinuses. This is called septoplasty, and will add an extra hour to the procedure.

At the end of the surgery, your sinuses will still be oozing a little blood. Nasal packings or foam are placed in your nostrils to stop the bleeding. If you have nasal packing (like a nasal tampon) the surgeon will see you back in a few days to take it out. You need to stop taking aspirin, ibuprofen (Advil or Motrin), naproxen (Alleve) and similar meds at least one week before surgery. These meds can cause bleeding.

Sinus surgery is usually safe. There is a 1 percent risk of a major complication. Problems that may happen due to sinus surgery can be: blindness, double vision, injury to brain tissue, and leakage of fluid from around the brain. More common minor problems are scarring, need for more surgery, decreased sense of smell, and nosebleeds.

You can go home the same day of surgery. You will need someone to drive you home.

After Your Surgery Instructions

Nosebleed Safety Measures

You may have a slow trickle of blood down your throat or out of the front of your nose for a few days. You need to see your surgeon right away if you are having a lot of bleeding or it seems too much to you. If you are having bothersome oozing, it can help to spray oxymetazoline (Afrin) 2 sprays in each nostril. You can use the spray up to 4 times a day during the first week. Only use the spray for 1 week. Oxymetazoline constricts blood vessels and can decrease bleeding. However, if used longer than a week it can hurt the lining of your nose and cause nasal congestion that is only relieved by more oxymetazoline. To decrease the risk of nosebleeds after surgery:

1. Sneeze with your mouth open.

2. Do not blow your nose for at least 1 week after surgery. You may gently wipe the front of your nose, or gently use a Sinus Rinse bottle to cleanse the inside of your nose.

3. Keep your head elevated to lessen swelling. This is especially important at night. You could raise the head of your bed, sleep with 2–3 pillows, or sleep in a recliner. Avoid bending over.

4. If you take meds to control your blood pressure, make sure to take them as ordered. High blood pressure will make nosebleeds more likely.

5. Do not lift anything more than 10 pounds. Do not strain yourself in any way with vigorous activity, sex, or exercise for 2 weeks after surgery.

6. You need to stop taking aspirin, ibuprofen (Advil or Motrin), naproxen (Alleve) and similar meds at least one week after surgery. These meds can increase risk of nosebleeds.

Nasal / Sinus Rinses

After surgery you need to keep your nasal cavities moist, to help blood clots dissolve and loosen crusting. Your surgeon may ask you to use nasal saline (salt water). You should use it as often during the day as you remember, or at least 4–5 times per day.

Your surgeon may ask you to do saline sinus rinses after surgery. Start rinses gently the evening after surgery. If the nose seems to be blocked, stop rinsing and gently try again the next day. This will really help dissolve clots and help nasal breathing and healing.

Activity

You need to avoid activity that raises your blood pressure for two weeks. Things that can raise your blood pressure are heavy lifting, hard exercise, and sex. This could cause a nosebleed.

Diet

You may eat your regular diet after surgery, as long as your stomach is not upset from the anesthesia. If it is, wait until you feel better before you start eating solid foods.

Pain

Pain is usually mild to moderate the first 24–48 hours. Then it will decrease. You may not need a strong narcotic pain med. The sooner you reduce your narcotic pain med use, the faster you will heal. As your pain lessens, try using extra-strength acetaminophen (Tylenol) instead of your narcotic med. It is best to reduce your pain to a level you can manage, rather than to get rid of the pain completely. Please start at a lower of narcotic pain med, and increase the dose only if the pain remains uncontrolled. Decrease the dose if the side effects are too severe.

Do not drive, operate dangerous machinery, or do anything dangerous if you are taking narcotic pain medication (such as oxycodone, hydrocodone, morphine, etc.) This medication affects your reflexes and responses, just like alcohol.

When to Call Your Surgeon

If you have:

1. Any concerns. Surgeons would much rather that you call them then worry at home, or get into trouble.

2. Fever over 101.5°F.

3. Any changes in your vision.

4. Headaches.

5. Leakage of clear fluid from your nose.

6. Excessive bleeding.

7. Pain that continues to increase instead of decrease.

8. Problem urinating.

9. If you have chest pain or difficulty breathing, don't call—go to the nearest emergency room right away.

Postoperative Appointment

You will need to have your nasal cavities and sinuses checked and possibly cleaned out at your postoperative visit. Usually you need to visit clinic in about 7–10 days after surgery.

Section 22.6

Tonsillectomy and Adenoidectomy

This section includes text excerpted from "Tonsillectomy and Adenoidectomy," U.S. Department of Veterans Affairs (VA), July 2013. Reviewed June 2017.

Tonsils

A tonsillectomy is surgery to remove your tonsils. The tonsils are 2 large lumps of tissue in the back of your throat. Tonsils are part of the immune system. Your body can do fine without them. Your tonsils may need to be taken out if you have frequent tonsil infections, if the tonsils are too large, or if there is concern for cancer.

You will be asleep under general anesthesia while your tonsils are being taken out. The doctor places tools inside your mouth to keep it open and to keep your tongue out of the way. Your doctor uses tools to take your tonsils out. The doctor uses tools to stop the bleeding in the areas where tissue was removed. Rarely, a tooth can be chipped or dislodged even though tooth protectors are used during surgery. You may have tongue numbness or taste change after surgery which sometimes can takes weeks to improve. The biggest risk from tonsillectomy is bleeding. Up to 10 percent of adults will need to come back and be treated for bleeding after tonsillectomy. Very rarely, a patient can have severe bleeding after surgery that leads to death.

The surgery usually lasts an hour or less. Having tonsils removed as an adult is more painful than it is for a child. You may have a very severe sore throat for two weeks or more after surgery. You will usually go home the same day of surgery. You will need someone to drive you home. If your tonsillectomy was done because of concerns about tonsil cancer, your surgeon or a resident surgeon will call you with the result of the biopsy as soon as it is available. If you have not heard the results within that time, please call the ENT clinic to request the results.

Adenoids

Adenoids are small lumps of tissue on the top of your throat. Many people no longer have adenoids by the time they are adults. Adenoids are removed in a similar way to tonsils. The pain after this surgery is usually less than after tonsillectomy. You may have ear pain after adenoidectomy.

Activity

No straining, heavy lifting, or vigorous exercise for 2 weeks after surgery.

Diet

You should follow a soft diet for two weeks. This means nothing sharp, for example, no Doritos, popcorn, nuts, etc. Any liquid or soft food is fine.

Pain

Throat pain may be moderate to severe. Do not drive, operate dangerous machinery, or do anything dangerous if you are a taking narcotic pain med (examples are oxycodone, hydrocodone, morphine, etc.). These drugs affect your reflexes and responses, just like alcohol.

Healing Process

It is normal to have bad breath as your throat heals after surgery. This may last several weeks. It is also normal to have a grey/white coating where your tonsils were as you heal. This will clear up within a few weeks.

When to Call Your Surgeon

If you have:

1. Any concerns. Surgeons would much rather that you call them then worry at home, or get into trouble.

2. Persistent fever over 101.5°F.

3. Unable to eat or drink.

4. Difficulty urinating.

5. Neck stiffness.

6. If you have chest pain or difficulty breathing, don't call—you will need to go to the nearest emergency room immediately.

Bleeding

The time that you are most risk for bleeding is within 24 hours after surgery, and again 5–7 days after surgery. At 5–7 days after surgery, scabs in your throat can peel off and cause serious bleeding. If you have a tiny amount of blood in your saliva, you can stay at home and keep an eye on it. Go back to a liquid diet for the remainder of the day. If you have bright red blood from your mouth or throat, you will need to be seen by your surgeon. If it is severe, go to the nearest emergency room.

Postoperative Appointment

The surgeon will usually schedule an appointment about 1 month after your tonsillectomy and/or adenoidectomy.

Section 22.7

Thyroid Surgery

This section includes text excerpted from
"Thyroidectomy," U.S. Department of Veterans
Affairs (VA), July 2013. Reviewed June 2017.

Thyroid Gland

Your thyroid gland is in the front lower part of your neck. It makes hormones that help make your body work right. Your thyroid gland has 2 sections. Each section has parathyroid glands.

Thyroidectomy

Thyroid nodules (round hard lump of cells) are common. If a nodule has cancer in it, then the half of the thyroid gland with the nodule must be taken out. The surgery is needed to find out if it is cancer. If you have cancer, your thyroid gland, as well as tissue and lymph nodes around the gland may be taken out. Some people have a big thyroid that causes problems swallowing or breathing. This is called a goiter and is not cancer. If you have a goiter you may need surgery to take it out.

Your surgeon makes an incision (cut) in the lower area of your neck. The exact size of the cut varies, so you may ask your surgeon to show you. The surgeon then carefully cuts out the thyroid lobe(s.) Your surgeon will find your vocal cord nerve and work around it. There are tiny glands called parathyroid glands that are carefully cut away from the gland and left in the neck. If your whole thyroid needs to be taken out, the same process is carried out on the other side.

Your vocal cord is usually not harmed by the surgery. Your voice may be hoarse or weak after surgery. Only 10–30 percent will be hoarse after surgery. Less than 5 percent will always be hoarse after the surgery. The surgeon will check your vocal cords at your postoperative visit so try not to worry about it until then.

Your parathyroid glands may not work as well as they should after surgery. This can cause your calcium blood levels to drop too low. This can be life-threatening. This may be a problem for a short time, or it may be long lasting. Up to 30 percent of patients will have problems with their parathyroid glands. It is rare to have long lasting problems with your parathyroid.

If you have just one half of your thyroid removed (thyroid lobectomy, or hemithyroidectomy) then you may go home the same day of surgery. You will need someone to drive you home. You will stay in the hospital at least 1 night if you had to have your whole thyroid taken out (total thyroidectomy). Your blood calcium levels will be checked every 6 hours. If they are stable, you can go home the next day. If they are too low, you will be given calcium and vitamin D until your levels become stable. This may take 2–3 days, rarely more.

If you have had your whole thyroid taken out, you will have to take a thyroid hormone pill every day for the rest of your life. The exact dose of the med may need to be adjusted over time. The surgeon will ask your primary care doctor or endocrinologist (a doctor that treats diseases that affect your glands) to check blood tests 6 weeks after starting your thyroid hormone. Your dose of the thyroid hormone med will be adjusted as needed. Sometimes, your endocrinologist does not want you to start taking this hormone until the tests come back showing you do not have cancer. Your surgeon will let you know.

You should be called by your surgeon as soon as the lab doctor looks at your thyroid for cancer. This can take 5–7 business days or more. Please call if you have not heard the results and it has been 7 business days since surgery.

Postoperative Instructions

Incision

Please keep the incision dry for 3 days, and then you may shower and pat the incision dry. You may use Q-tips or gauze dipped in a ½ hydrogen peroxide and ½ water mixture to remove any dried blood over the incision. After washing, apply a thin film of an antibacterial ointment such as Polysporin. Apply the ointment 2 times a day. However, if your surgeon used skin glue you may shower right away, and you do not need to use antibiotic ointment. The skin glue will slowly peel off after 1–2 weeks. If it has not all come off by your postoperative appointment, it will be removed at that time.

Please avoid any activity that pulls across the incision, such as shaving, for at least 2 weeks. The rest of the face may be shaved. The staples and/or stitches will be taken out 1–2 weeks after surgery at your postoperative appointment in the Ear Nose Throat (ENT) clinic.

Drain

Some patients go home with a thin drain tube and an egg shaped collecting bulb called a Jackson-Pratt (JP) drain. The tube should be gently stripped every 4 hours. A nurse will teach you how to do this before you leave the hospital. When the JP drain looks half full or at least 2 times a day, please empty the bulb into a small plastic measuring cup. Then write down the amount in the cup. Pour the fluid in the sink or toilet. When the amount of fluid emptied from the drain is 30 ml (or 2 tablespoons) or less in a 24-hour period, the drain is ready to be taken out. If the drain is in place for 1 week it needs to be taken out no matter how much fluid drained. Call the ENT clinic to have the drain taken out. If it is a weekend or holiday, call the ENT resident doctor on call to have the drain taken out.

The fluid from the JP drain should be red, pink, or straw colored (yellow.) If it is milky or looks like pus, you need to be seen by your surgeon right away.

Head of Bed

Please raise the head of your bed 30–45 degrees or sleep in a recliner for the first 3–4 days to decrease swelling. The skin above the incision may look swollen after lying down for a few hours.

Activity

No straining, heavy lifting, or vigorous exercise for 2 weeks after surgery.

Diet

You may eat your regular diet after surgery.

Pain

Your pain can be mild to moderate the first 24–48 hours. The pain usually lessens after that. Many patients complain more about a sore throat from the breathing tube used during surgery then about pain from the surgery itself. Your pain will get better in 1–2 days and is best treated with throat lozenges.

You may not need strong narcotic pain medication. The sooner you reduce your narcotic pain medication use, the faster you will heal. As your pain lessens, try using extra-strength acetaminophen (Tylenol) instead of your narcotic med. It is best to reduce your pain to a level you can manage, rather than to get rid of the pain completely. Please start at a lower of narcotic pain med, and increase the dose only if the pain remains uncontrolled. Decrease the dose if the side effects are too severe.

Do not drive, operate dangerous machinery, or do anything dangerous if you are taking narcotic pain medication (such as oxycodone, hydrocodone, morphine, etc.) This medication affects your reflexes and responses, just like alcohol.

When to Call Your Surgeon

If you have:

1. Any concerns. Surgeons would much rather that you call them then worry at home, or get into trouble.

2. Any numbness or tingling around your mouth, in your fingers or toes, or anywhere. This may be a sign of low blood calcium levels. If you have muscle cramping and or curling of your fingers or toes, this could be even more seriously low blood calcium levels. This can be a life-threatening problem. You must go have your blood calcium levels drawn immediately. You should not drive if you are having these symptoms. You need to have someone drive you to the nearest Emergency Room (ER), if possible have the ER staff call your surgeon after drawing your blood calcium and giving you extra calcium if needed. Bring these postoperative instructions with you to show to them. If your blood calcium gets too low, you could have seizures or your heart could stop, so you must take this seriously!

3. Fever over 101.5°F.

4. Foul smelling discharge from your incision.

5. Large amount of bleeding.

6. More than expected swelling of your neck.

7. Increase warmth or redness around the incision.

8. Problems urinating.

9. Pain that continues to increase instead of decrease.

10. Choking or coughing with food or liquid.

Postoperative Appointment

If you have stitches, you will need to have them taken out at your postoperative visit 7–10 days after surgery. If you have skin glue, you need to be seen about 2–3 weeks after surgery.

Chapter 23

Eye Surgery

Chapter Contents

Section 23.1

Cataract Surgery

This section includes text excerpted from "Facts about Cataract," National Eye Institute (NEI), September 2015.

About Cataracts

What Is the Lens?

The lens is a clear part of the eye that helps to focus light, or an image, on the retina. The retina is the light-sensitive tissue at the back of the eye. In a normal eye, light passes through the transparent lens to the retina. Once it reaches the retina, light is changed into nerve signals that are sent to the brain. The lens must be clear for the retina to receive a sharp image. If the lens is cloudy from a cataract, the image you see will be blurred

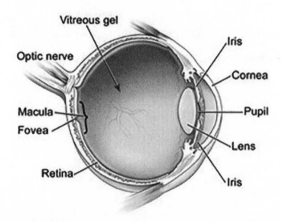

Figure 23.1. *Eye*

What Is a Cataract?

A cataract is a clouding of the lens in the eye that affects vision. Most cataracts are related to aging. Cataracts are very common in older people. By age 80, more than half of all Americans either have a cataract or have had cataract surgery. A cataract can occur in either or both eyes. It cannot spread from one eye to the other.

What Causes Cataracts?

The lens lies behind the iris and the pupil. It works much like a camera lens. It focuses light onto the retina at the back of the eye, where an image is recorded. The lens also adjusts the eye's focus, letting us see things clearly both up close and far away. The lens is made of mostly water and protein. The protein is arranged in a precise way that keeps the lens clear and lets the light pass through it.

But as we age, some of the protein may clump together and start to cloud a small area of the lens. This is a cataract. Over time, the cataract may grow larger and cloud more of the lens, making it harder to see.

Researchers suspect that there are several causes of cataract, such as smoking and diabetes. Or, it may be that the protein in the lens just changes from the wear and tear it takes over the years.

Who Is at Risk for Cataract?

The risk of cataract increases as you get older. Other risk factors for cataract include:

- Certain diseases (for example, diabetes).
- Personal behavior (smoking, alcohol use).
- The environment (prolonged exposure to ultraviolet sunlight).

What Are the Symptoms of a Cataract?

The most common symptoms of a cataract are:

- Cloudy or blurry vision.
- Colors seem faded.
- Glare. Headlights, lamps, or sunlight may appear too bright. A halo may appear around lights.
- Poor night vision.
- Double vision or multiple images in one eye. (This symptom may clear as the cataract gets larger.)
- Frequent prescription changes in your eyeglasses or contact lenses.

These symptoms also can be a sign of other eye problems. If you have any of these symptoms, check with your eye care professional.

Are There Different Types of Cataract?

Yes. Although most cataracts are related to aging, there are other types of cataract:

- **Secondary cataract.** Cataracts can form after surgery for other eye problems, such as glaucoma. Cataracts also can develop in people who have other health problems, such as diabetes. Cataracts are sometimes linked to steroid use.

- **Traumatic cataract.** Cataracts can develop after an eye injury, sometimes years later.

- **Congenital cataract.** Some babies are born with cataracts or develop them in childhood, often in both eyes. These cataracts may be so small that they do not affect vision. If they do, the lenses may need to be removed.

- **Radiation cataract.** Cataracts can develop after exposure to some types of radiation.

How Is a Cataract Detected?

Cataract is detected through a comprehensive eye exam that includes:

1. **Visual acuity test.** This eye chart test measures how well you see at various distances.

2. **Dilated eye exam.** Drops are placed in your eyes to widen, or dilate, the pupils. Your eye care professional uses a special magnifying lens to examine your retina and optic nerve for signs of damage and other eye problems. After the exam, your close-up vision may remain blurred for several hours.

3. **Tonometry.** An instrument measures the pressure inside the eye. Numbing drops may be applied to your eye for this test.

Your eye care professional also may do other tests to learn more about the structure and health of your eye.

Treatment for Cataracts

How Is a Cataract Treated?

The symptoms of early cataract may be improved with new eyeglasses, brighter lighting, anti-glare sunglasses, or magnifying lenses. If these measures do not help, surgery is the only effective treatment. Surgery involves removing the cloudy lens and replacing it with an artificial lens.

A cataract needs to be removed only when vision loss interferes with your everyday activities, such as driving, reading, or watching TV. You and your eye care professional can make this decision together. Once you understand the benefits and risks of surgery, you can make an informed decision about whether cataract surgery is right for you. In most cases, delaying cataract surgery will not cause long-term damage to your eye or make the surgery more difficult. You do not have to rush into surgery.

Sometimes a cataract should be removed even if it does not cause problems with your vision. For example, a cataract should be removed if it prevents examination or treatment of another eye problem, such as age-related macular degeneration or diabetic retinopathy.

If you choose surgery, your eye care professional may refer you to a specialist to remove the cataract.

If you have cataracts in both eyes that require surgery, the surgery will be performed on each eye at separate times, usually four weeks apart.

Is Cataract Surgery Effective?

Cataract removal is one of the most common operations performed in the United States. It also is one of the safest and most effective types of surgery. In about 90 percent of cases, people who have cataract surgery have better vision afterward.

What Are the Risks of Cataract Surgery?

As with any surgery, cataract surgery poses risks, such as infection and bleeding. Before cataract surgery, your doctor may ask you to temporarily stop taking certain medications that increase the risk of bleeding during surgery. After surgery, you must keep your eye clean, wash your hands before touching your eye, and use the prescribed medications to help minimize the risk of infection. Serious infection can result in loss of vision.

Cataract surgery slightly increases your risk of retinal detachment. Other eye disorders, such as high myopia (nearsightedness), can further increase your risk of retinal detachment after cataract surgery. One sign of a retinal detachment is a sudden increase in flashes or floaters. Floaters are little "cobwebs" or specks that seem to float about in your field of vision. If you notice a sudden increase in floaters or flashes, see an eye care professional immediately. A retinal detachment is a medical emergency. If necessary, go to an emergency service or hospital. Your eye must be examined by an eye surgeon as soon as possible. A retinal detachment causes no pain. Early treatment for retinal detachment often can prevent permanent loss of vision. The sooner you get treatment, the more likely you will regain good vision. Even if you are treated promptly, some vision may be lost.

Talk to your eye care professional about these risks. Make sure cataract surgery is right for you.

What If I Have Other Eye Conditions and Need Cataract Surgery?

Many people who need cataract surgery also have other eye conditions, such as age-related macular degeneration or glaucoma. If you have other eye conditions in addition to cataract, talk with your doctor. Learn about the risks, benefits, alternatives, and expected results of cataract surgery.

What Happens before Surgery?

A week or two before surgery, your doctor will do some tests. These tests may include measuring the curve of the cornea and the size and shape of your eye. This information helps your doctor choose the right type of intraocular lens (IOL).

You may be asked not to eat or drink anything 12 hours before your surgery.

What Happens during Surgery?

At the hospital or eye clinic, drops will be put into your eye to dilate the pupil. The area around your eye will be washed and cleansed.

The operation usually lasts less than one hour and is almost painless. Many people choose to stay awake during surgery. Others may need to be put to sleep for a short time. If you are awake, you will have an anesthetic to numb the nerves in and around your eye.

216

After the operation, a patch may be placed over your eye. You will rest for a while. Your medical team will watch for any problems, such as bleeding. Most people who have cataract surgery can go home the same day. You will need someone to drive you home.

What Happens after Surgery?

Itching and mild discomfort are normal after cataract surgery. Some fluid discharge is also common. Your eye may be sensitive to light and touch. If you have discomfort, your doctor can suggest treatment. After one or two days, moderate discomfort should disappear.

For a few weeks after surgery, your doctor may ask you to use eyedrops to help healing and decrease the risk of infection. Ask your doctor about how to use your eyedrops, how often to use them, and what effects they can have. You will need to wear an eye shield or eyeglasses to help protect your eye. Avoid rubbing or pressing on your eye.

When you are home, try not to bend from the waist to pick up objects on the floor. Do not lift any heavy objects. You can walk, climb stairs, and do light household chores.

In most cases, healing will be complete within eight weeks. Your doctor will schedule exams to check on your progress.

Can Problems Develop after Surgery?

Problems after surgery are rare, but they can occur. These problems can include infection, bleeding, inflammation (pain, redness, swelling), loss of vision, double vision, and high or low eye pressure. With prompt medical attention, these problems can usually be treated successfully.

Sometimes the eye tissue that encloses the IOL becomes cloudy and may blur your vision. This condition is called an after-cataract. An after-cataract can develop months or years after cataract surgery.

An after-cataract is treated with a laser. Your doctor uses a laser to make a tiny hole in the eye tissue behind the lens to let light pass through. This outpatient procedure is called a YAG laser capsulotomy. It is painless and rarely results in increased eye pressure or other eye problems. As a precaution, your doctor may give you eyedrops to lower your eye pressure before or after the procedure.

When will My Vision Be Normal Again?

You can return quickly to many everyday activities, but your vision may be blurry. The healing eye needs time to adjust so that it can focus properly with the other eye, especially if the other eye has a cataract. Ask your doctor when you can resume driving.

If you received an IOL, you may notice that colors are very bright. The IOL is clear, unlike your natural lens that may have had a yellowish/brownish tint. Within a few months after receiving an IOL, you will become used to improved color vision. Also, when your eye heals, you may need new glasses or contact lenses.

What Can I Do If I Already Have Lost Some Vision from Cataract?

If you have lost some vision, speak with your surgeon about options that may help you make the most of your remaining vision.

What Can I Do to Protect My Vision?

Wearing sunglasses and a hat with a brim to block ultraviolet sunlight may help to delay cataract. If you smoke, stop. Researchers also believe good nutrition can help reduce the risk of age-related cataract. They recommend eating green leafy vegetables, fruit, and other foods with antioxidants.

If you are age 60 or older, you should have a comprehensive dilated eye exam at least once every two years. In addition to cataract, your eye care professional can check for signs of age-related macular degeneration, glaucoma, and other vision disorders. Early treatment for many eye diseases may save your sight.

Section 23.2

Glaucoma Surgery

This section includes text excerpted from "Facts about Glaucoma," National Eye Institute (NEI), November 14, 2014.

Glaucoma Defined

What Is Glaucoma?

Glaucoma is a group of diseases that damage the eye's optic nerve and can result in vision loss and blindness. However, with early detection and treatment, you can often protect your eyes against serious vision loss.

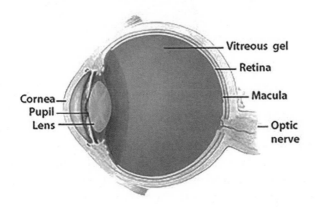

Figure 23.2. *The Optic Nerve*

The optic nerve. The optic nerve is a bundle of more than 1 million nerve fibers. It connects the retina to the brain. (See Figure 23.2) The retina is the light-sensitive tissue at the back of the eye. A healthy optic nerve is necessary for good vision.

How Does the Optic Nerve Get Damaged by Open-Angle Glaucoma?

Several large studies have shown that eye pressure is a major risk factor for optic nerve damage. In the front of the eye is a space called the anterior chamber. A clear fluid flows continuously in and out of the chamber and nourishes nearby tissues. The fluid leaves the chamber at the open angle where the cornea and iris meet. (See Figure 23.3.) When the fluid reaches the angle, it flows through a spongy meshwork, like a drain, and leaves the eye.

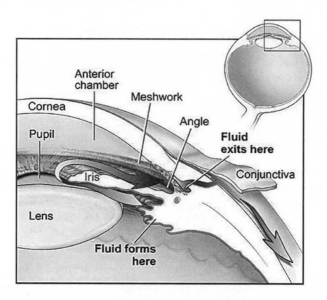

Figure 23.3. *Fluid Flow in the Eye*

In open-angle glaucoma, even though the drainage angle is "open," the fluid passes too slowly through the meshwork drain. Since the fluid builds up, the pressure inside the eye rises to a level that may damage the optic nerve. When the optic nerve is damaged from increased pressure, open-angle glaucoma—and vision loss—may result. That's why controlling pressure inside the eye is important.

Another risk factor for optic nerve damage relates to blood pressure. Thus, it is important to also make sure that your blood pressure is at a proper level for your body by working with your medical doctor.

Can I Develop Glaucoma If I Have Increased Eye Pressure?

Not necessarily. Not every person with increased eye pressure will develop glaucoma. Some people can tolerate higher levels of eye pressure better than others. Also, a certain level of eye pressure may be high for one person but normal for another.

Whether you develop glaucoma depends on the level of pressure your optic nerve can tolerate without being damaged. This level is different for each person. That's why a comprehensive dilated eye exam is very important. It can help your eye care professional determine what level of eye pressure is normal for you.

Can I Develop Glaucoma without an Increase in My Eye Pressure?

Yes. Glaucoma can develop without increased eye pressure. This form of glaucoma is called low-tension or normal-tension glaucoma. It is a type of open-angle glaucoma.

Who Is at Risk for Open-Angle Glaucoma?

Anyone can develop glaucoma. Some people, listed below, are at higher risk than others:

- African Americans over age 40
- Everyone over age 60, especially Mexican Americans
- People with a family history of glaucoma

A comprehensive dilated eye exam can reveal more risk factors, such as high eye pressure, thinness of the cornea, and abnormal optic nerve anatomy. In some people with certain combinations of these high-risk factors, medicines in the form of eyedrops reduce the risk of developing glaucoma by about half.

Glaucoma Symptoms

At first, open-angle glaucoma has no symptoms. It causes no pain. Vision stays normal. Glaucoma can develop in one or both eyes.

Without treatment, people with glaucoma will slowly lose their peripheral (side) vision. As glaucoma remains untreated, people may miss objects to the side and out of the corner of their eye. They seem to be looking through a tunnel. Over time, straight-ahead (central) vision may decrease until no vision remains.

How Is Glaucoma Detected?

Glaucoma is detected through a comprehensive dilated eye exam that includes the following:

- **Visual acuity test.** This eye chart test measures how well you see at various distances.

- **Visual field test.** This test measures your peripheral (side vision). It helps your eye care professional tell if you have lost peripheral vision, a sign of glaucoma.

- **Dilated eye exam.** In this exam, drops are placed in your eyes to widen, or dilate, the pupils. Your eye care professional uses a special magnifying lens to examine your retina and optic nerve for signs of damage and other eye problems. After the exam, your close-up vision may remain blurred for several hours.

- **Tonometry** is the measurement of pressure inside the eye by using an instrument called a tonometer. Numbing drops may be applied to your eye for this test. A tonometer measures pressure inside the eye to detect glaucoma.

- **Pachymetry** is the measurement of the thickness of your cornea. Your eye care professional applies a numbing drop to your eye and uses an ultrasonic wave instrument to measure the thickness of your cornea.

Can Glaucoma Be Cured?

No. There is no cure for glaucoma. Vision lost from the disease cannot be restored.

Glaucoma Treatments

Immediate treatment for early-stage, open-angle glaucoma can delay progression of the disease. That's why early diagnosis is very important.

Glaucoma treatments include medicines, laser trabeculoplasty, conventional surgery, or a combination of any of these. While these treatments may save remaining vision, they do not improve sight already lost from glaucoma.

Medicines. Medicines, in the form of eyedrops or pills, are the most common early treatment for glaucoma. Taken regularly, these eye drops lower eye pressure. Some medicines cause the eye to make less fluid. Others lower pressure by helping fluid drain from the eye.

Before you begin glaucoma treatment, tell your eye care professional about other medicines and supplements that you are taking. Sometimes the drops can interfere with the way other medicines work.

Glaucoma medicines need to be taken regularly as directed by your eye care professional. Most people have no problems. However, some medicines can cause headaches or other side effects. For example, drops may cause stinging, burning, and redness in the eyes.

Many medicines are available to treat glaucoma. If you have problems with one medicine, tell your eye care professional. Treatment with a different dose or a new medicine may be possible.

Because glaucoma often has no symptoms, people may be tempted to stop taking, or may forget to take, their medicine. You need to use the drops or pills as long as they help control your eye pressure. Regular use is very important.

Make sure your eye care professional shows you how to put the drops into your eye.

Laser trabeculoplasty. Laser trabeculoplasty helps fluid drain out of the eye. Your doctor may suggest this step at any time. In many cases, you will need to keep taking glaucoma medicines after this procedure.

Laser trabeculoplasty is performed in your doctor's office or eye clinic. Before the surgery, numbing drops are applied to your eye. As you sit facing the laser machine, your doctor holds a special lens to your eye. A high-intensity beam of light is aimed through the lens and reflected onto the meshwork inside your eye. You may see flashes of bright green or red light. The laser makes several evenly spaced burns that stretch the drainage holes in the meshwork. This allows the fluid to drain better.

Like any surgery, laser surgery can cause side effects, such as inflammation. Your doctor may give you some drops to take home for any soreness or inflammation inside the eye. You will need to make several follow-up visits to have your eye pressure and eye monitored.

If you have glaucoma in both eyes, usually only one eye will be treated at a time. Laser treatments for each eye will be scheduled several days to several weeks apart.

Studies show that laser surgery can be very good at reducing the pressure in some patients. However, its effects can wear off over time. Your doctor may suggest further treatment.

Conventional surgery. Conventional surgery makes a new opening for the fluid to leave the eye. Your doctor may suggest this treatment at any time. Conventional surgery often is done after medicines and laser surgery have failed to control pressure.

Conventional surgery, called trabeculectomy, is performed in an operating room. Before the surgery, you are given medicine to help you relax. Your doctor makes small injections around the eye to numb it. A small piece of tissue is removed to create a new channel for the fluid to drain from the eye. This fluid will drain between the eye tissue layers and create a blister-like "filtration bleb."

For several weeks after the surgery, you must put drops in the eye to fight infection and inflammation. These drops will be different from those you may have been using before surgery.

Conventional surgery is performed on one eye at a time. Usually the operations are four to six weeks apart.

Conventional surgery is about 60 to 80 percent effective at lowering eye pressure. If the new drainage opening narrows, a second operation may be needed. Conventional surgery works best if you have not had previous eye surgery, such as a cataract operation.

Sometimes after conventional surgery, your vision may not be as good as it was before conventional surgery. Conventional surgery can cause side effects, including cataract, problems with the cornea, inflammation, infection inside the eye, or low eye pressure problems. If you have any of these problems, tell your doctor so a treatment plan can be developed.

What Are Some Other Forms of Glaucoma and How Are They Treated?

Open-angle glaucoma is the most common form. Some people have other types of the disease.

In low-tension or normal-tension glaucoma, optic nerve damage and narrowed side vision occur in people with normal eye pressure. Lowering eye pressure at least 30 percent through medicines slows the disease in some people. Glaucoma may worsen in others despite low pressures.

A comprehensive medical history is important to identify other potential risk factors, such as low blood pressure, that contribute to low-tension glaucoma. If no risk factors are identified, the treatment options for low-tension glaucoma are the same as for open-angle glaucoma.

In angle-closure glaucoma, the fluid at the front of the eye cannot drain through the angle and leave the eye. The angle gets blocked by part of the iris. People with this type of glaucoma may have a sudden increase in eye pressure. Symptoms include severe pain and nausea, as well as redness of the eye and blurred vision. If you have these symptoms, you need to seek treatment immediately. This is a medical emergency. If your doctor is unavailable, go to the nearest hospital or clinic. Without treatment to restore the flow of fluid, the eye can become blind. Usually, prompt laser surgery and medicines can clear the blockage, lower eye pressure, and protect vision.

In congenital glaucoma, children are born with a defect in the angle of the eye that slows the normal drainage of fluid. These children usually have obvious symptoms, such as cloudy eyes, sensitivity to light, and excessive tearing. Conventional surgery typically is the suggested treatment, because medicines are not effective and can cause more serious side effects in infants and be difficult to administer. Surgery is safe and effective. If surgery is done promptly, these children usually have an excellent chance of having good vision.

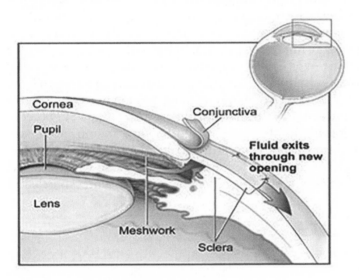

Figure 23.4. *Conventional Surgery for Eye*

Conventional surgery makes a new opening for the fluid to leave the eye.

Secondary glaucomas can develop as complications of other medical conditions. For example, a severe form of glaucoma is called neovascular glaucoma, and can be a result from poorly controlled diabetes or high blood pressure. Other types of glaucoma sometimes occur with cataract, certain eye tumors, or when the eye is inflamed or irritated by a condition called uveitis. Sometimes glaucoma develops after other eye surgeries or serious eye injuries. Steroid drugs used to treat eye inflammations and other diseases can trigger glaucoma in some people. There are two eye conditions known to cause secondary forms of glaucoma.

- **Pigmentary glaucoma** occurs when pigment from the iris sheds off and blocks the meshwork, slowing fluid drainage.

- **Pseudoexfoliation glaucoma** occurs when extra material is produced and shed off internal eye structures and blocks the meshwork, again slowing fluid drainage.

Depending on the cause of these secondary glaucomas, treatment includes medicines, laser surgery, or conventional or other glaucoma surgery.

What You Can Do

If you are being treated for glaucoma, be sure to take your glaucoma medicine every day. See your eye care professional regularly. You also can help protect the vision of family members and friends who may be at high risk for glaucoma—African Americans over age 40; everyone over age 60, especially Mexican Americans; and people with a family history of the disease. Encourage them to have a comprehensive dilated eye exam at least once every two years. Remember that lowering eye pressure in the early stages of glaucoma slows progression of the disease and helps save vision. Medicare covers an annual comprehensive dilated eye exam for some people at high risk for glaucoma. These people include those with diabetes, those with a family history of glaucoma, and African Americans age 50 and older.

Section 23.3

Macular Degeneration Surgery

This section includes text excerpted from "Age-Related Macular Degeneration: About AMD," NIHSeniorHealth, National Institute on Aging (NIA), December 2016.

About Age-Related Macular Degeneration (AMD)

Age-related macular degeneration (AMD) is a common eye condition and a leading cause of vision loss among people age 60 and older. It causes damage to the macula, a small spot near the center of the retina and the part of the eye needed for sharp, central vision, which lets us see objects that are straight ahead.

In some people, AMD advances so slowly that vision loss does not occur for a long time. In others, the disease progresses faster and may lead to a loss of vision in one or both eyes. As AMD progresses, a blurred area near the center of vision is a common symptom. Over time, the blurred area may grow larger or you may develop blank spots in your central vision. Objects also may not appear to be as bright as they used to be.

AMD by itself does not lead to complete blindness, with no ability to see. However, the loss of central vision in AMD can interfere with simple everyday activities, such as the ability to see faces, drive, read, write, or do close work, such as cooking or fixing things around the house.

Who Is at Risk?

Age is a major risk factor for AMD. The disease is most likely to occur after age 60, but it can occur earlier. Other risk factors for AMD include:

- **Smoking.** Research shows that smoking doubles the risk of AMD.

- **Race.** AMD is more common among Caucasians than among African-Americans or Hispanics/Latinos.

- **Family history and genetics.** People with a family history of AMD are at higher risk. At last count, researchers had identified nearly 20 genes that can affect the risk of developing AMD. Many more genetic risk factors are suspected.

Does Lifestyle Make a Difference?

Researchers have found links between AMD and some lifestyle choices, such as smoking. You might be able to reduce your risk of AMD or slow its progression by making these healthy choices.

- Eat a healthy diet high in green leafy vegetables and fish.

- Don't smoke.

- Maintain normal blood pressure and cholesterol levels.

- Watch your weight.

- Exercise.

Treatment of AMD

Early AMD

Currently, no treatment exists for early AMD, which in many people shows no symptoms or loss of vision. Your eye care professional may recommend that you get a comprehensive dilated eye exam at least once a year. The exam will help determine if your condition is advancing.

AMD occurs less often in people who exercise, avoid smoking, and eat nutritious foods including green leafy vegetables and fish. If you already have AMD, adopting some of these habits may help you keep your vision longer.

Intermediate and Late AMD

Researchers at the National Eye Institute (NEI) tested whether taking nutritional supplements could protect against AMD in the Age-Related Eye Disease Studies (AREDS and AREDS2). They found that daily intake of certain high-dose vitamins and minerals can slow progression of the disease in people who have intermediate AMD, and those who have late AMD in one eye.

Findings from the AREDS Trials

The first AREDS trial showed that a combination of vitamin C, vitamin E, beta-carotene, zinc, and copper can reduce the risk of late AMD by 25 percent. The AREDS2 trial tested whether this formulation could be improved by adding lutein, zeaxanthin or omega-3 fatty acids. Omega-3 fatty acids are nutrients enriched in fish oils. Lutein, zeaxanthin and beta-carotene all belong to the same family of vitamins, and are abundant in green leafy vegetables.

The AREDS2 trial found that adding lutein and zeaxanthin or omega-3 fatty acids to the original AREDS formulation (with beta-carotene) had no overall effect on the risk of late AMD. However, the trial also found that replacing beta-carotene with a 5-to-1 mixture of lutein and zeaxanthin may help further reduce the risk of late AMD. While beta-carotene has been linked to an increased risk of lung cancer in current and former smokers, lutein and zeaxanthin appear to be safe regardless of smoking status.

Here are the clinically effective doses tested in AREDS and AREDS2.

- 500 milligrams (mg) of vitamin C

- 400 international units of vitamin E

- 80 mg zinc as zinc oxide (25 mg in AREDS2)

- 2 mg copper as cupric oxide

- 15 mg beta-carotene, OR 10mg lutein and 2mg zeaxanthin

A number of companies offer nutritional supplements that were formulated based on these studies. The label may refer to "AREDS" or "AREDS2."

Taking AREDS Supplements

If you have intermediate or late AMD, you might benefit from taking such supplements. But first, be sure to review and compare the labels. Many of the supplements have different ingredients, or different doses, from those tested in the AREDS trials. Also, consult your doctor or eye care professional about which supplement, if any, is right for you. For example, if you smoke regularly, or used to, your doctor may recommend that you avoid supplements containing beta-carotene.

Even if you take a daily multivitamin, you should consider taking an AREDS supplement if you are at risk for late AMD. The formulations tested in the AREDS trials contain much higher doses of vitamins and minerals than what is found in multivitamins. Tell your doctor or eye care professional about any multivitamins you are taking when you are discussing possible AREDS formulations.

Genetic Makeup and AREDS Supplements

You may see claims that your specific genetic makeup (genotype) can influence how you will respond to AREDS supplements. Some studies have claimed that, depending on genotype, some patients will benefit from AREDS supplements and others could be harmed. These claims are based on a portion of data from the AREDS research. NEI investigators analyzed the complete AREDS data. Their findings to date indicate that AREDS supplements are beneficial for patients of all tested genotypes. Based on the overall data, the American Academy of Ophthalmology (AAO) does not support the use of genetic testing to guide treatment for AMD.

Not a Cure

Finally, remember that the AREDS formulation is not a cure. It does not help people with early AMD, and will not restore vision already lost from AMD. But it may delay the onset of late AMD. It also may help slow vision loss in people who already have late AMD.

Advanced Neovascular AMD

Neovascular AMD typically results in severe vision loss. However, eye care professionals can try different therapies to stop further vision loss. You should remember that the therapies described below are not a cure. The condition may progress even with treatment.

Injections. One option to slow the progression of neovascular AMD is to inject drugs into the eye. With neovascular AMD, abnormally high levels of vascular endothelial growth factor (VEGF) are secreted in your eyes. VEGF is a protein that promotes the growth of new abnormal blood vessels. Anti-VEGF injection therapy blocks this growth. If you get this treatment, you may need multiple monthly injections. Before each injection, your eye will be numbed and cleaned with antiseptics. To further reduce the risk of infection, you may be prescribed antibiotic drops. A few different anti-VEGF drugs are available. They vary in cost and in how often they need to be injected, so you may wish to discuss these issues with your eye care professional.

Photodynamic therapy. In this technique selected areas of the retina are treated with laser. First, a drug called verteporfin will be injected into a vein in your arm. The drug travels through the blood vessels in your body, and is absorbed by new, growing blood vessels. Your eye care professional then shines a laser beam into your eye to activate the drug in the new abnormal blood vessels, while sparing normal ones. Once activated, the drug closes off the new blood vessels, slows their growth, and slows the rate of vision loss. This procedure is less common than anti-VEGF injections, and is often used in combination with them for specific types of neovascular AMD.

Laser surgery. Eye care professionals treat certain cases of neovascular AMD with laser surgery, though this is less common than other treatments. It involves aiming an intense "hot" laser at the abnormal blood vessels in your eyes to destroy them. This laser is not the same one used in photodynamic therapy which may be referred to as a "cold" laser. This treatment is more likely to be used when blood vessel growth is limited to a compact area in your eye, away from the center of the macula that can be easily targeted with the laser. Even so, laser treatment also may destroy some surrounding healthy tissue. This often results in a small blind spot where the laser has scarred the retina. In some cases, vision immediately after the surgery may be worse than it was before. But the surgery may also help prevent more severe vision loss from occurring years later.

Section 23.4

Laser Eye Surgery (LASIK) for Refractive Disorders

This section includes text excerpted from "LASIK," U.S. Food and Drug Administration (FDA), September 6, 2016.

What Is LASIK?

The Eye and Vision Errors

The cornea is a part of the eye that helps focus light to create an image on the retina. It works in much the same way that the lens of a camera focuses light to create an image on film. The bending and focusing of light is also known as refraction. Usually the shape of the cornea and the eye are not perfect and the image on the retina is out-of-focus (blurred) or distorted. These imperfections in the focusing power of the eye are called refractive errors. There are three primary types of refractive errors: myopia, hyperopia and astigmatism. Persons with myopia, or nearsightedness, have more difficulty seeing distant objects as clearly as near objects. Persons with hyperopia, or farsightedness, have more difficulty seeing near objects as clearly as distant objects. Astigmatism is a distortion of the image on the retina caused by irregularities in the cornea or lens of the eye. Combinations of myopia and astigmatism or hyperopia and astigmatism are common. Glasses or contact lenses are designed to compensate for the eye's imperfections. Surgical procedures aimed at improving the focusing power of the eye are called refractive surgery. In LASIK surgery, precise and controlled removal of corneal tissue by a special laser reshapes the cornea changing its focusing power.

Other Types of Refractive Surgery

Radial Keratotomy (RK) and Photorefractive Keratectomy (PRK) are other refractive surgeries used to reshape the cornea. In RK, a very

231

sharp knife is used to cut slits in the cornea changing its shape. PRK was the first surgical procedure developed to reshape the cornea, by sculpting, using a laser. Later, LASIK was developed. The same type of laser is used for LASIK and PRK. Often the exact same laser is used for the two types of surgery. The major difference between the two surgeries is the way that the stroma, the middle layer of the cornea, is exposed before it is vaporized with the laser. In PRK, the top layer of the cornea, called the epithelium, is scraped away to expose the stromal layer underneath. In LASIK, a flap is cut in the stromal layer and the flap is folded back.

Another type of refractive surgery is thermokeratoplasty in which heat is used to reshape the cornea. The source of the heat can be a laser, but it is a different kind of laser than is used for LASIK and PRK. Other refractive devices include corneal ring segments that are inserted into the stroma and special contact lenses that temporarily reshape the cornea (orthokeratology).

Before, during, and after Surgery

Before Surgery

If you decide to go ahead with LASIK surgery, you will need an initial or baseline evaluation by your eye doctor to determine if you are a good candidate. This is what you need to know to prepare for the exam and what you should expect:

If you wear contact lenses, it is a good idea to stop wearing them before your baseline evaluation and switch to wearing your glasses full-time. Contact lenses change the shape of your cornea for up to several weeks after you have stopped using them depending on the type of contact lenses you wear. Not leaving your contact lenses out long enough for your cornea to assume its natural shape before surgery can have negative consequences. These consequences include inaccurate measurements and a poor surgical plan, resulting in poor vision after surgery. These measurements, which determine how much corneal tissue to remove, may need to be repeated at least a week after your initial evaluation and before surgery to make sure they have not changed, especially if you wear RGP or hard lenses. If you wear:

- soft contact lenses, you should stop wearing them for 2 weeks before your initial evaluation.

- toric soft lenses or rigid gas permeable (RGP) lenses, you should stop wearing them for at least 3 weeks before your initial evaluation.

- hard lenses, you should stop wearing them for at least 4 weeks before your initial evaluation.

You should tell your doctor:

- about your past and present medical and eye conditions
- about all the medications you are taking, including over-the-counter medications and any medications you may be allergic to

Your doctor should perform a thorough eye exam and discuss:

- whether you are a good candidate
- what the risks, benefits, and alternatives of the surgery are
- what you should expect before, during, and after surgery
- what your responsibilities will be before, during, and after surgery

You should have the opportunity to ask your doctor questions during this discussion. Give yourself plenty of time to think about the risk/benefit discussion, to review any informational literature provided by your doctor, and to have any additional questions answered by your doctor before deciding to go through with surgery and before signing the informed consent form.

You should not feel pressured by your doctor, family, friends, or anyone else to make a decision about having surgery. Carefully consider the pros and cons.

The day before surgery, you should stop using:

- creams
- lotions
- makeup
- perfumes

These products as well as debris along the eyelashes may increase the risk of infection during and after surgery. Your doctor may ask you to scrub your eyelashes for a period of time before surgery to get rid of residues and debris along the lashes.

Also before surgery, arrange for transportation to and from your surgery and your first follow-up visit. On the day of surgery, your doctor may give you some medicine to make you relax. Because this medicine impairs your ability to drive and because your vision may be blurry, even if you don't drive make sure someone can bring you home after surgery.

During Surgery

The surgery should take less than 30 minutes. You will lie on your back in a reclining chair in an exam room containing the laser system. The laser system includes a large machine with a microscope attached to it and a computer screen.

A numbing drop will be placed in your eye, the area around your eye will be cleaned, and an instrument called a lid speculum will be used to hold your eyelids open.

Your doctor may use a mechanical microkeratome (a blade device) to cut a flap in the cornea.

If a mechanical microkeratome is used, a ring will be placed on your eye and very high pressures will be applied to create suction to the cornea. Your vision will dim while the suction ring is on and you may feel the pressure and experience some discomfort during this part of the procedure. The microkeratome, a cutting instrument, is attached to the suction ring. Your doctor will use the blade of the microkeratome to cut a flap in your cornea. Microkeratome blades are meant to be used only once and then thrown out. The microkeratome and the suction ring are then removed.

Your doctor may use a laser keratome (a laser device), instead of a mechanical microkeratome, to cut a flap on the cornea.

If a laser keratome is used, the cornea is flattened with a clear plastic plate. Your vision will dim and you may feel the pressure and experience some discomfort during this part of the procedure. Laser energy is focused inside the cornea tissue, creating thousands of small bubbles of gas and water that expand and connect to separate the tissue underneath the cornea surface, creating a flap. The plate is then removed.

You will be able to see, but you will experience fluctuating degrees of blurred vision during the rest of the procedure. The doctor will then lift the flap and fold it back on its hinge, and dry the exposed tissue.

The laser will be positioned over your eye and you will be asked to stare at a light. This is not the laser used to remove tissue from the cornea. This light is to help you keep your eye fixed on one spot once the laser comes on. If you cannot stare at a fixed object for at least 60 seconds, you may not be a good candidate for this surgery.

When your eye is in the correct position, your doctor will start the laser. At this point in the surgery, you may become aware of new sounds and smells. The pulse of the laser makes a ticking sound. As the laser removes corneal tissue, some people have reported a smell similar to burning hair. A computer controls the amount of laser energy delivered to your eye. Before the start of surgery, your doctor will have programmed the computer to vaporize a particular amount of tissue based on the measurements taken at your initial evaluation. After the pulses of laser energy vaporize the corneal tissue, the flap is put back into position.

A shield should be placed over your eye at the end of the procedure as protection, since no stitches are used to hold the flap in place. It is important for you to wear this shield to prevent you from rubbing your eye and putting pressure on your eye while you sleep, and to protect your eye from accidentally being hit or poked until the flap has healed.

After Surgery

Immediately after the procedure, your eye may burn, itch, or feel like there is something in it. You may experience some discomfort, or in some cases, mild pain and your doctor may suggest you take a mild pain reliever. Both your eyes may tear or water. Your vision will probably be hazy or blurry. You will instinctively want to rub your eye, but don't! Rubbing your eye could dislodge the flap, requiring further treatment. In addition, you may experience sensitivity to light, glare, starbursts or halos around lights, or the whites of your eye may look red or bloodshot. These symptoms should improve considerably within the first few days after surgery. You should plan on taking a few days off from work until these symptoms subside. You should contact your doctor immediately and not wait for your scheduled visit, if you experience severe pain, or if your vision or other symptoms get worse instead of better.

You should see your doctor within the first 24 to 48 hours after surgery and at regular intervals after that for at least the first six months. At the first postoperative visit, your doctor will remove the eye shield, test your vision, and examine your eye. Your doctor may give you one or more types of eye drops to take at home to help prevent infection and/or inflammation. You may also be advised to use artificial tears to help lubricate the eye. Do not resume wearing a contact lens in the operated eye, even if your vision is blurry.

You should wait one to three days following surgery before beginning any non-contact sports, depending on the amount of activity required, how you feel, and your doctor's instructions.

To help prevent infection, you may need to wait for up to two weeks after surgery or until your doctor advises you otherwise before using lotions, creams, or makeup around the eye. Your doctor may advise you to continue scrubbing your eyelashes for a period of time after surgery. You should also avoid swimming and using hot tubs or whirlpools for 1–2months.

Strenuous contact sports such as boxing, football, karate, etc., should not be attempted for at least four weeks after surgery. It is important to protect your eyes from anything that might get in them and from being hit or bumped.

During the first few months after surgery, your vision may fluctuate.

- It may take up to three to six months for your vision to stabilize after surgery.

- Glare, haloes, difficulty driving at night, and other visual symptoms may also persist during this stabilization period. If further correction or enhancement is necessary, you should wait until your eye measurements are consistent for two consecutive visits at least 3 months apart before re-operation.

- It is important to realize that although distance vision may improve after re-operation, it is unlikely that other visual symptoms such as glare or halos will improve.

- It is also important to note that no laser company has presented enough evidence for the U.S. Food and Drug Administration (FDA) to make conclusions about the safety or effectiveness of enhancement surgery.

Contact your eye doctor immediately, if you develop any new, unusual or worsening symptoms at any point after surgery. Such symptoms could signal a problem that, if not treated early enough, may lead to a loss of vision.

Section 23.5

Phakic Intraocular Lens Implantation Surgery

This section includes text excerpted from
"Phakic Intraocular Lenses," U.S. Food and Drug
Administration (FDA), October 20, 2015.

What Are Phakic Lenses?

Phakic intraocular lenses, or phakic lenses, are lenses made of plastic or silicone that are implanted into the eye permanently to reduce a person's need for glasses or contact lenses. Phakic refers to the fact that the lens is implanted into the eye without removing the eye's natural lens. During phakic lens implantation surgery, a small incision is made in the front of the eye. The phakic lens is inserted through the incision and placed just in front of or just behind the iris.

Before Surgery

Initial Visit

Before deciding to have phakic intraocular lens implantation surgery, you will need an initial examination to make sure your eye is healthy and suitable for surgery. Your doctor will take a complete history about your medical and eye health and perform a thorough examination of both eyes, which will include measurements of your pupils, anterior chamber depth (the distance between your cornea and iris), and endothelial cell counts (the number of cells on the back of your cornea).

If you wear contact lenses, your doctor may ask you to stop wearing them before your initial examination (from the day of, to a few weeks before), so that your refraction (measure of how much your eye bends light) and central keratometry readings (measure of how much the cornea curves) are more accurate.

At this time, you should tell your doctor if you:

- take any medications, including over-the-counter medications, vitamins, and other supplements

237

- have any allergies
- have had any eye conditions
- have undergone any previous eye surgery
- have had any medical conditions

Deciding to Have Surgery

To help you decide whether phakic lenses are right for you, talk to your doctor about your expectations and whether there are elements of your medical history, eye history, or eye examination that might increase your risk or prevent you from having the outcome you expect. Before you sign an informed consent document (a form giving permission to your doctor to operate on your eye), you should discuss with your doctor:

- whether you are a good candidate,
- what are the risks, benefits, and alternatives of the surgery,
- what you should expect before, during, and after surgery, and
- what your responsibilities will be before, during, and after surgery.

You should have the opportunity to ask your doctor questions during this discussion. Ask your doctor for the Patient Labeling of the lens that he or she recommends for you. Give yourself plenty of time to think about the risk/benefit discussion, to review any informational literature provided by your doctor, and to have any additional questions answered by your doctor before deciding to go through with surgery and before signing the informed consent document. You should not feel pressured by anyone to make a decision about having surgery. Carefully consider the pros and cons.

Within Weeks of Surgery

About one to two weeks before surgery, your eye doctor may schedule you for a laser iridotomy to prepare your eye for implantation of the phakic lens. Before the procedure, your eye doctor may put drops in your eye to make the pupil small and to numb the eye. While you are seated, you doctor will rest a large lens on your eye. He or she will then make a small hole (or holes) in the extreme outer edge of the iris (the colored part of your eye) with a laser. This hole (holes) are to prevent fluid buildup and pressure in the back chamber of your eye after phakic lens implantation surgery. This procedure is usually performed in an office or clinic setting, not in an operating room, and usually only takes a few minutes.

After the iridotomy procedure, the doctor may have you wait around awhile before checking your eye pressure and letting you go home. The procedure should not prevent you from driving home, but you should check with your eye doctor when you schedule your appointment. You will be given a prescription for steroid drops to put in your eye at home for several days to reduce inflammation from the iridotomy procedure. It is important that you follow all instructions your doctor gives you after the iridotomy procedure.

Possible complications of laser iridotomy include:

- iritis (inflammation in the front part of the eye)

- increase in eye pressure (usually within 1 to 4 hours after the procedure)

- cataract (clouding of the natural lens) from the laser

- hyphema (bleeding into the anterior chamber of the eye, behind the cornea and in front of the iris, that can cause high pressure inside the eye)

- injury to the cornea from the laser that can result in clouding of the cornea

- incomplete opening of the hole all the way through the iris

- closure of the new opening

- rarely, retinal burns

Your doctor may ask you to stop wearing contact lenses before your surgery (anywhere from the day of the surgery to a few weeks before).

Before your surgery, your eye doctor may ask you to temporarily stop taking certain medications that increase the risk of bleeding during surgery. How long before surgery you may need to stop these medications depends upon which medications you are using and the conditions they are treating. You and your eye doctor may need to discuss stopping certain medications with the doctor who prescribed them, since you may need some of these medications to prevent life-threatening events. For example, you may need medications that stop blood clotting to keep from having a stroke.

Within Days of Surgery

Your doctor may give you prescriptions for antibiotic drops to prevent infection and/or anti-inflammatory drops to prevent inflammation to put in your eye for a few days before surgery. Arrange for transportation to and from surgery and to your follow-up doctor's appointment the day after surgery, since you will be unable to drive. Your doctor will let you know when it is safe for you to drive again. Your eye doctor will probably tell you not to eat or drink anything after midnight the night before your surgery.

During Surgery: The Day of Surgery

Just before surgery, drops will be put in your eye. You will have to lie down for the surgery and remain still. If you cannot lie down flat on your back, you may not be a good candidate for this surgery. Usually, patients are not put to sleep for this type of surgery, but you may be given a sedative or other medication to make you relax and an I.V. (intravenous) may be started. Your doctor may inject medication around the eye to numb the eye. The doctor also may give you an injection around the eye to also prevent you from being able to move your eye or see out of your eye. You will have to ask your doctor to find out exactly which of these types of anesthesia will be used in your case. Your eye and the surrounding area will be cleaned and an instrument called a lid speculum will be used to hold your eyelids open.

The doctor will make an incision in your cornea, sclera (the white part of your eye), or limbus (where the cornea meets the sclera). He or she will place a lubricant into your eye to help protect the back of the cornea (the endothelial cells) during the insertion of the phakic lens. The doctor will insert the phakic lens through the incision in the eye into the anterior chamber, behind the cornea and in front of the iris. Depending upon the type of phakic lens, the doctor will either attach the lens to the front of the iris in the anterior chamber of the eye or move it through the pupil into position behind the iris and in front of the lens in the posterior chamber of the eye. The doctor will remove the lubricant and may close the incision with tiny stitches, depending upon the type of incision. Your doctor will place some eye drops or ointment in your eye and cover your eye with a patch and/or a shield. The surgery will probably take around 30 minutes.

After the surgery is over, you may be brought to a recovery room for a couple of hours before you will be allowed to go home. You will be given prescriptions for antibiotic and anti-inflammatory drops to use at home as directed. You will be given an Implant Identification Card, which you should keep as a permanent record of the lens that was implanted in your eye. Make sure you show this card to anyone who takes care of your eyes in the future. You will be asked to go home and take it easy for the rest of the day.

After Surgery

Immediately after Surgery

After the surgical procedure, you may be sensitive to light and have a feeling that something is in your eye. You may experience minor discomfort after the procedure. Your doctor may prescribe pain medication to make you more comfortable during the first few days after the surgery. You should contact your eye doctor immediately if you have severe pain.

You should see your eye doctor the day after surgery. Your doctor will remove the patch and/or shield and will check your vision and the condition of your eye. Your doctor will instruct you on how to use the eye drops that you were prescribed for after the surgery. You will need to take these drops for up to a few weeks after surgery to decrease inflammation and help prevent infection. Your doctor may instruct you to continue wearing the shield all day and all night or just at night. You should wear the shield until your doctor tells you that you no longer have to do so. The shield is meant to prevent you from rubbing your eye or putting pressure on your eye while you sleep and to protect your eye from accidentally being hit or poked while it is healing.

As You Recover

Your vision will probably be somewhat hazy or blurry for the first several days after surgery. Your vision should start to improve after the first several days, but may continue to fluctuate for the next several weeks. It usually takes about 2 to 4 weeks for the vision to stabilize. Do NOT rub your eyes, especially for the first 3 to 5 days. You may also experience sensitivity to light, glare, starbursts or halos around lights, or the whites of your eye may look red or bloodshot. These symptoms should decrease as your eye recovers over the next several weeks.

You should contact your doctor immediately if you develop severe pain or if your vision or other symptoms get worse instead of better. Follow all postoperative instructions given to you by your surgeon and surgical center.

Remember to:

- Wash your hands before putting drops in your eye.

- Use the prescribed medications to help minimize the risk of infection and inflammation. Serious infection or inflammation can result in loss of vision.

- Try not to get water in your eyes until your doctor says it is okay to do so.

- Try not to bend from the waist to pick up objects on the floor, as this can cause undue pressure to your eyes. Do not lift any heavy objects.

- Do not engage in any strenuous activity until your doctor says it is okay to do so. It will take about 8 weeks for your eye to heal.

Long-Term Care

Your doctor will instruct you to return for additional follow-up visits to monitor your progress. Initially, these visits will be closer together (a few days to a few weeks apart) and then they will be spread out (several weeks to several months apart). It is important to go to all these appointments, even if you think you are doing well, so that the doctor can check for complications that you may not be aware of.

Because you will have a permanent implant in your eye with long-term risks, and especially since all these risks are not known at this time, you will need to be followed by an eye doctor on a regular basis for the rest of your life. Endothelial cell counts will have to be performed on a regular basis. You and/or your doctor should maintain records of these measurements, so as to be able to estimate the rate of cell loss. It is especially important for you to have your endothelial cells counted before you and your eye doctor consider any other intraocular procedures, such as cataract surgery, that will decrease the endothelial cell count even further.

Annual eye exams are usually recommended. However, if you have any problems with your vision or your eyes, such as flashing lights, floating spots, or blank spots in your vision (symptoms of a retinal detachment), you should see an eye doctor right away and inform him or her that you have a phakic lens implant. When participating in sports or other activities during which you might injure your eye, like home improvement work, always wear protective eyewear, such as safety goggles.

Chapter 24

Dental and Endodontic Surgery

Chapter Contents

Section 24.1

Oral Surgical Procedures

This section includes text excerpted from "Oral Surgical Procedures," Centers for Disease Control and Prevention (CDC), March 25, 2016.

What Are Oral Surgical Procedures?

Oral surgical procedures involve the incision, excision, or reflection of tissue that exposes the normally sterile areas of the oral cavity. Examples are biopsy, periodontal surgery, apical surgery, implant surgery, and surgical extractions of teeth (removal of erupted or nonerupted tooth requiring elevation of mucoperiosteal flap, removal of bone or section of tooth, and suturing if needed).

Recommended Infection Prevention Measures

Oral surgical procedures raise the risk of local or systemic infection because microorganisms from inside or outside the mouth can enter the vascular system and other normally sterile areas of the oral cavity (e.g., bone or subcutaneous tissue). These procedures require a higher level of infection prevention than routine procedures, including the following:

- Surgical hand antisepsis using an antimicrobial agent that is fast-acting, has a broad spectrum of activity, and has a persistent effect

- Use of sterile surgeon's gloves

- Use of sterile irrigating solutions and devices designed for delivering sterile irrigating fluids such as a sterile bulb syringe, sterile single-use disposable products, or sterilizable tubing

Sterile Gloves for Performing Surgical Procedures

Sterile gloves minimize transmission of microorganisms from the hands of surgical dental healthcare personnel (DHCP) to patients and prevent contamination of the hands of surgical DHCP with the patient's blood and body fluids. In addition, sterile surgeon's gloves are more rigorously regulated by the U.S. Food and Drug Administration (FDA) and therefore might provide an increased level of protection for the provider if exposure to blood is likely.

Sterile Water for Performing Surgery

Appropriate delivery devices (e.g., sterile bulb syringe or sterile, single-use disposable irrigating syringes) should be used to deliver sterile water. Alternatively, oral surgery and implant handpieces, as well as ultrasonic scalers, are available that bypass the dental unit to deliver sterile water or other solutions by using sterile single-use disposable or sterilizable tubing.

Section 24.2

Periodontal (Gum) Disease

This section includes text excerpted from "Periodontal (Gum) Disease: Causes, Symptoms, and Treatments," National Institute of Dental and Craniofacial Research (NIDCR), September 2013. Reviewed June 2017.

If you have been told you have periodontal (gum) disease, you're not alone. Many adults in the United States have some form of the disease. Periodontal diseases range from simple gum inflammation to serious disease that results in major damage to the soft tissue and bone that support the teeth. In the worst cases, teeth are lost.

Whether your gum disease is stopped, slowed, or gets worse depends a great deal on how well you care for your teeth and gums every day, from this point forward.

Causes of Gum Disease

Our mouths are full of bacteria. These bacteria, along with mucus and other particles, constantly form a sticky, colorless "plaque" on teeth. Brushing and flossing help get rid of plaque. Plaque that is not removed can harden and form "tartar" that brushing doesn't clean. Only a professional cleaning by a dentist or dental hygienist can remove tartar.

Gingivitis

The longer plaque and tartar are on teeth, the more harmful they become. The bacteria cause inflammation of the gums that is called "gingivitis." In gingivitis, the gums become red, swollen and can bleed easily. Gingivitis is a mild form of gum disease that can usually be reversed with daily brushing and flossing, and regular cleaning by a dentist or dental hygienist. This form of gum disease does not include any loss of bone and tissue that hold teeth in place.

Periodontitis

When gingivitis is not treated, it can advance to "periodontitis" (which means "inflammation around the tooth"). In periodontitis, gums pull away from the teeth and form spaces (called "pockets") that become infected. The body's immune system fights the bacteria as the plaque spreads and grows below the gum line. Bacterial toxins and the body's natural response to infection start to break down the bone and connective tissue that hold teeth in place. If not treated, the bones, gums, and tissue that support the teeth are destroyed. The teeth may eventually become loose and have to be removed.

Risk Factors of Gum Disease

The risk factors for gum disease includes:

- Smoking
- Hormonal changes in girls/women
- Diabetes
- Other illnesses and their treatments
- Medications
- Genetic susceptibility

Symptoms of Gum Disease

Symptoms of gum disease include:

- Bad breath that won't go away

- Red or swollen gums

- Tender or bleeding gums

- Painful chewing

- Loose teeth

- Sensitive teeth

- Receding gums or longer appearing teeth

Any of these symptoms may be a sign of a serious problem, which should be checked by a dentist. At your dental visit the dentist or hygienist should:

- Ask about your medical history to identify underlying conditions or risk factors (such as smoking) that may contribute to gum disease.

- Examine your gums and note any signs of inflammation.

- Use a tiny ruler called a "probe" to check for and measure any pockets. In a healthy mouth, the depth of these pockets is usually between 1 and 3 millimeters. This test for pocket depth is usually painless.

Treatment for Gum Disease

The main goal of treatment is to control the infection. The number and types of treatment will vary, depending on the extent of the gum disease. Any type of treatment requires that the patient keep up good daily care at home. The doctor may also suggest changing certain behaviors, such as quitting smoking, as a way to improve treatment outcome.

Deep Cleaning (Scaling and Root Planing)

The dentist, periodontist, or dental hygienist removes the plaque through a deep-cleaning method called scaling and root planing. Scaling means scraping off the tartar from above and below the gum line. Root planing gets rid of rough spots on the tooth root where the germs gather, and helps remove bacteria that contribute to the disease. In some cases a laser may be used to remove plaque and tartar. This procedure can result in less bleeding, swelling, and discomfort compared to traditional deep cleaning methods.

247

Medications

Medications may be used with treatment that includes scaling and root planning, but they cannot always take the place of surgery. Depending on how far the disease has progressed, the dentist or periodontist may still suggest surgical treatment. Long-term studies are needed to find out if using medications reduces the need for surgery and whether they are effective over a long period of time.

Surgical Treatments

Flap surgery. Surgery might be necessary if inflammation and deep pockets remain following treatment with deep cleaning and medications. A dentist or periodontist may perform flap surgery to remove tartar deposits in deep pockets or to reduce the periodontal pocket and make it easier for the patient, dentist, and hygienist to keep the area clean. This common surgery involves lifting back the gums and removing the tartar. The gums are then sutured back in place so that the tissue fits snugly around the tooth again. After surgery the gums will heal and fit more tightly around the tooth. This sometimes results in the teeth appearing longer.

Bone and tissue grafts. In addition to flap surgery, your periodontist or dentist may suggest procedures to help regenerate any bone or gum tissue lost to periodontitis. Bone grafting, in which natural or synthetic bone is placed in the area of bone loss, can help promote bone growth. A technique that can be used with bone grafting is called guided tissue regeneration. In this procedure, a small piece of mesh-like material is inserted between the bone and gum tissue. This keeps the gum tissue from growing into the area where the bone should be, allowing the bone and connective tissue to regrow. Growth factors—proteins that can help your body naturally regrow bone—may also be used. In cases where gum tissue has been lost, your dentist or periodontist may suggest a soft tissue graft, in which synthetic material or tissue taken from another area of your mouth is used to cover exposed tooth roots.

Since each case is different, it is not possible to predict with certainty which grafts will be successful over the long-term. Treatment results depend on many things, including how far the disease has progressed, how well the patient keeps up with oral care at home, and certain risk factors, such as smoking, which may lower the chances of success. Ask your periodontist what the level of success might be in your particular case.

Gum Disease Cause Health Problems beyond the Mouth

In some studies, researchers have observed that people with gum disease (when compared to people without gum disease) were more likely to develop heart disease or have difficulty controlling blood sugar. Other studies showed that women with gum disease were more likely than those with healthy gums to deliver preterm, low birth weight babies. But so far, it has not been determined whether gum disease is the cause of these conditions.

There may be other reasons people with gum disease sometimes develop additional health problems. For example, something else may be causing both the gum disease and the other condition, or it could be a coincidence that gum disease and other health problems are present together. More research is needed to clarify whether gum disease actually causes health problems beyond the mouth, and whether treating gum disease can keep other health conditions from developing. In the meantime, it's a fact that controlling gum disease can save your teeth—a very good reason to take care of your teeth and gums.

Section 24.3

Endodontic Conditions and Treatment

"Endodontic Conditions and Treatment,"
© 2017 Omnigraphics. June 2017.

Endodontics

Endodontics is a dental specialty that studies and treats the pulp of teeth. The word endodontic is derived from the Greek words endo, which means "inside," and odont, which translates as "tooth." To understand endodontic treatment, it helps know a bit about dental anatomy. The tooth is covered by a hard layer of enamel. Another hard layer, called dentin, lies under the enamel and covers soft tissue known as the pulp, a collection of blood vessels, nerves, and connective tissue that is responsible for nourishing the tooth. The pulp is located in the center of the tooth and extends from under the crown down to the tissue under the root. Pulp is especially important during tooth growth and development, but once the tooth is fully grown, it can survive without the pulp because the surrounding tissues are able to provide nourishment.

Almost all teeth can be treated endodontically. However, in some cases treatment may not be possible. For example, this might be the case if the chambers that contain the root (called root canals) are not accessible, if the tooth is badly fractured, or if there is inadequate bone support. Endodontics has advanced so much that teeth that would have been considered lost a few years ago, can be saved today.

Root Canal Treatment

The most common type of endodontic procedure is a root canal treatment, often called simply a root canal. It is a routine procedure that relieves pain, saves millions of teeth every year, and can help improve appearance.

This procedure becomes necessary when a tooth's pulp becomes inflamed or infected. The infection may arise as a result conditions such as tooth decay, repeated dental work, or a crack in the tooth. If left untreated, the infection may lead to an abscess, a more serious infection that can be life-threatening.

In root canal treatment, the pulp is fully removed from the tooth. The pulp chamber is cleaned and shaped, and the empty space is filled and sealed with an inert material. In subsequent visits, the dentist generally fixes a crown on the tooth or performs some other type of restorative work to return the tooth to its full function and appearance.

Symptoms Indicating That Root Canal May Be Necessary

Signs that root canal treatment may be needed include tooth pain, sensitivity to heat and cold, and tenderness to touch and chewing. You should also look for tooth discoloration and tenderness of lymph nodes, gum tissue, and bone. But sometimes infection requiring a root canal can be present with virtually no symptoms at all.

Root Canal Procedure

Root canal treatment generally consists of the following steps:

- The endodontist examines the tooth and X-rays it. A local anesthetic is then administered, and a sheet known as a dental dam may be placed in the mouth to isolate the tooth and keep it free of saliva.

- The endodontist drills through the crown of the tooth and uses various tools to remove the pulp.

- The space is then shaped and cleaned before it is filled with a biocompatible material, such as a rubber-like substance called gutta-percha. It is placed with adhesive cement, completely sealing the chamber. The tooth is then covered with a temporary filling, which remains in place until the next office visit.

- In the next step, the dentist or endodontist will prepare the tooth for a crown or will perform other restorative work to provide normal tooth function.

- If the tooth is incapable of holding the restoration on its own, the endodontist will fix a post inside the tooth, which will serve as an anchor.

Root Canal Treatment and Pain

Modern anesthetics and techniques are generally able to ensure that little pain is felt during a root canal procedure. But after a root canal, the tooth and surrounding area may be sensitive. This can be treated by prescription medication or by over-the-counter pain relievers. However, if pain persists for more than a few days after the treatment, consult your endodontist immediately.

Cost of Root Canal Treatment

As with any medical treatment, the cost of a root canal can depend on the complexity of the procedure. For example, molars tend to be more difficult to treat than other teeth and thus might cost more. But most dental insurance policies cover endodontic procedures, and in any case, endodontic treatment and tooth restoration is likely to be less expensive than tooth extraction, because the latter involves the additional cost of fixing an implant or bridge at the site of the extraction to restore chewing function and prevent teeth from shifting.

After Root Canal Treatment

To avoid fracture or other damage, you must not bite or chew on food with the tooth that has undergone endodontic treatment until the restoration work has been done. After the procedure is complete, it is important to practice good, basic dental hygiene, like brushing, flossing, dental checkups, and cleaning.

The restored tooth should last for a long time. But in some cases, the treated tooth might not heal and could become infected again in the future. In some cases, new trauma, decay, or a crack may result in an infection in the treated tooth. Or the endodontist may discover that complicating factors caused the tooth to be treated improperly to begin with. In such cases, a second endodontic procedure may be able to save the tooth.

Endodontic Surgery

In cases where root canal treatment will not suffice, an endodontist may recommend surgery, which can often save a tooth by providing better access for treatment. Surgery can also help the endodontist make a diagnosis that might otherwise not be possible, since some conditions do not show up in diagnostics, such as X-rays. And in some cases, a tiny fracture or canal may remain undetected in nonsurgical treatment. With surgery, the endodontist will be able to make a more thorough inspection of the area and provide the required treatment.

In addition, it can become difficult to reach the end of the root with instruments in a root canal procedure if there is calcification in the canal. With endodontic surgery, a dentist will be able to reach the end of the root to clean and seal it properly. Or, after a root canal, the tooth might not heal fully and become infected. This could occur quite some time after successful treatment. Endodontic surgery is often required to save the tooth in such cases.

Finally, endodontic surgery is often performed to treat damage to the root surface or the surrounding bone when no other type of treatment would be effective.

Apicoectomy

An apicoectomy, also called a root-end resection or root-end filling, is the most common type of oral surgery. It generally involves the following steps:

- The gum tissue around the tooth is opened and the underlying bone is exposed.

- Any inflamed or infected tissue is then removed, along with the end of the root.

- The end of the root canal is often sealed with a filling, and the gum tissue is sutured.

- The gum tissue generally heals in a few weeks, while it may take a few months for the bone to heal fully.

Other Types of Endodontic Surgery

Other endodontic surgical procedures include dividing a tooth in half, repairing injured roots, and removing the root. Another type of endodontic surgery, intentional replantation, involves extracting the tooth, then replacing it in the socket after an endodontic procedure has been completed.

Endodontic Surgery and Pain

Endodontic surgeries are usually done under local anesthesia and are generally not painful during the procedure. However, pain is typically felt during healing process. The endodontist will likely prescribe medication to alleviate the pain. You will also be given postoperative instructions to follow. Talk to your endodontist if you have any queries after surgery or if the pain does not respond to medication.

After Endodontic Surgery

In many cases, patients are able to drive themselves home after endodontic surgery. But if your surgeon suggests otherwise, be sure that you make suitable arrangements for transportation.

Most patients find that they are able return to work the next day, however recovery time and postoperative effects vary from individual to individual. The endodontist will discuss recovery time with you during your consultation.

Although successful healing and full recovery are typical, there are, of course, no guarantees with any type of medical or dental treatment, including surgery. A particular procedure is recommended by an endodontist because he or she believes it offers the best possible treatment option for saving your natural tooth. An endodontist will discuss the chances of success so that you are able to make an informed decision.

Cost of Endodontic Surgery

As with root canal treatment, the cost of endodontic surgery varies with the complexity of the procedure and a number of other factors.

Some insurance plans cover certain types of treatment, while others do not. Talk to your employer or insurance company to learn if your particular surgery is covered under your plan.

Endodontic Retreatment

A tooth that has undergone endodontic treatment can last a lifetime with proper care. But when a treated tooth does not heal properly, becomes infected, and causes pain, a second procedure may be needed to save the tooth. If you experience pain or discomfort in a tooth that was previously treated, talk to your endodontist about retreatment.

Retreatment Procedure

The endodontist will first discuss the procedure with you. If retreatment is required, the endodontist will generally follow these steps:

- Reopen the tooth to get access to the filling in the root canals by disassembling the crown, post, and filling material.

- Once the filling has been removed, the endodontist examines the canals with magnification and illumination to assess their condition.

- The canals are then cleaned and sealed with a temporary filling. If the canals are very narrow or blocked, the endodontist may suggest endodontic surgery.

- Once the retreatment is complete, you will need to make additional visits for restoration procedures in order to regain full tooth function and appearance.

Need for Endodontic Retreatment

The best possible option always is to save your natural teeth. So even if initial treatment fails, retreatment may be able to allow teeth to function properly for many years. Technological improvements are always being made in endodontics, and it is possible that retreatment may be able to employ tools and techniques that didn't even exist just a few years ago.

If nonsurgical retreatment will be ineffective, then surgical retreatment may be necessary. This will entail a process similar to that of an initial endodontic surgery, including incision, assessment, cleaning, and stitches. Your endodontist will discuss the options and necessary treatment with you.

Cost of Endodontic Retreatment

Understandably, the cost of retreatment depends on the complexity of the condition. The endodontist will need to remove the filling, assess the previous work and the underlying structures, and then redo the procedure, or use an entirely different procedure. Therefore, retreatment will likely cost more than the initial procedure, especially if surgical retreatment is necessary.

Dental insurance may cover the expenses for all or part of retreatment, but some plans cover just the initial endodontic procedure. Your employer or insurance company can help clarify this.

Alternatives to Endodontic Treatment

Tooth extraction is generally the only alternative to endodontic treatment. Once a tooth has been extracted, it must be replaced with a bridge, implant, or a partially removable denture to restore chewing function and to prevent adjacent teeth from shifting. Since extraction involves additional procedures to maintain tooth function, endodontic treatment is usually the best option, from a cost perspective, as well as for utility and appearance. Although, artificial teeth can be very effective, nothing is better than having natural teeth, and an endodontic procedure can help you retain those teeth for a long time.

References

1. "Endodontic Surgery Explained," American Association of Endodontists, n.d.

2. "Root Canals Explained," American Association of Endodontists, n.d.

3. "Endodontic Retreatment Explained," American Association of Endodontists, n.d.

4. "An Overview of Root Canals," WebMD, June 10, 2016.

5. Horne, Steven B., DDS. "Root Canal," MedicineNet, n.d.

6. "Oral Surgery," WebMD, July 28, 2016.

Chapter 25

Breast Surgeries

Chapter Contents

Section 25.1

Surgery Choices for Women with Ductal Carcinoma in Situ (DCIS) or Breast Cancer

This section includes text excerpted from "Surgery Choices for Women with DCIS or Breast Cancer," National Cancer Institute (NCI), January 19, 2015.

Are You Facing a Decision about Surgery for Ductal Carcinoma in Situ (DCIS) or Breast Cancer?

Do you have ductal carcinoma in situ (DCIS) or breast cancer that can be removed with surgery? If so, you may be able to choose which type of breast surgery to have. Often, your choice is between breast-sparing surgery (surgery that takes out the cancer and leaves most of the breast) and a mastectomy (surgery that removes the whole breast).

Once you are diagnosed, treatment will usually not begin right away. There should be enough time for you to meet with breast cancer surgeons, learn the facts about your surgery choices, and think about what is important to you. Learning all you can will help you make a choice you can feel good about.

Talk with Your Doctor

Talk with a breast cancer surgeon about your choices. Find out:

- what happens during surgery
- the types of problems that sometimes occur
- any treatment you might need after surgery

Be sure to ask a lot of questions and learn as much as you can. You may also wish to talk with family members, friends, or others who have had surgery.

Get a Second Opinion

After talking with a surgeon, think about getting a second opinion. A second opinion means getting the advice of another surgeon. This surgeon might tell you about other treatment options. Or, he or she may agree with the advice you got from the first doctor.

Some people worry about hurting their surgeon's feelings if they get a second opinion. But, it is very common and good surgeons don't mind. Also, some insurance companies require it. It is better to get a second opinion than worry that you made the wrong choice.

If you think you might have a mastectomy, this is also a good time to learn about breast reconstruction. Think about meeting with a reconstructive plastic surgeon to learn about this surgery and if it seems like a good option for you.

Check with Your Insurance Company

Each insurance plan is different. Knowing how much your plan will pay for each type of surgery, including reconstruction, special bras, prostheses, and other needed treatments can help you decide which surgery is best for you.

Learn about the Types of Surgery

Most women with DCIS or breast cancer that can be treated with surgery have three surgery choices.

Breast-Sparing Surgery, Followed by Radiation Therapy

Breast-sparing surgery means the surgeon removes only the DCIS or cancer and some normal tissue around it. If you have cancer, the surgeon will also remove one or more lymph nodes from under your arm. Breast-sparing surgery usually keeps your breast looking much like it did before surgery. Other words for breast-sparing surgery include:

- Lumpectomy

- Partial mastectomy

- Breast-conserving surgery

- Segmental mastectomy

After breast-sparing surgery, most women also receive radiation therapy. The main goal of this treatment is to keep cancer from coming back in the same breast. Some women will also need chemotherapy, hormone therapy, and/or targeted therapy.

Mastectomy

In a mastectomy, the surgeon removes the whole breast that contains the DCIS or cancer. There are two main types of mastectomy. They are:

- **Total (simple) mastectomy.** The surgeon removes your whole breast. Sometimes, the surgeon also takes out one or more of the lymph nodes under your arm.

- **Modified radical mastectomy.** The surgeon removes your whole breast, many of the lymph nodes under your arm, and the lining over your chest muscles.

Some women will also need radiation therapy, chemotherapy, hormone therapy, and/or targeted therapy. If you have a mastectomy, you may choose to wear a prosthesis (breast-like form) in your bra or have breast reconstruction surgery.

Mastectomy with Breast Reconstruction Surgery

You can have breast reconstruction at the same time as the mastectomy, or anytime after. This type of surgery is done by a plastic surgeon with experience in reconstruction surgery. The surgeon uses an implant or tissue from another part of your body to create a breast-like shape that replaces the breast that was removed. The surgeon may also make the form of a nipple and add a tattoo that looks like the areola (the dark area around your nipple).

There are two main types of breast reconstruction surgery:

1. **Breast Implant**. Breast reconstruction with an implant is often done in steps. The first step is called tissue expansion. This is when the plastic surgeon places a balloon expander under the chest muscle. Over many weeks, saline (salt water) will be added to the expander to stretch the chest muscle and the skin on top of it. This process makes a pocket for the implant.

   Once the pocket is the correct size, the surgeon will remove the expander and place an implant (filled with saline or silicone gel) into the pocket. This creates a new breast-like shape. Although this shape looks like a breast, you will not have the same feeling in it because nerves were cut during your mastectomy.

   Breast implants do not last a lifetime. If you choose to have an implant, chances are you will need more surgery later on to remove or replace it. Implants can cause problems such as breast hardness, pain, and infection. The implant may also break, move, or shift. These problems can happen soon after surgery or years later.

2. **Tissue Flap**. In tissue flap surgery, a reconstructive plastic surgeon builds a new breast-like shape from muscle, fat, and skin taken from other parts of your body (usually your belly, back, or buttock). This new breast-like shape should last the rest of your life. Women who are very thin or obese, smoke, or have serious health problems often cannot have tissue flap surgery.

Healing after tissue flap surgery often takes longer than healing after breast implant surgery. You may have other problems, as well. For example, if you have a muscle removed, you might lose strength in the area from which it was taken. Or, you may get an infection or have trouble healing. Tissue flap surgery is best done by a reconstructive plastic surgeon who has special training in this type of surgery and has done it many times before.

Compare the Types of Surgery

The charts in this section can help you compare the different surgeries with each other. See how the surgeries are alike and how they are different.

Before Surgery

Table 25.1. Determining the Right Surgery Choice

Breast-Sparing Surgery	Most women with DCIS or breast cancer can choose to have breast-sparing surgery, usually followed by radiation therapy.
Mastectomy	Most women with DCIS or breast cancer can choose to have a mastectomy. A mastectomy may be a better choice for you if: • You have small breasts and a large area of DCIS or cancer. • You have DCIS or cancer in more than one part of your breast. • The DCIS or cancer is under the nipple. • You are not able to receive radiation therapy.

Table 25.1. Continued

Mastectomy with Reconstruction	If you have a mastectomy, you might also want breast reconstruction surgery. You can choose to have reconstruction surgery at the same time as your mastectomy or wait and have it later.

Recovering from Surgery

Will I Have Pain?

Most people have some pain after surgery.

Talk with your doctor or nurse before surgery about ways to control pain after surgery. Also, tell them if your pain control is not working.

Table 25.2. Time Required for Returning to Normal Activities

Breast-Sparing Surgery	Most women are ready to return to most of their usual activities within 5 to 10 days.
Mastectomy	It may take 3 to 4 weeks to feel mostly normal after a mastectomy.
Mastectomy with Reconstruction	Your recovery will depend on the type of reconstruction you have. It can take 6 to 8 weeks or longer to fully recover from breast reconstruction.

Table 25.3. Other Problems

Breast-Sparing Surgery	You may feel very tired and have skin changes from radiation therapy.
Mastectomy	You may feel out of balance if you had large breasts and do not have reconstruction surgery. This may also lead to neck and shoulder pain.
Mastectomy with Reconstruction	You may not like how your breast-like shape looks. If you have an implant: • Your breast may harden and can become painful • You will likely need more surgery if your implant breaks or leaks If you have flap surgery, you may lose strength in the part of your body where a muscle was removed.

What Other Types of Treatment Might I Need?

If you chose to have breast sparing surgery, you will usually need radiation therapy. Radiation treatments are usually given 5 days a week for 5 to 8 weeks.

If you have a mastectomy, you may still need radiation therapy. No matter which surgery you choose, you might need:

- Chemotherapy

- Hormone therapy

- Targeted therapy

Life after Surgery

Table 25.4. Breast Shape Post Surgery

Breast-Sparing Surgery	Your breast should look a lot like it did before surgery. But if your tumor is large, your breast may look different or smaller after breast-sparing surgery. You will have a small scar where the surgeon cut to remove the DCIS or cancer. The length of the scar will depend on how large an incision the surgeon needed to make.
Mastectomy	Your breast and nipple will be removed. You will have a flat chest on the side of your body where the breast was removed. You will have a scar over the place where your breast was removed. The length of the scar will depend on the size of your breast. If you have smaller breasts, your scar is likely to be smaller than if you have larger breasts.
Mastectomy with Reconstruction	You will have a breast-like shape, but your breast will not look or feel like it did before surgery. And, it will not look or feel like your other breast. You will have scars where the surgeon stitched skin together to make the new breast-like shape. If you have tissue flap reconstruction, you will have scars around the new breast, as well as the area where the surgeon removed the muscle, fat, and skin to make the new breast-like shape.

To get a better idea of what to expect, ask your surgeon if you can see before and after pictures of other women who have had different types of surgery.

Remember, even though surgery leaves scars where the surgeon cut the skin and stitched it back together, they tend to fade over time.

Table 25.5. Feelings Post Surgery

Breast-Sparing Surgery	Yes. You should still have feeling in your breast, nipple, and areola (the dark area around your nipple).
Mastectomy	Maybe. After surgery, the skin around where the surgeon cut and maybe the area under your arm will be numb (have no feeling). This numb feeling may improve over 1 to 2 years, but it will never feel like it once did. Also, the skin where your breast was may feel tight.
Mastectomy with Reconstruction	No. The area around your breast will not have feeling.

Table 25.6. Further Surgery Requirements

Breast-Sparing Surgery	If the surgeon does not remove all the DCIS or cancer the first time, you may need more surgery.
Mastectomy	If you have problems after your mastectomy, you may need more surgery.
Mastectomy with Reconstruction	You will need more than one surgery to build a new breast-like shape. The number of surgeries you need will depend on the type of reconstruction you have and if you choose to have a nipple or areola added. Some women may also decide to have surgery on the opposite breast to help it match the new breast-like shape better. If you have an implant, you are likely to need surgery many years later to remove or replace it.

With all three surgeries, you may need more surgery to remove lymph nodes from under your arm. Having your lymph nodes removed can cause lymphedema.

Will the Type of Surgery I Have Affect How Long I Live?

No. Research has shown that women who have breast-sparing surgery live as long as women who have a mastectomy. This does not change if you also have reconstruction.

Table 25.7. Chances of Recurrence

Breast-Sparing Surgery	There is a chance that your cancer will come back in the same breast. But if it does, it is not likely to affect how long you live. About 10 percent of women (1 out of every 10) who have breast-sparing surgery along with radiation therapy get cancer in the same breast within 12 years. If this happens, you can be effectively treated with a mastectomy.
Mastectomy	There is a smaller chance that your cancer will return in the same area than if you have breast-sparing surgery. About 5 percent of women (1 out of every 20) who have a mastectomy will get cancer on the same side of their chest within 12 years.
Mastectomy with Reconstruction	Your chances are the same as mastectomy, since breast reconstruction surgery does not affect the chances of the cancer returning.

Think about What Is Important to You

After you have talked with a breast cancer surgeon and learned the facts, you may also want to talk with your spouse or partner, family, friends, or other women who have had breast cancer surgery.

Then, think about what is important to you. Thinking about these questions and talking them over with others might help.

About surgery choices:

- If I have breast-sparing surgery, am I willing and able to have radiation therapy 5 days a week for 5 to 8 weeks?

- If I have a mastectomy, do I also want breast reconstruction surgery?

- If I have breast reconstruction surgery, do I want it at the same time as my mastectomy?

- What treatment does my insurance cover? What do I have to pay for?

Life after surgery:

- How important is it to me how my breast looks after cancer surgery?

- How important is it to me how my breast feels after cancer surgery?

- If I have a mastectomy and do not have reconstruction, will my insurance cover my prostheses and special bras?

- Where can I find breast prostheses and special bras?

Learning more:

- Do I want a second opinion?

- Is there someone else I should talk with about my surgery choices?

- What else do I want to learn or do before I make my choice about breast cancer surgery?

Section 25.2

Breast Biopsy

This section includes text excerpted from "Having a Breast Biopsy: A Review of the Research for Women and Their Families," Agency for Healthcare Research and Quality (AHRQ), U.S. Department of Health and Human Services (HHS), May 26, 2016.

What Is a Breast Biopsy?

A biopsy is the only test that can tell for sure if a shadow or lump is breast cancer. During a breast biopsy, the doctor removes a small amount of tissue from the breast.

There are two main kinds of breast biopsy: core-needle biopsy and open surgical biopsy. The kind of breast biopsy a doctor recommends may depend on what the shadow or lump looks like on the mammogram. It may also depend on the size of the shadow or lump and where it is located in the breast. After the biopsy, a doctor will look at the tissue under a microscope. This doctor, called a pathologist, looks for changes in the tissue. The doctor's report will tell if there is cancer or not. It takes about a week to get the report.

Kinds of Breast Biopsies

Core-Needle Biopsy

Your doctor will probably suggest a core-needle biopsy. It is done using local anesthesia, which means that the breast will be numbed.

The doctor puts a hollow needle into the breast and takes out a small amount of tissue. The doctor may place a tiny marker inside the breast to mark the spot where the biopsy was done.

There are several ways to do core-needle biopsies. Some of these use different types of imaging equipment.

- **Ultrasound-guided core-needle biopsy** uses ultrasound to guide the needle to the lump. Ultrasound uses sound waves to create a picture of the inside of the breast. It is like the ultrasound used to look at the baby in the womb while a woman is pregnant. You will lie on your back or side for this procedure. The doctor will hold the ultrasound device against your breast to guide the needle.

- **Stereotactic-guided core-needle biopsy** uses X-ray equipment and a computer to guide the needle. Usually for this kind of biopsy, you lie on your stomach on a special table. The table will have an opening for your breast. Your breast may be squeezed and flattened as it is for a mammogram.

- **Magnetic resonance imaging (MRI)-guided core-needle biopsy** is similar to stereotactic-guided core-needle biopsy, but MRI equipment is used to guide the needle.

- **Freehand core-needle biopsy** does not use ultrasound, X-ray, or MRI equipment. It is used less often and only for lumps that can be felt through the skin.

Open Surgical Biopsy

An open surgical biopsy is usually done only if you have a high risk of cancer or if the lump is in an area of the breast that cannot be reached with a core-needle biopsy. It is done using general anesthesia. You will be given medicine to make you sleepy through an IV needle placed in a vein in your arm.

The surgeon makes a 1-inch to 2-inch cut in the breast and removes part or all of the lump. Some of the tissue around the lump also may be taken out. If the lump can be seen on a mammogram or an ultrasound but cannot be felt, a radiologist (a doctor who specializes in medical imaging) usually inserts a thin wire to mark the spot for the surgeon before the biopsy.

Biopsy Results

After the biopsy, the pathologist who looked at the tissue will send a report to your doctor. The report will tell if the lump is cancer or not.

Your doctor will go over the report with you. Waiting for these results can be difficult. It can take about a week to get the results

- **If no cancer is found,** the biopsy result is called benign. Benign means it is not cancer. Some benign results need follow-up. Talk with your doctor or nurse about what is recommended for you.

- **If cancer is found,** the report will tell you the kind of cancer you have. It will help you and your doctor talk about the next steps. Often, this may include seeing a breast cancer specialist. You also may need more imaging tests or surgery. All this information will help you and your doctor think through your treatment options.

Take time to think. Most women with breast cancer have time to think about their options.

Questions for Your Doctor or Nurse

Talking about options:

- What kind of biopsy do you recommend? Why?
- Are there any other options?
- How long will the biopsy take?
- What are the possible side effects?
- Could the biopsy cause scarring or bruising?

Preparing for a biopsy:

- How many days before my biopsy should I stop taking aspirin? Are there other medicines I should avoid?
- Can I have someone in the room with me during the biopsy?
- Do I need someone to drive me home?
- When will I get the results?
- Who will give me the results?

If my biopsy does not show cancer:

- What kind of follow-up do I need?
- When should I have my next mammogram?

If my biopsy shows cancer:

- What are the next steps?

- What are my options for treatment?

- Can you tell me about support groups for women with breast cancer?

Section 25.3

Lumpectomy

This section includes text excerpted from "Early-Stage Breast Cancer Treatment Fact Sheet," Office on Women's Health (OWH), U.S. Department of Health and Human Services (HHS), July 16, 2012. Reviewed June 2017.

Questions about Breast-Sparing Surgery with Radiation

If I choose breast-sparing surgery, how much of my breast has to be taken out?

In a lumpectomy the surgeon removes the cancer and a small amount of surrounding normal tissue but leaves most of the breast intact. With other types of breast-sparing surgery, somewhat larger areas of the healthy breast are removed. This distance between the outer edge of the tumor and outer edge of the normal tissue surrounding it is known as the *margin*. The goal of breast-sparing surgery is to obtain *clear*, or *clean*, *margins*—that is, a band of normal breast tissue around the entire tumor that is completely free of cancer. This dictates how much breast is ultimately removed.

Will breast-sparing surgery affect the look of my breast? What will the scar look like?

How the breast looks after surgery will depend on the size of the cancer compared to the size of the breast and the amount of healthy breast tissue that is removed. The appearance of the scar depends on the type of surgery and the location of the cancer. Your doctor can give you an idea of how breast-sparing surgery may affect the look of your breast. If your doctor says that breast-sparing surgery is an option for you, then he or she expects that the cancer plus a margin of normal tissue can be removed with a good cosmetic outcome.

Will I still have feeling in my breast after breast-sparing surgery?

Most women who have breast-sparing surgery followed by radiation therapy will still have sensation in the breast.

What does radiation therapy after breast-sparing surgery involve?

Radiation therapy is usually performed as an outpatient procedure over a period of at least 5 weeks. Some women are not able to make that commitment. Some women live far from radiation facilities or can't afford to take the time for daily treatments. Others may have health conditions such as pregnancy, lupus, or heart disease, that prevent them from undergoing radiation. Since radiation therapy lowers the risk of recurrence for women who choose breast-sparing surgery, patients and their doctors must consider the requirements for radiation therapy before deciding which surgical option is best for them.

Why do I need radiation therapy if the tumor is removed with clear margins?

Women who have radiation therapy after breast-sparing surgery are less likely to have cancer come back in the same breast than women who have breast-sparing surgery without radiation.

What are the chances of the cancer coming back if I have breast-sparing surgery with radiation? If I decide on a breast-sparing surgery with radiation, how can you be sure there are no other "spots" in the breast?

Most women who have breast-sparing surgery followed by radiation will not have cancer recur in the same breast. In studies, recurrence rates within 10 years of breast-sparing surgery followed by radiation range from 4 percent to 20 percent. This might seem like a big range. But keep in mind that cancer that recurs in the same breast can be treated and does not affect chances of a healthy recovery compared to mastectomy. Another thing to keep in mind is that doctors suggest breast-sparing surgery only if they feel it offers a very good chance of removing all of the cancer. Obtaining a clear margin is one way the surgeon can lower the risk of recurrence. Radiation also lowers the risk of the cancer recurring in the same breast.

What are the side effects of breast-sparing surgery? What about the side effects of radiation? I hear it makes the breast hard.

When considering what kind of surgery to have, it is important to know that there are potential side effects common to all surgical procedures. Any surgical procedure carries a risk of infection, poor wound healing, bleeding, or a reaction to the anesthesia. Also, pain and tenderness in the affected area is common, usually only in the short term. Because nerves may be injured or cut during surgery, most women will experience numbness and tingling in the chest, underarm, shoulder, and/or upper arm. Women who undergo breast-sparing surgery usually find these changes in sensation improve over 1 or 2 years, but they may never go away completely.

Radiation therapy can cause side effects, such as fatigue or skin irritation. These side effects tend to be mild. Radiation therapy can cause a skin condition that looks like sunburn. This usually fades, but in some women it never goes away completely. Some women do find that radiation makes their breast feel hard or firm. Again, this may last just a few months, or longer.

Removal of lymph nodes under the arms may be performed. This can lead to pain and arm swelling, called *lymphedema*, which can last a long time and be debilitating.

Keep in mind that the side effects of treatment vary for each person. Some women may have many side effects or complications, others may have very few. Pain medication, physical therapy, and other strategies can help women manage side effects and recovery.

I heard that radiation can cause cancer. Will it increase my risk for other cancers?

Radiation therapy has improved greatly through the years, and the doses are much lower than they used to be. The risk of another cancer due to radiation therapy to the breast is very small. The bottom line is that women who have radiation therapy after breast-sparing surgery are less likely to have cancer recur in the same breast, and they live just as long as women who undergo mastectomy without radiation.

271

If cancer recurs in the same breast after having breast-sparing surgery followed by radiation, will I need a mastectomy then? Will I be able to have breast reconstruction even though I have had radiation?

Cancer that recurs in the same breast usually is removed with surgery. Most often a mastectomy is performed at that time, because radiation is not recommended a second time. Breast reconstruction is possible after previous radiation therapy, but the surgery may be harder to perform. This issue should be discussed with a plastic surgeon.

Section 25.4

Breast Reconstruction

This section includes text excerpted from "Breast Reconstruction after Mastectomy," National Cancer Institute (NCI), February 24, 2017.

Many women who have a mastectomy—surgery to remove an entire breast to treat or prevent breast cancer—have the option of having the shape of the removed breast rebuilt. Women who choose to have their breasts rebuilt have several options for how it can be done. Breasts can be rebuilt using implants (saline or silicone). They can also be rebuilt using autologous tissue (that is, tissue from elsewhere in the body). Sometimes both implants and autologous tissue are used to rebuild the breast. Surgery to reconstruct the breasts can be done (or started) at the time of the mastectomy (which is called immediate reconstruction) or it can be done after the mastectomy incisions have healed and breast cancer therapy has been completed (which is called delayed reconstruction). Delayed reconstruction can happen months or even years after the mastectomy.

In a final stage of breast reconstruction, a nipple and areola may be re-created on the reconstructed breast, if these were not preserved during the mastectomy.

Sometimes breast reconstruction surgery includes surgery on the other, or contralateral, breast so that the two breasts will match in size and shape.

Reconstructing a Woman's Breast Using Implants

Implants are inserted underneath the skin or chest muscle following the mastectomy. (Most mastectomies are performed using a technique called skin-sparing mastectomy, in which much of the breast skin is saved for use in reconstructing the breast.)

Implants are usually placed as part of a two-stage procedure.

- In the first stage, the surgeon places a device, called a tissue expander, under the skin that is left after the mastectomy or under the chest muscle. The expander is slowly filled with saline during periodic visits to the doctor after surgery.

- In the second stage, after the chest tissue has relaxed and healed enough, the expander is removed and replaced with an implant. The chest tissue is usually ready for the implant 2 to 6 months after mastectomy.

In some cases, the implant can be placed in the breast during the same surgery as the mastectomy—that is, a tissue expander is not used to prepare for the implant. Surgeons are increasingly using material called acellular dermal matrix as a kind of scaffold or "sling" to support tissue expanders and implants. Acellular dermal matrix is a kind of mesh that is made from donated human or pig skin that has been sterilized and processed to remove all cells to eliminate the risks of rejection and infection.

Reconstruct the Breast Using Body Tissue

In autologous tissue reconstruction, a piece of tissue containing skin, fat, blood vessels, and sometimes muscle is taken from elsewhere in a woman's body and used to rebuild the breast. This piece of tissue is called a flap. Different sites in the body can provide flaps for breast reconstruction. Flaps used for breast reconstruction most often come from the abdomen or back. However, they can also be taken from the thigh or buttocks.

Depending on their source, flaps can be pedicled or free.

- **With a pedicled flap,** the tissue and attached blood vessels are moved together through the body to the breast area. Because the blood supply to the tissue used for reconstruction is left intact, blood vessels do not need to be reconnected once the tissue is moved.

- **With free flaps,** the tissue is cut free from its blood supply. It must be attached to new blood vessels in the breast area, using a technique called microsurgery. This gives the reconstructed breast a blood supply.

Abdominal and back flaps include:

- **DIEP flap.** Tissue comes from the abdomen and contains only skin, blood vessels, and fat, without the underlying muscle. This type of flap is a free flap.

- **Latissimus dorsi (LD) flap.** Tissue comes from the middle and side of the back. This type of flap is pedicled when used for breast reconstruction. (LD flaps can be used for other types of reconstruction as well.)

- **SIEA flap (also called SIEP flap).** Tissue comes from the abdomen as in a DIEP flap but includes a different set of blood vessels. It also does not involve cutting of the abdominal muscle and is a free flap. This type of flap is not an option for many women because the necessary blood vessels are not adequate or do not exist.

- **TRAM flap.** Tissue comes from the lower abdomen as in a DIEP flap but includes muscle. It can be either pedicled or free.

Flaps taken from the thigh or buttocks are used for women who have had previous major abdominal surgery or who don't have enough abdominal tissue to reconstruct a breast. These types of flaps are free flaps. With these flaps an implant is often used as well to provide sufficient breast volume.

- **IGAP flap.** Tissue comes from the buttocks and contains only skin, blood vessels, and fat.

- **PAP flap.** Tissue, without muscle, that comes from the upper inner thigh.

- **SGAP flap.** Tissue comes from the buttocks as in an IGAP flap, but includes a different set of blood vessels and contains only skin, blood vessels, and fat.

- **TUG flap.** Tissue, including muscle, that comes from the upper inner thigh.

In some cases, an implant and autologous tissue are used together. For example, autologous tissue may be used to cover an implant when there isn't enough skin and muscle left after mastectomy to allow for expansion and use of an implant.

Reconstructing the Nipple and Areola?

After the chest heals from reconstruction surgery and the position of the breast mound on the chest wall has had time to stabilize, a surgeon can reconstruct the nipple and areola. Usually, the new nipple is created by cutting and moving small pieces of skin from the reconstructed breast to the nipple site and shaping them into a new nipple. A few months after nipple reconstruction, the surgeon can re-create the areola. This is usually done using tattoo ink. However, in some cases, skin grafts may be taken from the groin or abdomen and attached to the breast to create an areola at the time of the nipple reconstruction.

Some women who do not have surgical nipple reconstruction may consider getting a realistic picture of a nipple created on the reconstructed breast from a tattoo artist who specializes in 3D nipple tattooing. A mastectomy that preserves a woman's own nipple and areola, called nipple-sparing mastectomy, may be an option for some women, depending on the size and location of the breast cancer and the shape and size of the breasts.

Factors That Can Affect the Timing of Breast Reconstruction

One factor that can affect the timing of breast reconstruction is whether a woman will need radiation therapy. Radiation therapy can sometimes cause wound healing problems or infections in reconstructed breasts, so some women may prefer to delay reconstruction until after radiation therapy is completed. However, because of improvements in surgical and radiation techniques, immediate reconstruction with an implant is usually still an option for women who will need radiation therapy. Autologous tissue breast reconstruction is usually reserved for after radiation therapy, so that the breast and chest wall tissue damaged by radiation can be replaced with healthy tissue from elsewhere in the body.

Another factor is the type of breast cancer. Women with inflammatory breast cancer usually require more extensive skin removal. This can make immediate reconstruction more challenging, so it may be recommended that reconstruction be delayed until after completion of adjuvant therapy.

Even if a woman is a candidate for immediate reconstruction, she may choose delayed reconstruction. For instance, some women prefer not to consider what type of reconstruction to have until after they have recovered from their mastectomy and subsequent adjuvant treatment. Women who delay reconstruction (or choose not to undergo the procedure at all) can use external breast prostheses, or breast forms, to give the appearance of breasts.

Factors That Can Affect the Choice of Breast Reconstruction Method

Several factors can influence the type of reconstructive surgery a woman chooses. These include the size and shape of the breast that is being rebuilt, the woman's age and health, her history of past surgeries, surgical risk factors (for example, smoking history and obesity), the availability of autologous tissue, and the location of the tumor in the breast. Women who have had past abdominal surgery may not be candidates for an abdominally based flap reconstruction. Each type of reconstruction has factors that a woman should think about before making a decision. Some of the more common considerations are listed below.

Reconstruction with Implants

Surgery and recovery:

- Enough skin and muscle must remain after mastectomy to cover the implant
- Shorter surgical procedure than for reconstruction with autologous tissue; little blood loss
- Recovery period may be shorter than with autologous reconstruction
- Many follow-up visits may be needed to inflate the expander and insert the implant

Possible complications:

- Infection
- Accumulation of clear fluid causing a mass or lump (seroma) within the reconstructed breast
- Pooling of blood (hematoma) within the reconstructed breast
- Blood clots
- Extrusion of the implant (the implant breaks through the skin)
- Implant rupture (the implant breaks open and saline or silicone leaks into the surrounding tissue)

- Formation of hard scar tissue around the implant (known as a contracture)

- Obesity, diabetes, and smoking may increase the rate of complications

- Possible increased risk of developing a very rare form of immune system cancer called anaplastic large cell lymphoma

Other considerations:

- May not be an option for patients who have previously undergone radiation therapy to the chest

- May not be adequate for women with very large breasts

- Will not last a lifetime; the longer a woman has implants, the more likely she is to have complications and to need to have her implants removed or replaced

- Silicone implants may feel more natural than saline implants to the touch

- The U.S. Food and Drug Administration (FDA) recommends that women with silicone implants undergo periodic magnetic resonance imaging (MRI) screenings to detect possible "silent" rupture of the implants

Reconstruction with Autologous Tissue

Surgery and recovery:

- Longer surgical procedure than for implants

- The initial recovery period may be longer than for implants

- Pedicled flap reconstruction is usually a shorter operation than free flap reconstruction and usually requires a shorter hospitalization

- Free flap reconstruction is a longer, highly technical operation compared with pedicled flap reconstruction that requires a surgeon who has experience with microsurgery to reattach blood vessels

Possible complications:

- Necrosis (death) of the transferred tissue

- Blood clots may be more frequent with some flap sources

- Pain and weakness at the site from which the donor tissue was taken

- Obesity, diabetes, and smoking may increase the rate of complications

Other considerations:

- May provide a more natural breast shape than implants

- May feel softer and more natural to the touch than implants

- Leaves a scar at the site from which the donor tissue was taken

- Can be used to replace tissue that has been damaged by radiation therapy

All women who undergo mastectomy for breast cancer experience varying degrees of breast numbness and loss of sensation (feeling) because nerves that provide sensation to the breast are cut when breast tissue is removed during surgery. However, a woman may regain some sensation as the severed nerves grow and regenerate, and breast surgeons continue to make technical advances that can spare or repair damage to nerves.

Any type of breast reconstruction can fail if healing does not occur properly. In these cases, the implant or flap will have to be removed. If an implant reconstruction fails, a woman can usually have a second reconstruction using an alternative approach.

Will Health Insurance Pay for Breast Reconstruction?

The Women's Health and Cancer Rights Act of 1998 (WHCRA) is a federal law that requires group health plans and health insurance companies that offer mastectomy coverage to also pay for reconstructive surgery after mastectomy. This coverage must include all stages of reconstruction and surgery to achieve symmetry between the breasts, breast prostheses, and treatment of complications that result from the mastectomy, including lymphedema. Some health plans sponsored by religious organizations and some government health plans may be exempt from WHCRA. Also, WHCRA does not apply to Medicare and Medicaid.

However, Medicare may cover breast reconstruction surgery as well as external breast prostheses (including a postsurgical bra) after a medically necessary mastectomy. Medicaid benefits vary by state; a woman should contact her state Medicaid office for information on whether, and to what extent, breast reconstruction is covered. A woman considering breast reconstruction may want to discuss costs and health insurance coverage with her doctor and insurance company before choosing to have the surgery. Some insurance companies require a second opinion before they will agree to pay for a surgery.

Follow-Up Care and Rehabilitation after Breast Reconstruction

Any type of reconstruction increases the number of side effects a woman may experience compared with those after a mastectomy alone. A woman's medical team will watch her closely for complications, some of which can occur months or even years after surgery. Women who have either autologous tissue or implant-based reconstruction may benefit from physical therapy to improve or maintain shoulder range of motion or help them recover from weakness experienced at the site from which the donor tissue was taken, such as abdominal weakness. A physical therapist can help a woman use exercises to regain strength, adjust to new physical limitations, and figure out the safest ways to perform everyday activities.

Breast Reconstruction and Checking for Breast Cancer Recurrence

Studies have shown that breast reconstruction does not increase the chances of breast cancer coming back or make it harder to check for recurrence with mammography. Women who have one breast removed by mastectomy will still have mammograms of the other breast. Women who have had a skin-sparing mastectomy or who are at high risk of breast cancer recurrence may have mammograms of the reconstructed breast if it was reconstructed using autologous tissue.

However, mammograms are generally not performed on breasts that are reconstructed with an implant after mastectomy. A woman with a breast implant should tell the radiology technician about her implant before she has a mammogram. Special procedures may be necessary to improve the accuracy of the mammogram and to avoid damaging the implant.

What Are Some Developments in Breast Reconstruction after Mastectomy?

- **Oncoplastic surgery.** In general, women who have lumpectomy or partial mastectomy for early-stage breast cancer do not have reconstruction. However, for some of these women the surgeon may use plastic surgery techniques to reshape the breast at the time of cancer surgery. This type of breast-conserving surgery, called oncoplastic surgery, may use local tissue rearrangement, reconstruction through breast reduction surgery, or transfer of tissue flaps. Long-term outcomes of this type of surgery are comparable to those for standard breast-conserving surgery.

- **Autologous fat grafting.** A newer type of breast reconstruction technique involves the transfer of fat tissue from one part of the body (usually the thighs, abdomen, or buttocks) to the reconstructed breast. The fat tissue is harvested by liposuction, washed, and liquified so that it can be injected into the area of interest. Fat grafting is mainly used to correct deformities and asymmetries that may appear after breast reconstruction. It is also sometimes used to reconstruct an entire breast. Although concern has been raised about the lack of long-term outcome studies, this technique is considered safe.

Section 25.5

Breast Implant Surgery

This section includes text excerpted from "Breast Implant Surgery," U.S. Food and Drug Administration (FDA), March 21, 2017.

Breast implant surgery can be performed in a hospital, surgery center or doctor's office. Breast implant surgery patients may have to stay overnight in the hospital (inpatient surgery) or may be able to go home afterward (outpatient surgery). The surgery can be done under local anesthesia, where the patient remains awake and only the breast is numbed to block the pain, or under general anesthesia, where medicine is given to make the patient sleep. Most women receive general anesthesia for this surgery. Breast implant surgery can last from one to several hours depending on the procedure and personal circumstances.

If the surgery is done in a hospital, the length of the hospital stay will vary based on the type of surgery, the development of any complications after surgery and your general health. The length of the hospital stay may also depend on the type of coverage your insurance provides.

Surgical Consultation

Before surgery you should have a consultation with your surgeon. Be prepared to ask questions about the surgeon's experience, your surgery and expected outcomes. The surgeon should be able to discuss whether you are a good candidate for breast implants, the different type of implants, options for size, shape, surface texture, and placement based on your particular circumstances, as well as the risks and benefits of implant surgery. The surgeon should also be able to provide you with before and after pictures of other patients to help you better understand your expectations and potential outcomes from surgery.

During the consultation you will need to discuss your medical history, including any medical conditions or drug allergies you may have. You should also discuss any previous surgeries you've had, especially to the breast, and what drugs you are currently taking, including supplements, herbal and over-the-counter (OTC) medications.

It is important to tell the surgeon if you think you may be pregnant. If you are undergoing breast implant surgery for reconstruction, you will also need to speak with your surgeon about your personal circumstances, including being treated with chemotherapy and/or radiation therapy, as these can affect your risks of complication and the appearance of the reconstructed breast. The surgeon should also speak to you about the amount of breast tissue that will remain after surgery and future screening for breast implant ruptures and breast cancer.

During the consultation be sure to ask the surgeon for a copy of the patient labeling for the breast implant s/he plans to use. You have the right to request this information, and your physician is expected to provide it. Be sure to read the patient labeling entirely prior to surgery. It will provide you with information specific to your breast implants, including how to take care of them. Make sure you read and understand the informed consent form before you sign it.

Breast implant manufacturers conduct clinical studies to evaluate new types of breast implants and to understand the long-term experiences of women who receive breast implants. If you are interested in participating in a clinical study, be sure to ask your surgeon what specific steps you will need to take.

Before Surgery

Your surgeon may ask that you have a mammogram or breast X-rays prior to surgery in order to identify any breast abnormality and so the surgeon has a preoperative image of your breast tissue. You will usually be asked to not eat or drink anything after midnight the night before surgery and to bring loose clothing, including a loose-fitting bra without underwire, to wear after surgery. If you are going home the same day as the surgery, you will need to plan for someone to drive you home. Your surgeon should discuss with you the extent of surgery, the estimated time it will take and how they plan to treat for pain and nausea.

During Surgery

After surgery you will be taken to a recovery area to be monitored. Your breasts will be wrapped in gauze or a surgical bra. Your surgeon should describe the usual after surgery (postoperative) recovery process, the possible complications that may occur, and the recovery period. Following the operation, as with any surgery, you can expect some pain, swelling, bruising and tenderness. These effects may last for a month or longer, but should disappear with time. Scarring is a natural result of surgery. Prior to surgery, ask your surgeon to describe the location, size and appearance of any expected scars. For most women, scars will fade over time into thin lines. The darker your skin, the more prominent the scars are likely to be.

Your surgeon may prescribe medications for pain and/or nausea. If you experience bleeding, fever, warmth, redness of the breast, or other symptoms of infection, you should immediately report these symptoms to your surgeon. Your surgeon should tell you about wound healing and how to care for your wound. You may need a postoperative bra, compression bandage or jogging bra for extra support as you heal. At your surgeon's recommendation you will most likely be able to return to work within one to two weeks, but you should avoid any strenuous activities that could raise your pulse and blood pressure for at least two weeks.

Ask your surgeon about a schedule for follow-up visits, limits on your activities, precautions you should take, and when you can return to your normal activities, including exercising. If you received silicone gel-filled breast implants, the FDA recommends that you receive magnetic resonance imaging (MRI) screening for silent rupture 3 years after receiving your implant and every 2 years after that. Continue to get mammograms to screen for breast cancer. Be sure to tell the person giving your mammogram that you have breast implants. Breast implants may make it difficult to see breast tissue on standard mammograms, so they may need to use different techniques.

If you are enrolled in a clinical study, be sure to ask your surgeon for a schedule of follow-up examinations set by the study plan.

After Surgery

After surgery you will be taken to a recovery area to be monitored. Your breasts will be wrapped in gauze or a surgical bra. Your surgeon should describe the usual after surgery (postoperative) recovery process, the possible complications that may occur, and the recovery period. Following the operation, as with any surgery, you can expect some pain, swelling, bruising and tenderness. These effects may last for a month or longer, but should disappear with time. Scarring is a natural result of surgery. Prior to surgery, ask your surgeon to describe the location, size and appearance of any expected scars. For most women, scars will fade over time into thin lines. The darker your skin, the more prominent the scars are likely to be.

Your surgeon may prescribe medications for pain and/or nausea. If you experience bleeding, fever, warmth, redness of the breast, or other symptoms of infection, you should immediately report these symptoms to your surgeon. Your surgeon should tell you about wound healing and how to care for your wound. You may need a postoperative bra, compression bandage or jogging bra for extra support as you heal. At your surgeon's recommendation you will most likely be able to return to work within one to two weeks, but you should avoid any strenuous activities that could raise your pulse and blood pressure for at least two weeks.

Ask your surgeon about a schedule for follow-up visits, limits on your activities, precautions you should take, and when you can return to your normal activities, including exercising. If you received silicone gel-filled breast implants, the FDA recommends that you receive magnetic resonance imaging (MRI) screening for silent rupture 3 years after receiving your implant and every 2 years after that.

Continue to get mammograms to screen for breast cancer. Be sure to tell the person giving your mammogram that you have breast implants. Breast implants may make it difficult to see breast tissue on standard mammograms, so they may need to use different techniques. If you are enrolled in a clinical study, be sure to ask your surgeon for a schedule of follow-up examinations set by the study plan.

Questions to Ask before Having Breast Implant Surgery

When choosing a surgeon for a breast implant procedure, you may want to consider their years of experience, their board certification, their patient follow-up, and your own comfort level with the surgeon. Most breast implant procedures are performed by board-certified plastic and reconstructive surgeons. The following questions can help guide your discussion with your surgeon regarding breast implant surgery.

Questions to Ask

About your surgeon:

1. How many breast implant procedures do you do each year?

2. What percentage of your practice is dedicated to breast augmentation? To breast reconstruction?

3. What type of implants do you use? Saline or silicone? What is your experience with each?

4. What is the most common complication you encounter with breast implant surgery?

5. What is your rate of complications in general (capsule contracture, infection, etc.)?

6. What is your reoperation rate?

7. What is the most common type of reoperation you perform?

About breast implants and expected outcomes:

1. What shape, size, and surface texture are you recommending for my implants?

2. Why are you recommending one type of breast implant over another? Why do you recommend this one for me?

3. How long will my breast implants last?

4. What incision site and placement are you recommending for me?

5. Do you have before and after photos I can look at for each procedure?

6. What results are reasonable for me to expect?

7. How will breast implants feel? Will they alter my breast skin or nipple sensation?

8. What are the risks and complications associated with having breast implants?

9. Can I still get breast implants for augmentation if I have a strong family history of breast cancer?

10. How many additional operations on my breast implants can I expect to have over my lifetime?

11. How will I be able to tell if my breast implant has ruptured or if there is a problem with my breast implants?

12. How will my breasts look if I decide to have the implants removed and not replaced?

13. How easy or difficult is it to remove the implants?

14. How easy or difficult is it to increase the size of the implants after the breast implants have been placed?

15. What can I expect my breasts to look like over time? What do I need to do to maintain them?

16. What kind of additional follow-up will I need?

17. What are the long-term consequences of breast implants?

18. What will my breasts look like after pregnancy? After breastfeeding?

19. Will the breast implants affect my ability to breastfeed a baby?

20. What are my options if I am dissatisfied with the outcome of my breast implants?

21. Can I still get mammograms with breast implants in place?

22. Will the mammogram rupture my breast implant?

23. What alternate procedures or products are available besides breast implants?

About the breast implant operation:

1. How long will I be in pain after the surgery?

2. What is my expected recovery time?

3. Will I need help at home for normal activities after the surgery and if so for about how long?

4. How long do you expect my operation to take?

5. What (if any) secondary procedures associated with my breast augmentation/breast reconstruction will be required?

6. How likely is it that I will get an infection after the surgery?

7. How much risk is there from the anesthesia?

8. What can I do to minimize the risk of short-term and long-term complications?

9. Where will my scar be?

Things to Consider before Getting Breast Implants

There are several important things to consider before deciding to undergo breast implant surgery, including understanding your own expectations and reasons for having the surgery. Below are some things the FDA thinks you should consider before undergoing breast augmentation, reconstruction or revision surgery.

- Breast implants are not lifetime devices; the longer you have your implants, the more likely it will be for you to have them removed.

- The longer you have breast implants, the more likely you are to experience local complications and adverse outcomes.

- The most common local complications and adverse outcomes are capsular contracture, reoperation and implant removal. Other complications include rupture or deflation, wrinkling, asymmetry, scarring, pain, and infection at the incision site.

- You should assume that you will need to have additional surgeries (reoperations).

- Many of the changes to your breast following implantation may be cosmetically undesirable and irreversible.

- If you have your implants removed but not replaced, you may experience changes to your natural breasts such as dimpling, puckering, wrinkling, breast tissue loss, or other undesirable cosmetic changes.

- If you have breast implants, you will need to monitor your breasts for the rest of your life. If you notice any abnormal changes in your breasts, you will need to see a doctor promptly.

- If you have silicone gel-filled breast implants, you will need to undergo periodic MRI examinations in order to detect ruptures that do not cause symptoms ("silent ruptures"). For early detection of silent rupture, the FDA recommends that women with silicone gel-filled breast implants receive MRI screenings 3 years after they receive a new implant and every 2 years after that. MRI screening for implant rupture is costly and may not be covered by your insurance.

- If you have breast implants, you have a low risk of developing a rare type of cancer called breast implant-associated anaplastic large cell lymphoma (BIA-ALCL) in the breast tissue surrounding the implant. BIA-ALCL is not breast cancer. Women diagnosed with BIA-ALCL may need to be treated with surgery, chemotherapy and/or radiation therapy.

Chapter 26

Respiratory Tract and Lung Surgeries

Chapter Contents

Section 26.1

Treating Recurrent Respiratory Papillomatosis (RRP)

This section includes text excerpted from "Recurrent
Respiratory Papillomatosis or Laryngeal Papillomatosis,"
National Institute on Deafness and Other Communication
Disorders (NIDCD), March 6, 2017.

What Is Recurrent Respiratory Papillomatosis (RRP)?

Recurrent respiratory papillomatosis (RRP) is a disease in which
tumors grow in the air passages leading from the nose and mouth into
the lungs (respiratory tract). Although the tumors can grow anywhere
in the respiratory tract, their presence in the larynx (voice box) causes
the most frequent problems, a condition called laryngeal papillomatosis. The tumors may vary in size and grow very quickly. They often
grow back even when removed.

What Is the Cause of RRP?

RRP is caused by two types of human papilloma virus (HPV), called
HPV 6 and HPV 11. There are more than 150 types of HPV and they
do not all have the same symptoms.

Most people who encounter HPV never develop any illness. However, many HPVs can cause small wart-like, noncancerous tumors
called papillomas. The most common illness caused by HPV 6 and
HPV 11 is genital warts. Although scientists are uncertain how
people are infected with HPV 6 or HPV 11, the virus is thought to
be spread through sexual contact or when a mother with genital
warts passes it to her baby during childbirth. HPV 6 and HPV 11
can also cause disease of the uterine cervix and, in rare cases, cervical cancer.

According to the Centers for Disease Control and Prevention (CDC),
the incidence of RRP is rare. Fewer than 2,000 children get RRP each
year.

Who Is Affected by RRP?

RRP affects adults as well as infants and small children who may have contracted the virus during childbirth. According to the RRP Foundation (www.rrpf.org), there are roughly 20,000 cases in the United States. Among children, the incidence of RRP is approximately 4.3 per 100,000; among adults, it's about 1.8 per 100,000.

What Are the Symptoms of RRP?

Normally, voice is produced when air from the lungs is pushed past two side-by-side elastic muscles—called vocal folds or vocal cords—with sufficient pressure to cause them to vibrate. When the tumors interfere with the normal vibrations of the vocal folds, it causes hoarseness, which is the most common symptom of RRP. Eventually, the tumors may block the airway passage and cause difficulty breathing.

**Parts of the respiratory tract
affected by RRP**

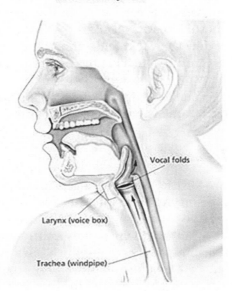

Figure 26.1. *Parts of the Respiratory Tract Affected by RRP*

Because the tumors grow quickly, young children with the disease may find it difficult to breathe when sleeping, or they may experience difficulty swallowing. Adults and children may experience hoarseness, chronic coughing, or breathing problems. The symptoms tend to be more severe in children than in adults; however, some children experience some relief or remission of the disease when they begin puberty. Because of the similarity of the symptoms, RRP is sometimes misdiagnosed as asthma or chronic bronchitis.

How Is RRP Diagnosed?

Two routine tests for RRP are indirect and direct laryngoscopy. In an indirect laryngoscopy, an otolaryngologist—a doctor who specializes in diseases of the ear, nose, throat, head, and neck—or speech-language pathologist will typically insert a flexible fiberoptic telescope, called an endoscope, into a patient's nose or mouth and then view the larynx on a monitor. Some medical professionals use a video camera attached to a flexible tube to examine the larynx. An older, less common method is for the otolaryngologist to place a small mirror in the back of the throat and angle the mirror down toward the larynx to inspect it for tumors.

- A direct laryngoscopy is conducted in the operating room with the use of general anesthesia. This method allows the otolaryngologist to view the vocal folds and other parts of the larynx under high magnification. This procedure is usually used to minimize discomfort, especially with children, or to enable the doctor to collect tissue samples from the larynx or other parts of the throat to examine them for abnormalities.

How Is RRP Treated?

There is no cure for RRP. Surgery is the primary method for removing tumors from the larynx or airway. Because traditional surgery can result in problems due to scarring of the larynx tissue, many surgeons are now using laser surgery, which uses an intense laser light as the surgical tool. Carbon dioxide lasers—which pass electricity through a tube containing carbon dioxide and other gases to generate light—are currently the most popular type used for this purpose. In the past 10 years, surgeons have begun using a device called a microdebrider, which uses suction to hold the tumor while a small internal rotary blade removes the growth.

Once the tumors have been removed, they have a tendency to return unpredictably. It is common for patients to require repeat surgery. With some patients, surgery may be required every few weeks in order to keep the breathing passage open, while others may require surgery only once a year. In the most extreme cases where tumor growth is aggressive, a tracheotomy may be performed. A tracheotomy is a surgical procedure in which an incision is made in the front of the patient's neck and a breathing tube (trach tube) is inserted through an opening, called a stoma, into the trachea (windpipe). Rather than breathing through the nose and mouth, the patient will now breathe through the trach tube. Although the trach tube keeps the breathing passage open, doctors try to remove it as soon as it is feasible.

Some patients may be required to keep a trach tube indefinitely in order to keep the breathing passage open. In addition, because the trach tube re-routes all or some of the exhaled air away from the vocal folds, the patient may find it difficult to speak. With the help of a voice specialist or speech-language pathologist who specializes in voice, the patient can learn how to use his or her voice.

Adjuvant therapies—therapies that are used in addition to surgery—have been used to treat more severe cases of RRP. Drug treatments may include antivirals such as interferon and cidofovir, which block the virus from making copies of itself, and indole-3-carbinol, a cancer-fighting compound found in cruciferous vegetables, such as broccoli and Brussels sprouts. To date, the results of these and other adjuvant therapies have been mixed or not yet fully proven.

Section 26.2

Tracheostomy

This section includes text excerpted from "Tracheostomy," National Heart, Lung, and Blood Institute (NHLBI), December 9, 2016.

A tracheostomy is a surgically made hole that goes through the front of your neck into your trachea, or windpipe. A breathing tube, called a trach tube, is placed through the hole and directly into your windpipe to help you breathe. A tracheostomy may be used to help people who need to be on ventilators for more than a couple of weeks or who have conditions that block the upper airways.

The Procedure

A surgeon can make a tracheostomy in a hospital operating room when you are asleep from general anesthesia. A doctor or emergency medical technician can make a tracheostomy safely at a patient's bedside, such as in the intensive care unit (ICU), or elsewhere in a life-threatening situation. A tracheostomy usually takes 20 to 45 minutes to perform. The surgeon or other healthcare professional will make a cut through the lower front part of your neck and then cut into your windpipe. Cuffed trach tubes may be used. These tubes use air to widen or narrow the tube to fit the hole. After inserting and placing the trach tube into the windpipe, the surgeon or other healthcare professional will use stitches, surgical tape, or a Velcro band to hold the tube in place.

After the Surgery

After getting the tracheostomy, you may stay in the hospital to recover depending on your health. It can take up to two weeks for a tracheostomy to fully form, or mature. During this time, you will not be able to eat normally and will likely receive nutrients through a feeding tube. You may have difficulty talking after your tracheostomy. A speech therapist can help you to regain normal swallowing ability and use your voice to speak clearly. Your trach tube will be removed when you no longer need it. The hole usually closes on its own, but surgery can close the hole if needed.

Tracheostomy is a fairly common and simple procedure, especially for critical care patients in hospitals. Soon after the procedure, it is possible to have bleeding, infection, pneumothorax or collapsed lung, or subcutaneous emphysema. Over time, complications may include windpipe scarring or an abnormal connection, called a fistula, between the windpipe and esophagus that causes food and saliva to enter your lungs. It is also possible to have complications that affect the function of the trach tube, such as the tube slipping or falling out of place, or that affect the windpipe or other airway structures. Proper care and handling of the tracheostomy, the tubes, and other related supplies can help reduce risks.

Section 26.3

Treating Atelectasis (Collapsed Lung)

This section includes text excerpted from "Atelectasis," National
Heart, Lung, and Blood Institute (NHLBI), January 13, 2012.
Reviewed June 2017.

What Is Atelectasis?

Atelectasis is a condition in which one or more areas of your lungs
collapse or don't inflate properly. If only a small area or a few small
areas of the lungs are affected, you may have no signs or symptoms.

If a large area or several large areas of the lungs are affected, they
may not be able to deliver enough oxygen to your blood. This can cause
symptoms and complications.

What Causes Atelectasis?

Atelectasis can occur if the lungs can't fully expand and fill with
air. Atelectasis has many causes.

Conditions and Factors That Prevent Deep Breathing and Coughing

Conditions and factors that prevent deep breathing and coughing
can cause atelectasis. For example, if you're taking shallow breaths
or breathing with the help of a ventilator, your lungs don't fill with
air in the normal way.

Normally, when you take a deep breath, the base (bottom) and the
back of your lungs fill with air first. However, if you're taking shallow
breaths or using a ventilator, air may not make it all the way to the
air sacs at the bottom of your lungs. Thus, these air sacs won't inflate
properly.

Atelectasis is very common after surgery. The medicine used during
surgery to temporarily put you to sleep can decrease or stop your
normal effort to breathe and urge to cough. Sometimes, especially
after chest or abdominal surgery, pain may keep you from wanting to

take deep breaths. As a result, part of your lung may collapse or not inflate right.

Pressure from outside the lungs also may make it hard to take deep breaths. A number of factors can cause pressure outside the lungs. Examples include a tumor, a tight body cast, a bone deformity, or pleural effusion (fluid buildup between the ribs and the lungs).

Lung conditions and other medical disorders that affect your ability to breathe deeply or cough and clear mucus from your lungs also may lead to atelectasis. One example is respiratory distress syndrome (RDS).

RDS is a breathing disorder that affects some newborns. It's more common in premature infants because their lungs aren't able to make enough surfactant. Surfactant is a liquid that coats the inside of the lungs and helps keep the air sacs open. Without enough surfactant, part of the lungs may collapse.

Other lung conditions and medical disorders that can cause atelectasis include pneumonia, lung cancer, and neuromuscular diseases. Rarely, asthma, chronic obstructive pulmonary disease (COPD), and cystic fibrosis are associated with atelectasis.

Migrating atelectasis in newborns is rare and may be caused by neuromuscular diseases. "Migrating" means that the part of the lung that collapses will change depending on the position of the baby.

An Airway Blockage

An airway blockage also can cause atelectasis. A blockage may be due to a foreign object (such as an inhaled peanut), a mucus plug, lung cancer, or a poorly placed breathing tube from a ventilator.

When a blockage occurs, the air that's already in the air sacs is absorbed into the bloodstream. New air can't get past the blockage to refill the air sacs, so the affected area of lung deflates.

Who Is at Risk for Atelectasis?

You might be at risk for atelectasis if you can't take deep breaths or cough, or if you have an airway blockage.

Conditions that can increase your risk for atelectasis include:

- Surgery in which you're given medicine to make you sleep. This medicine can decrease or stop your normal effort to breathe and urge to cough.

- Any condition or factor that causes pain when you breathe. Examples include surgery on your chest or abdomen, trauma, broken ribs, or pleurisy (inflammation of the membrane that surrounds your lungs and lines your chest cavity).

- Being on a ventilator (a machine that supports breathing).
- A blockage in your airway due to a foreign object, a mucus plug, lung cancer, or a poorly placed breathing tube.
- Lung conditions and other medical disorders that affect your ability to breathe deeply or cough. Examples include respiratory distress syndrome, pneumonia, lung cancer, and neuromuscular diseases. Rarely, asthma, COPD (chronic obstructive pulmonary disease), and cystic fibrosis are associated with atelectasis.

People who have one of the conditions above and who smoke or are obese are at greater risk for atelectasis than people who don't smoke or aren't obese.

Infants and toddlers (birth to 3 years old) who have risk factors for atelectasis seem to develop the condition more easily than adults.

What Are the Signs and Symptoms of Atelectasis?

Atelectasis likely won't cause signs or symptoms if it only affects a small area of lung.

If atelectasis affects a large area of lung, especially if it occurs suddenly, it may cause a low level of oxygen in your blood. As a result, you may feel short of breath. Your heart rate and breathing rate may increase, and your skin and lips may turn blue.

Other symptoms might be related to the underlying cause of the atelectasis (for example, chest pain due to surgery).

If your child has atelectasis, you may notice that he or she seems agitated, anxious, or scared.

How Is Atelectasis Diagnosed?

Your doctor will diagnose atelectasis based on your signs and symptoms and the results from tests and procedures. Atelectasis might be detected as a result of a chest X-ray done for an underlying lung condition.

Atelectasis usually is diagnosed by a radiologist, pulmonologist (lung specialist), emergency medicine physician, or a primary care doctor (such as a pediatrician, internal medicine specialist, or family practitioner).

Diagnostic Tests and Procedures

The most common test used to diagnose atelectasis is a chest X-ray. A chest X-ray is a painless test that creates pictures of the structures inside your chest, such as your heart, lungs, and blood vessels.

Your doctor also may recommend a chest computed tomography scan, or chest CT scan. This test creates precise pictures of the structures in your chest. A chest CT scan is a type of X-ray. However, the pictures from a chest CT scan show more details than pictures from a standard chest X-ray.

Atelectasis often resolves without treatment. If the condition is severe or lasts a long time and your doctor thinks it's caused by an airway blockage, he or she may use bronchoscopy. This procedure is used to look inside your airway.

During the procedure, your doctor passes a thin, flexible tube called a bronchoscope through your nose (or sometimes your mouth), down your throat, and into your airway. If you have a breathing tube, the bronchoscope can be passed through the tube to your airway.

A light and small camera on the bronchoscope allow your doctor to see inside your airway. Your doctor also can remove blockages during the procedure.

How Is Atelectasis Treated?

The main goals of treating atelectasis are to treat the cause of the condition and to re-expand the collapsed lung tissue. Treatment may vary based on the underlying cause of the atelectasis.

Atelectasis Caused by Surgery

If atelectasis is caused by surgery, your doctor may recommend that you take the following steps to fully expand your lungs:

- Perform deep breathing exercises. This is very important after surgery. While in the hospital, you may use a device called an incentive spirometer. This device measures how much air you're breathing in and how fast you're breathing in. Using this device encourages you to breathe in deeply and slowly.

- Change your position. Sit up or walk around as soon as possible after surgery with your doctor's permission.

- Make an effort to cough. Coughing helps clear mucus and other substances from your airways.

Your doctor also may suggest using positive end-expiratory pressure (PEEP) or continuous positive airway pressure (CPAP). Both devices use mild air pressure to help keep the airways and air sacs open.

Atelectasis Caused by Pressure from outside the Lungs

If pressure from outside the lungs causes atelectasis, your doctor will treat the cause of the pressure. For example, if the cause is a tumor or fluid buildup, your doctor will remove the tumor or fluid. This will allow your lung to fully expand.

Atelectasis Caused by a Blockage

If a blockage causes atelectasis, you'll receive treatment to remove the blockage or relieve it. If the blockage is from an inhaled object, such as a peanut, your doctor will remove it during bronchoscopy.

If a mucus plug is blocking your airways, your doctor may use suction to remove it. Other treatments also can help clear excess mucus from the lungs, such as:

- **Chest clapping or percussion**. This treatment involves pounding your chest and back over and over with your hands or a device to loosen the mucus from your lungs so you can cough it up.
- **Postural drainage**. For this treatment, your bed may be tilted so that your head is lower than your chest. This allows mucus to drain more easily.
- **Medicines**. Your doctor may prescribe medicines to help open your airways or to loosen mucus.

Atelectasis Caused by a Lung Condition or Other Medical Disorder

If a lung condition or other medical disorder causes atelectasis, your doctor will treat the underlying cause with medicines, procedures, or other therapies.

How Can Atelectasis Be Prevented?

Not smoking before surgery can lower your risk of atelectasis. If you smoke, ask your doctor how far in advance of your surgery you should quit smoking.

After surgery, your doctor may recommend that you take the following steps to fully expand your lungs:

- **Perform deep breathing exercises**. These exercises are very important after surgery. While in the hospital, you may use a device called an incentive spirometer. This device measures how much air you're breathing in and how fast you're breathing in. Using this device encourages you to breathe deeply and slowly.

- **Change your position**. Sit up or walk around as soon as possible after surgery (with your doctor's permission).

- **Make an effort to cough**. Coughing helps clear mucus and other substances from your airways.

If deep breathing is painful, your doctor may prescribe medicines to control the pain. This can make it easier for you to take deep breaths and fully expand your lungs.

Your doctor also might suggest using positive end-expiratory pressure (PEEP) or continuous positive airway pressure (CPAP). Both devices use mild air pressure to help keep the airways and air sacs open.

Section 26.4

Lung Transplant

This section includes text excerpted from "Lung Transplant," National Heart, Lung, and Blood Institute (NHLBI), December 9, 2016.

Lung transplant is surgery to remove a diseased lung and replace it with a healthy lung. Lung transplants are used to improve the quality of life and extend the lifespan for people who have severe or advanced chronic lung conditions. In rare instances, a lung transplant may be performed at the same time as a heart transplant in patients who have severe heart and lung disease.

Eligibility for Lung Transplant Surgery

You may be eligible for lung transplant surgery if you have severe lung disease that does not respond to other treatments. If you are otherwise healthy enough for surgery, you will be placed on the National Organ Procurement and Transplantation Network's (OPTN) waiting list. This network handles the nation's organ-sharing process. If a match is found, you will need to have your lung transplant surgery right away.

The Procedure

This surgery will be performed in a hospital. You will have general anesthesia and will not be awake for the surgery. Tubes will help you breathe, give you medicine, and help with other bodily functions. A surgeon will open your chest, cut the main airway and blood vessels, and remove your diseased lung. The surgeon will connect the healthy donor lung, reconnect the blood vessels, and close your chest.

Recovering from Surgery

After the surgery, you will recover in the hospital's intensive care unit (ICU) before moving to a hospital room for one to three weeks. Your doctor may recommend pulmonary rehabilitation after your lung transplant surgery to help you regain and improve your breathing. Pulmonary rehabilitation may include exercise training, education, and counseling. Pulmonary function tests will help doctors monitor your breathing and recovery. After leaving the hospital, you will visit your doctor often to check for infection or rejection of your new lung, to test your lung function, and to make sure that you are recovering well.

The first year after lung transplant surgery is when you are most at risk for possibly life-threatening complications such as rejection and infection. To help prevent rejection, you will need to take medicines for the rest of your life that suppress your immune system and help prevent your body from rejecting your new lungs. These important medicines weaken your immune system and increase your chance for infections, and over time they can increase your risk for cancer, diabetes, osteoporosis, and kidney damage. Practicing good hygiene, obtaining routine vaccines, and adopting healthy lifestyle choices such as heart-healthy eating and not smoking are very important. Getting emotional support and following your doctor's advice will help you recover and stay as healthy as possible.

Chapter 27

Heart and Vascular Surgery

Chapter Contents

Section 27.1

An Overview of Heart Surgery

This section includes text excerpted from "Heart Surgery," National
Heart, Lung, and Blood Institute (NHLBI), November 8, 2013.
Reviewed June 2017.

Heart Surgery

Heart surgery is done to correct problems with the heart. Many
heart surgeries are done each year in the United States for various
heart problems.

Heart surgery is used for both children and adults. This section
discusses heart surgery for adults.

The most common type of heart surgery for adults is coronary artery
bypass grafting (CABG). During CABG, a healthy artery or vein from
the body is connected, or grafted, to a blocked coronary (heart) artery.

The grafted artery or vein bypasses (that is, goes around) the
blocked portion of the coronary artery. This creates a new path for
oxygen-rich blood to flow to the heart muscle. CABG can relieve chest
pain and may lower your risk of having a heart attack.

Doctors also use heart surgery to:

- Repair or replace heart valves, which control blood flow through
  the heart

- Repair abnormal or damaged structures in the heart

- Implant medical devices that help control the heartbeat or support heart function and blood flow

- Replace a damaged heart with a healthy heart from a donor

Traditional heart surgery, often called open-heart surgery, is done
by opening the chest wall to operate on the heart. The surgeon cuts
through the patient's breastbone (or just the upper part of it) to open
the chest.

Once the heart is exposed, the patient is connected to a heart-
lung bypass machine. The machine takes over the heart's pumping
action and moves blood away from the heart. This allows the surgeon

to operate on a heart that isn't beating and that doesn't have blood flowing through it.

Another type of heart surgery is called off-pump, or beating heart, surgery. It's like traditional open-heart surgery because the chest bone is opened to access the heart. However, the heart isn't stopped, and a heart-lung bypass machine isn't used. Off-pump heart surgery is limited to CABG.

Surgeons can now make small incisions (cuts) between the ribs to do some types of heart surgery. The breastbone is not opened to reach the heart. This is called minimally invasive heart surgery. This type of heart surgery may or may not use a heart-lung bypass machine.

Newer methods of heart surgery (such as off-pump and minimally invasive) may reduce risks and speed up recovery time. Studies are underway to compare these types of heart surgery with traditional open-heart surgery.

The results of these studies will help doctors decide the best surgery to use for each patient.

The results of heart surgery in adults often are excellent. Heart surgery can reduce symptoms, improve quality of life, and improve the chances of survival.

Types of Heart Surgery

Coronary Artery Bypass Grafting

CABG is the most common type of heart surgery. CABG improves blood flow to the heart. Surgeons use CABG to treat people who have severe coronary heart disease (CHD).

CHD is a disease in which a waxy substance called plaque builds up inside the coronary arteries. These arteries supply oxygen-rich blood to your heart.

Over time, plaque can harden or rupture (break open). Hardened plaque narrows the coronary arteries and reduces the flow of oxygen-rich blood to the heart. This can cause chest pain or discomfort called angina.

If the plaque ruptures, a blood clot can form on its surface. A large blood clot can mostly or completely block blood flow through a coronary artery. This is the most common cause of a heart attack. Over time, ruptured plaque also hardens and narrows the coronary arteries.

During CABG, a healthy artery or vein from the body is connected, or grafted, to the blocked coronary artery. The grafted artery or vein bypasses (that is, goes around) the blocked portion of the coronary artery. This creates a new path for oxygen-rich blood to flow to the heart muscle.

Surgeons can bypass multiple blocked coronary arteries during one surgery.

CABG isn't the only treatment for CHD. A nonsurgical procedure that opens blocked or narrow coronary arteries is percutaneous coronary intervention (PCI), also known as coronary angioplasty.

During PCI, a thin, flexible tube with a balloon at its tip is threaded through a blood vessel to the narrow or blocked coronary artery. Once in place, the balloon is inflated to push the plaque against the artery wall. This restores blood flow through the artery.

During PCI, a stent might be placed in the coronary artery to help keep it open. A stent is a small mesh tube that supports the inner artery wall.

If both CABG and PCI are options, your doctor can help you decide which treatment is right for you.

Transmyocardial Laser Revascularization

Transmyocardial laser revascularization, or TMR, is surgery used to treat angina.

TMR is most often used when no other treatments work. For example, if you've already had one CABG procedure and can't have another one, TMR might be an option. For some people, TMR is combined with CABG.

If TMR is done alone, the procedure may be performed through a small opening in the chest.

During TMR, a surgeon uses lasers to make small channels through the heart muscle and into the heart's lower left chamber (the left ventricle).

It isn't fully known how TMR relieves angina. The surgery may help the heart grow tiny new blood vessels. Oxygen-rich blood may flow through these vessels into the heart muscle, which could relieve angina.

Heart Valve Repair or Replacement

For the heart to work well, blood must flow in only one direction. The heart's valves make this possible. Healthy valves open and close in a precise way as the heart pumps blood.

Each valve has a set of flaps called leaflets. The leaflets open to allow blood to pass from one heart chamber into another or into the arteries. Then the leaflets close tightly to stop blood from flowing backward.

Heart surgery is used to fix leaflets that don't open as wide as they should. This can happen if they become thick or stiff or fuse together. As a result, not enough blood flows through the valve.

Heart surgery also is used to fix leaflets that don't close tightly. This problem can cause blood to leak back into the heart chambers, rather than only moving forward into the arteries as it should.

To fix these problems, surgeons either repair the valve or replace it with a man-made or biological valve. Biological valves are made from pig, cow, or human heart tissue and may have man-made parts as well.

To repair a mitral or pulmonary valve that's too narrow, a cardiologist (heart specialist) will insert a catheter (a thin, flexible tube) through a large blood vessel and guide it to the heart.

The cardiologist will place the end of the catheter inside the narrow valve. He or she will inflate and deflate a small balloon at the tip of the catheter. This widens the valve, allowing more blood to flow through it. This approach is less invasive than open-heart surgery.

Researchers also are testing new ways to use catheters in other types of valve surgeries. For example, catheters might be used to place clips on the mitral valve leaflets to hold them in place.

Catheters also might be used to replace faulty aortic valves. For this procedure, the catheter usually is inserted into an artery in the groin (upper thigh) and threaded to the heart.

In some cases, surgeons might make a small cut in the chest and left ventricle (the lower left heart chamber). They will thread the catheter into the heart through the small opening.

The catheter has a deflated balloon at its tip with a folded replacement valve around it. The balloon is used to expand the new valve so it fits securely within the old valve.

Currently, surgery to replace the valve is the traditional treatment for reasonably healthy people. However, catheter procedures might be a safer option for patients who have conditions that make open-heart surgery very risky.

Arrhythmia Treatment

An arrhythmia is a problem with the rate or rhythm of the heartbeat. During an arrhythmia, the heart can beat too fast, too slow, or with an irregular rhythm.

Many arrhythmias are harmless, but some can be serious or even life threatening. If the heart rate is abnormal, the heart may not be

307

able to pump enough blood to the body. Lack of blood flow can damage the brain, heart, and other organs.

Medicine usually is the first line of treatment for arrhythmias. If medicine doesn't work well, your doctor may recommend surgery. For example, surgery may be used to implant a pacemaker or an implantable cardioverter defibrillator (ICD).

A pacemaker is a small device that's placed under the skin of your chest or abdomen. Wires connect the pacemaker to your heart chambers. The device uses low-energy electrical pulses to control your heart rhythm. Most pacemakers have a sensor that starts the device only if your heart rhythm is abnormal.

An ICD is another small device that's placed under the skin of your chest or abdomen. This device also is connected to your heart with wires. An ICD checks your heartbeat for dangerous arrhythmias. If the device senses one, it sends an electric shock to your heart to restore a normal heart rhythm.

Another arrhythmia treatment is called maze surgery. For this surgery, the surgeon makes new paths for the heart's electrical signals to travel through. This type of surgery is used to treat atrial fibrillation, the most common type of serious arrhythmia.

Simpler, less invasive procedures also are used to treat atrial fibrillation. These procedures use high heat or intense cold to prevent abnormal electrical signals from moving through the heart.

Aneurysm Repair

An aneurysm is a balloon-like bulge in the wall of an artery or the heart muscle. This bulge can occur if the artery wall weakens. Pressure from blood moving through the artery or heart causes the weak area to bulge.

Over time, an aneurysm can grow and burst, causing dangerous, often fatal bleeding inside the body. Aneurysms also can develop a split in one or more layers of the artery wall. The split causes bleeding into and along the layers of the artery wall.

Aneurysms in the heart most often occur in the heart's lower left chamber (the left ventricle). Repairing an aneurysm involves surgery to replace the weak section of the artery or heart wall with a patch or graft.

Heart Transplant

A heart transplant is surgery to remove a person's diseased heart and replace it with a healthy heart from a deceased donor. Most heart transplants are done on patients who have end-stage heart failure.

Heart failure is a condition in which the heart is damaged or weak. As a result, it can't pump enough blood to meet the body's needs. "End-stage" means the condition is so severe that all treatments, other than heart transplant, have failed.

Patients on the waiting list for a donor heart receive ongoing treatment for heart failure and other medical conditions. Ventricular assist devices (VADs) or total artificial hearts (TAHs) might be used to treat these patients.

Surgery To Place Ventricular Assist Devices or Total Artificial Hearts

A VAD is a mechanical pump that is used to support heart function and blood flow in people who have weak hearts.

Your doctor may recommend a VAD if you have heart failure that isn't responding to treatment or if you're waiting for a heart transplant. You can use a VAD for a short time or for months or years, depending on your situation.

A TAH is a device that replaces the two lower chambers of the heart (the ventricles). You may benefit from a TAH if both of your ventricles don't work well due to end-stage heart failure.

Placing either device requires open-heart surgery.

Surgical Approaches

Surgeons can use different approaches to operate on the heart, including open-heart surgery, off-pump heart surgery, and minimally invasive heart surgery.

The surgical approach will depend on the patient's heart problem, general health, and other factors.

Open-Heart Surgery

Open-heart surgery is any kind of surgery in which a surgeon makes a large incision (cut) in the chest to open the rib cage and operate on the heart. "Open" refers to the chest, not the heart. Depending on the type of surgery, the surgeon also may open the heart.

Once the heart is exposed, the patient is connected to a heart-lung bypass machine. The machine takes over the heart's pumping action and moves blood away from the heart. This allows the surgeon to operate on a heart that isn't beating and that doesn't have blood flowing through it.

309

Open-heart surgery is used to do CABG, repair or replace heart valves, treat atrial fibrillation, do heart transplants, and place VADs and TAHs.

Off-Pump Heart Surgery

Surgeons also use off-pump, or beating heart, surgery to do CABG. This approach is like traditional open-heart surgery because the chest bone is opened to access the heart. However, the heart isn't stopped, and a heart-lung bypass machine isn't used.

Off-pump heart surgery isn't right for all patients. Work with your doctor to decide whether this type of surgery is an option for you. Your doctor will carefully consider your heart problem, age, overall health, and other factors that may affect the surgery.

Minimally Invasive Heart Surgery

For minimally invasive heart surgery, a surgeon makes small incisions (cuts) in the side of the chest between the ribs. This type of surgery may or may not use a heart-lung bypass machine.

Minimally invasive heart surgery is used to do some bypass and maze surgeries. It's also used to repair or replace heart valves, insert pacemakers or ICDs, or take a vein or artery from the body to use as a bypass graft for CABG.

One type of minimally invasive heart surgery that is becoming more common is robotic-assisted surgery. For this surgery, a surgeon uses a computer to control surgical tools on thin robotic arms.

The tools are inserted through small incisions in the chest. This allows the surgeon to do complex and highly precise surgery. The surgeon always is in total control of the robotic arms; they don't move on their own.

Who Needs Heart Surgery?

Heart surgery is used to treat many heart problems. For example, it's used to:

- Treat heart failure and coronary heart disease (CHD)

- Fix heart valves that don't work well

- Control abnormal heart rhythms

- Place medical devices

- Replace a damaged heart with a healthy one

If other treatments—such as lifestyle changes, medicines, and medical procedures—haven't worked or can't be used, heart surgery might be an option.

Specialists Involved

Your primary care doctor, a cardiologist, and a cardiothoracic surgeon will work with you to decide whether you need heart surgery.

A cardiologist specializes in diagnosing and treating heart problems. A cardiothoracic surgeon specializes in surgery on the heart and lungs.

These doctors will talk with you and do tests to learn about your general health and your heart problem. They'll discuss the test results with you and help you make decisions about the surgery.

Medical Evaluation

Your doctors will talk with you about:

- The kind of heart problem you have and the symptoms it's causing. Your doctor may ask you how long you've had symptoms.
- Your past treatment of heart problems, including surgeries, procedures, and medicines.
- Your family's history of heart problems.
- Your history of other health problems, such as diabetes or high blood pressure.
- Your age and general health.

You also may have blood tests, such as a complete blood count, a lipoprotein panel (cholesterol test), and other tests as needed.

Diagnostic Tests

Tests are done to find out more about your heart problem and your general health. This helps your doctors decide whether you need heart surgery, what type of surgery you need, and when to do it.

EKG (Electrocardiogram)

An EKG is a painless, noninvasive test that records the heart's electrical activity. "Noninvasive" means that no surgery is done and no instruments are inserted into your body.

The test shows how fast the heart is beating and its rhythm (steady or irregular). An EKG also records the strength and timing of electrical signals as they pass through the heart.

An EKG can show signs of heart damage due to CHD and signs of a previous or current heart attack.

Stress Test

Some heart problems are easier to diagnose when your heart is working hard and beating fast. During stress testing, you exercise to make your heart work hard and beat fast. If you can't exercise, you may be given medicine to raise your heart rate.

As part of the test, your blood pressure is checked and an EKG is done. Other heart tests also might be done.

Echocardiography

Echocardiography (echo) is a painless, noninvasive test. This test uses sound waves to create a moving picture of your heart. Echocardiography shows the size and shape of your heart and how well your heart chambers and valves are working.

The test also can show areas of poor blood flow to your heart, areas of heart muscle that aren't working well, and previous injury to your heart muscle caused by poor blood flow.

Coronary Angiography

Coronary angiography is a test that uses dye and special X-rays to show the insides of your coronary arteries.

To get the dye into your coronary arteries, your doctor will use a procedure called cardiac catheterization.

A thin, flexible tube called a catheter is put into a blood vessel in your arm, groin (upper thigh), or neck. The tube is threaded into your coronary arteries, and the dye is released into your bloodstream.

Special X-rays are taken while the dye is flowing through the coronary arteries. These X-rays are called angiograms.

The dye lets your doctor study blood flow through the heart and blood vessels. This helps your doctor find blockages that can cause a heart attack.

Aortogram

An aortogram is an angiogram of the aorta. The aorta is the main artery that carries blood from your heart to your body. An aortogram may show the location and size of an aortic aneurysm.

Chest X-Ray

A chest X-ray creates pictures of the structures inside your chest, such as your heart, lungs, and blood vessels.

This test gives your doctor information about the size and shape of your heart. A chest X-ray also shows the position and shape of the large arteries around your heart.

Cardiac Computed Tomography Scan

A cardiac computed tomography scan, or cardiac CT scan, is a painless test that uses an X-ray machine to take clear, detailed pictures of the heart.

Sometimes an iodine-based dye (contrast dye) is injected into one of your veins during the scan. The contrast dye highlights your coronary (heart) arteries on the X-ray pictures. This type of CT scan is called a coronary CT angiography, or CTA.

A cardiac CT scan can show whether plaque is narrowing your coronary arteries or whether you have an aneurysm. A CT scan also can find problems with the heart's function and valves.

Cardiac Magnetic Resonance Imaging

Magnetic resonance imaging (MRI) is a safe, noninvasive test that uses magnets, radio waves, and a computer to create pictures of your organs and tissues.

Cardiac MRI creates images of your heart as it is beating. The computer makes both still and moving pictures of your heart and major blood vessels.

Cardiac MRI shows the structure and function of your heart. This test can show the size and location of an aneurysm.

What to Expect before Heart Surgery

There are many types of heart surgery. One person's experience before surgery can be very different from another's.

Some people carefully plan their surgeries with their doctors. They know exactly when and how their surgeries will happen. Other people need emergency heart surgery. For example, they might be diagnosed with blocked coronary arteries and admitted to the hospital right away for surgery.

If you're having a planned surgery, your doctors and others on your healthcare team will meet with you to explain what will

313

happen. They'll tell you how to prepare for the surgery. You might be admitted to the hospital the afternoon or morning before your surgery.

You may have some tests before the surgery, such as an EKG (electrocardiogram), chest X-ray, or blood tests. An intravenous (IV) line will be placed into a blood vessel in your arm or chest to give you fluids and medicines.

A member of your healthcare team may shave the area where your surgeon will make the incision (cut). Also, your skin might be washed with special soap to reduce the risk of infection.

Just before the surgery, you'll be moved to the operating room. You'll be given medicine so that you fall asleep and don't feel pain during the surgery.

What to Expect during Heart Surgery

Heart surgery is done in a hospital, and a team of experts is involved. Cardiothoracic surgeons perform the surgery with other doctors and nurses who help.

How long the surgery takes will depend on the type of surgery you're having. CABG, the most common type of heart surgery, takes about 3–6 hours.

Traditional Open-Heart Surgery

For this type of surgery, you'll be given medicine to help you fall asleep. A doctor will check your heartbeat, blood pressure, oxygen levels, and breathing during the surgery.

A breathing tube will be placed in your lungs through your throat. The tube will connect to a ventilator (a machine that supports breathing).

Your surgeon will make a 6 to 8-inch incision (cut) down the center of your chest wall. Then, he or she will cut your breastbone and open your rib cage to reach your heart.

During the surgery, you'll receive medicine to thin your blood and keep it from clotting. A heart-lung bypass machine will be connected to your heart. The machine will take over your heart's pumping action and move blood away from your heart.

A specialist will oversee the heart-lung bypass machine. The machine will allow the surgeon to operate on a heart that isn't beating and that doesn't have blood flowing through it.

Heart-Lung Bypass Machine

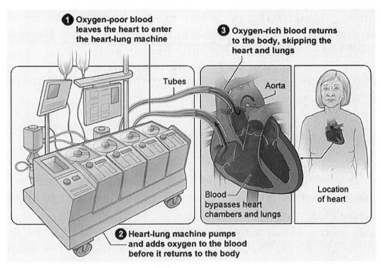

Figure 27.1. *Heart-Lung Bypass Machine*

The image shows how a heart-lung bypass machine works during surgery.

You'll be given medicine to stop your heartbeat once you're connected to the heart-lung bypass machine. A tube will be placed in your heart to drain blood to the machine.

The machine will remove carbon dioxide (a waste product) from your blood, add oxygen to your blood, and then pump the blood back into your body. Your surgeon will insert tubes into your chest to drain fluid.

Once the bypass machine starts to work, the surgeon will repair your heart problem. After the surgery is done, he or she will restore blood flow to your heart. Usually, your heart will start beating again on its own. Sometimes mild electric shocks are used to restart the heart.

Once your heart has started beating again, your surgeon will remove the tubes and stop the heart-lung bypass machine. You'll be given medicine to allow your blood to clot again.

The surgeon will use wires to close your breastbone. The wires will stay in your body permanently. After your breastbone heals, it will be as strong as it was before the surgery.

Stitches or staples will be used to close the skin incision. Your breathing tube will be removed when you're able to breathe without it.

Off-Pump Heart Surgery

Off-pump heart surgery is like traditional open-heart surgery because the chest bone is opened to access the heart. However, the heart isn't stopped, and a heart-lung bypass machine isn't used.

Instead, your surgeon will steady your heart with a mechanical device so he or she can work on it. Your heart will continue to pump blood to your body.

Minimally Invasive Heart Surgery

For this type of heart surgery, your surgeon will make small incisions in the side of your chest between the ribs. These cuts can be as small as 2–3 inches. The surgeon will insert surgical tools through these small cuts.

A tool with a small video camera at the tip also will be inserted through an incision. This tool will allow the surgeon to see inside your body.

Some types of minimally invasive heart surgery use a heart-lung bypass machine and others don't.

What to Expect after Heart Surgery

Recovery in the Hospital

You may spend a day or more in the hospital's intensive care unit (ICU), depending on the type of heart surgery you have. An intravenous (IV) needle might be inserted in a blood vessel in your arm or chest to give you fluids until you're ready to drink on your own.

Your healthcare team may give you extra oxygen through a face mask or nasal prongs that fit just inside your nose. They will remove the mask or prongs when you no longer need them.

When you leave the ICU, you'll be moved to another part of the hospital for several days before you go home. While you're in the hospital, doctors and nurses will closely watch your heart rate, blood pressure, breathing, and incision site(s).

Recovery at Home

People respond differently to heart surgery. Your recovery at home will depend on what kind of heart problem and surgery you had. Your doctor will tell you how to:

- Care for your healing incision(s)

- Recognize signs of infection or other complications
- Cope with the after-effects of surgery

You also will get information about follow-up appointments, medicines, and situations when you should call your doctor right away.

After-effects of heart surgery are normal. They may include muscle pain, chest pain, or swelling (especially if you have an incision in your leg from coronary artery bypass grafting, or CABG).

Other after-effects may include loss of appetite, problems sleeping, constipation, and mood swings and depression. After-effects usually go away over time.

Recovery time after heart surgery depends on the type of surgery you had, your overall health before the surgery, and any complications from the surgery.

Your doctor will let you know when you can go back to your daily routine, such as working, driving, and physical activity.

Ongoing Care

Ongoing care after your surgery will include checkups with your doctor. During these visits, you may have blood tests, an EKG (electrocardiogram), echocardiography, or a stress test. These tests will show how your heart is working after the surgery.

After some types of heart surgery, you'll need to take a blood-thinning medicine. Your doctor will do routine tests to make sure you're getting the right amount of medicine.

Your doctor also may recommend lifestyle changes and medicines to help you stay healthy. Lifestyle changes may include quitting smoking, changing your diet, being physically active, and reducing and managing stress.

Your doctor also may refer you to cardiac rehabilitation (rehab). Cardiac rehab is a medically supervised program that helps improve the health and well-being of people who have heart problems.

Cardiac rehab includes exercise training, education on heart healthy living, and counseling to reduce stress and help you recover. Your doctor can tell you where to find a cardiac rehab program near your home.

What Are the Risks of Heart Surgery?

Heart surgery has risks, even though its results often are excellent. Risks include:

- bleeding

- infection, fever, swelling, and other signs of inflammation

- a reaction to the medicine used to make you sleep during the surgery

- arrhythmias (irregular heartbeats)

- damage to tissues in the heart, kidneys, liver, and lungs

- stroke, which may cause short-term or permanent damage

- death (Heart surgery is more likely to be life threatening in people who are very sick before the surgery.)

Memory loss and other issues, such as problems concentrating or thinking clearly, may occur in some people.

These problems are more likely to affect older patients and women. These issues often improve within 6–12 months of surgery.

In general, the risk of complications is higher if heart surgery is done in an emergency situation (for example, during a heart attack). The risk also is higher if you have other diseases or conditions, such as diabetes, kidney disease, lung disease, or peripheral artery disease (P.A.D.).

Section 27.2

Percutaneous Coronary Intervention (Coronary Angioplasty)

This section includes text excerpted from "Percutaneous Coronary Intervention," National Heart, Lung, and Blood Institute (NHLBI), December 9, 2016.

Percutaneous coronary intervention (PCI), also known as coronary angioplasty, is a nonsurgical procedure that improves blood flow to your heart. PCI requires cardiac catheterization, which is the insertion of a catheter tube and injection of contrast dye, usually iodine-based, into your coronary arteries. Doctors use PCI to open coronary arteries that are narrowed or blocked by the buildup of atherosclerotic plaque.

PCI may be used to relieve symptoms of coronary heart disease or to reduce heart damage during or after a heart attack.

The Procedure

A cardiologist, or doctor who specializes in the heart, will perform PCI in a hospital cardiac catheterization laboratory. You will stay awake, but you will be given medicine to relax you. Before your procedure, you will receive medicines through an intravenous (IV) line in your arm to prevent blood clots. Your doctor will clean and numb an area on the wrist or groin where your doctor will make a small hole and insert the catheter into your blood vessel. Live X-rays will help your doctor guide the catheter into your heart to inject special contrast dye that will highlight the blockage. To open a blocked artery, your doctor will insert another catheter over a guidewire and inflate a balloon at the tip of that catheter. Your doctor may put a small mesh tube called a stent in your artery to help keep the artery open.

Recovering from Surgery

After PCI, your doctor will remove the catheters and close and bandage the opening on your wrist or groin. You may develop a bruise and soreness where the catheters were inserted. It also is common to have discomfort or bleeding where the catheters were inserted. You will recover in a special unit of the hospital for a few hours or overnight. You will get instructions on how much activity you can do and what medicines to take. You will need a ride home because of the medicines or anesthesia you received. Your doctor will check your progress during a follow-up visit. If a stent is implanted, you will have to take special anticlotting medicines exactly as prescribed, usually for at least three to 12 months.

Serious complications from PCI don't occur often, but they can happen. These complications may include bleeding, blood vessel damage, a treatable allergic reaction to the contrast dye, the need for emergency coronary artery bypass grafting during the procedure, arrhythmias, damaged arteries, kidney damage, heart attack, stroke, or blood clots. Sometimes chest pain can occur during PCI because the balloon briefly blocks blood supply to the heart. Restenosis, or tissue regrowth in the treated portion of the artery, may occur in the following months and cause the artery to become narrow or blocked again. The risk of complications is higher if you are older, have chronic kidney disease, are experiencing heart failure at the time of the procedure, or have extensive heart disease and multiple blockages in your coronary arteries.

Section 27.3

Coronary Artery Bypass Grafting Surgery

This section includes text excerpted from "Coronary
Artery Bypass Grafting," National Heart, Lung, and Blood
Institute (NHLBI), February 23, 2012. Reviewed June 2017.

Coronary artery bypass grafting (CABG) is a type of surgery that
improves blood flow to the heart. Surgeons use CABG to treat people
who have severe coronary heart disease (CHD).

CHD is a disease in which a waxy substance called plaque builds
up inside the coronary arteries. These arteries supply oxygen-rich
blood to your heart.

Over time, plaque can harden or rupture (break open). Hardened
plaque narrows the coronary arteries and reduces the flow of oxygen-rich blood to the heart. This can cause chest pain or discomfort
called angina.

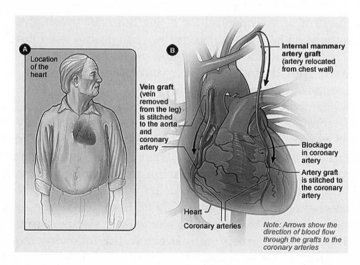

Figure 27.2. *Coronary Artery Bypass Grafting*

*Figure A shows the location of the heart. Figure B shows how vein and artery bypass
grafts are attached to the heart.*

If the plaque ruptures, a blood clot can form on its surface. A large blood clot can mostly or completely block blood flow through a coronary artery. This is the most common cause of a heart attack. Over time, ruptured plaque also hardens and narrows the coronary arteries.

CABG is one treatment for CHD. During CABG, a healthy artery or vein from the body is connected, or grafted, to the blocked coronary artery. The grafted artery or vein bypasses (that is, goes around) the blocked portion of the coronary artery. This creates a new path for oxygen-rich blood to flow to the heart muscle.

Surgeons can bypass multiple coronary arteries during one surgery.

Types of Coronary Artery Bypass Grafting

There are several types of CABG. Your doctor will recommend the best option for you based on your needs.

Traditional Coronary Artery Bypass Grafting

Traditional CABG is used when at least one major artery needs to be bypassed. During the surgery, the chest bone is opened to access the heart.

Medicines are given to stop the heart; a heart-lung bypass machine keeps blood and oxygen moving throughout the body during surgery. This allows the surgeon to operate on a still heart.

After surgery, blood flow to the heart is restored. Usually, the heart starts beating again on its own. Sometimes mild electric shocks are used to restart the heart.

Off-Pump Coronary Artery Bypass Grafting

This type of CABG is similar to traditional CABG because the chest bone is opened to access the heart. However, the heart isn't stopped, and a heart-lung bypass machine isn't used. Off-pump CABG sometimes is called beating heart bypass grafting.

Minimally Invasive Direct Coronary Artery Bypass Grafting

This type of surgery differs from traditional CABG because the chest bone isn't opened to reach the heart. Instead, several small cuts are made on the left side of the chest between the ribs. This type of surgery mainly is used to bypass blood vessels at the front of the heart.

Minimally invasive bypass grafting is a fairly new procedure. It isn't right for everyone, especially if more than one or two coronary arteries need to be bypassed.

Who Needs Coronary Artery Bypass Grafting?

CABG is used to treat people who have severe CHD that could lead to a heart attack. CABG also might be used during or after a heart attack to treat blocked arteries.

Your doctor may recommend CABG if other treatments, such as lifestyle changes or medicines, haven't worked. He or she also may recommend CABG if you have severe blockages in your large coronary (heart) arteries, especially if your heart's pumping action has already grown weak.

CABG also might be a treatment option if you have blockages in your coronary arteries that can't be treated with percutaneous coronary intervention (PCI), also known as coronary angioplasty.

Your doctor will decide whether you're a candidate for CABG based on factors such as:

- The presence and severity of CHD symptoms

- The severity and location of blockages in your coronary arteries

- Your response to other treatments

- Your quality of life

- Any other medical problems you have

Physical Exam and Diagnostic Tests

To find out whether you're a candidate for CABG, your doctor will give you a physical exam. He or she will check your heart, lungs, and pulse.

Your doctor also may ask you about any symptoms you have, such as chest pain or shortness of breath. He or she will want to know how often and for how long your symptoms occur, as well as how severe they are.

Your doctor will recommend tests to find out which arteries are clogged, how much they're clogged, and whether you have any heart damage.

EKG (Electrocardiogram)

An EKG is a simple test that detects and records your heart's electrical activity. The test shows how fast the heart is beating and its rhythm (steady or irregular). An EKG also records the strength and timing of electrical signals as they pass through each part of the heart.

An EKG can show signs of heart damage due to CHD and signs of a previous or current heart attack.

Echocardiography

Echocardiography (echo) uses sound waves to create a moving picture of your heart. The test shows the size and shape of your heart and how well your heart chambers and valves are working.

Echo also can show areas of poor blood flow to the heart, areas of heart muscle that aren't contracting normally, and previous injury to the heart muscle caused by poor blood flow.

There are several types of echo, including stress echo. This test is done both before and after a stress test. A stress echo usually is done to find out whether you have decreased blood flow to your heart, a sign of CHD.

Stress Test

Some heart problems are easier to diagnose when your heart is working hard and beating fast.

During stress testing, you exercise to make your heart work hard and beat fast while heart tests are done. If you can't exercise, you may be given medicine to raise your heart rate.

The heart tests done during stress testing may include nuclear heart scanning, echo, and positron emission tomography (PET) scanning of the heart.

Coronary Angiography and Cardiac Catheterization

Coronary angiography is a test that uses dye and special X-rays to show the insides of your coronary arteries.

To get the dye into your coronary arteries, your doctor will use a procedure called cardiac catheterization.

A thin, flexible tube called a catheter is put into a blood vessel in your arm, groin (upper thigh), or neck. The tube is threaded into your coronary arteries, and the dye is released into your bloodstream.

Special X-rays are taken while the dye is flowing through the coronary arteries. The dye lets your doctor study blood flow through the heart and blood vessels. This helps your doctor find blockages that can cause a heart attack.

Other Considerations

When deciding whether you're a candidate for CABG, your doctor also will consider your:

- History and past treatment of heart disease, including surgeries, procedures, and medicines
- History of other diseases and conditions
- Age and general health
- Family history of CHD, heart attack, or other heart diseases

Your doctor may recommend medicines and other medical procedures before CABG. For example, he or she may prescribe medicines to lower your cholesterol and blood pressure and improve blood flow through your coronary arteries.

PCI also might be tried. During this procedure, a thin, flexible tube with a balloon at its tip is threaded through a blood vessel to the narrow or blocked coronary artery.

Once in place, the balloon is inflated, pushing the plaque against the artery wall. This creates a wider path for blood to flow to the heart.

Sometimes a stent is placed in the artery during PCI. A stent is a small mesh tube that supports the inner artery wall.

Before Coronary Artery Bypass Grafting

You may have tests to prepare you for CABG. For example, you may have blood tests, an EKG (electrocardiogram), echocardiography, a chest X-ray, cardiac catheterization, and coronary angiography.

Your doctor will tell you how to prepare for CABG surgery. He or she will advise you about what you can eat or drink, which medicines to take, and which activities to stop (such as smoking). You'll likely be admitted to the hospital on the same day as the surgery.

If tests for coronary heart disease show that you have severe blockages in your coronary (heart) arteries, your doctor may admit you to the hospital right away. You may have CABG that day or the day after.

During Coronary Artery Bypass Grafting

CABG requires a team of experts. A cardiothoracic surgeon will do the surgery with support from an anesthesiologist, perfusionist (heart-lung bypass machine specialist), other surgeons, and nurses.

There are several types of CABG. They range from traditional surgery to newer, less-invasive methods.

Traditional Coronary Artery Bypass Grafting

This type of surgery usually lasts 3–6 hours, depending on the number of arteries being bypassed. Many steps take place during traditional CABG.

You'll be under general anesthesia for the surgery. The term "anesthesia" refers to a loss of feeling and awareness. General anesthesia temporarily puts you to sleep.

During the surgery, the anesthesiologist will check your heartbeat, blood pressure, oxygen levels, and breathing. A breathing tube will be placed in your lungs through your throat. The tube will connect to a ventilator (a machine that supports breathing).

The surgeon will make an incision (cut) down the center of your chest. He or she will cut your chest bone and open your rib cage to reach your heart.

You'll receive medicines to stop your heart. This allows the surgeon to operate on your heart while it's not beating. You'll also receive medicines to protect your heart function during the time that it's not beating.

A heart-lung bypass machine will keep oxygen-rich blood moving throughout your body during the surgery.

The surgeon will take an artery or vein from your body—for example, from your chest or leg—to use as the bypass graft. For surgeries with several bypasses, both artery and vein grafts are commonly used.

- **Artery grafts.** These grafts are much less likely than vein grafts to become blocked over time. The left internal mammary artery most often is used for an artery graft. This artery is located inside the chest, close to the heart. Arteries from the arm or other places in the body also are used.

- **Vein grafts.** Although veins are commonly used as grafts, they're more likely than artery grafts to become blocked over time. The saphenous vein—a long vein running along the inner side of the leg—typically is used.

When the surgeon finishes the grafting, he or she will restore blood flow to your heart. Usually, the heart starts beating again on its own. Sometimes mild electric shocks are used to restart the heart.

You'll be disconnected from the heart-lung bypass machine. Then, tubes will be inserted into your chest to drain fluid.

The surgeon will use wire to close your chest bone (much like how a broken bone is repaired). The wire will stay in your body permanently. After your chest bone heals, it will be as strong as it was before the surgery.

Stitches or staples will be used to close the skin incision. The breathing tube will be removed when you're able to breathe without it.

Nontraditional Coronary Artery Bypass Grafting

Nontraditional CABG includes off-pump CABG and minimally invasive CABG.

Off-Pump Coronary Artery Bypass Grafting

Surgeons can use off-pump CABG to bypass any of the coronary (heart) arteries. Off-pump CABG is similar to traditional CABG because the chest bone is opened to access the heart.

However, the heart isn't stopped and a heart-lung-bypass machine isn't used. Instead, the surgeon steadies the heart with a mechanical device.

Off-pump CABG sometimes is called beating heart bypass grafting.

Minimally Invasive Direct Coronary Artery Bypass Grafting

There are several types of minimally invasive direct coronary artery bypass (MIDCAB) grafting. These types of surgery differ from traditional bypass surgery because the chest bone isn't opened to reach the heart. Also, a heart-lung bypass machine isn't always used for these procedures.

MIDCAB procedure. This type of surgery mainly is used to bypass blood vessels at the front of the heart. Small incisions are made between your ribs on the left side of your chest, directly over the artery that needs to be bypassed.

The incisions usually are about 3 inches long. (The incision made in traditional CABG is at least 6 to 8 inches long.) The left internal mammary artery most often is used for the graft in this procedure. A heart-lung bypass machine isn't used during MIDCAB grafting.

Port-access coronary artery bypass procedure. The surgeon does this procedure through small incisions (ports) made in your chest. Artery or vein grafts are used. A heart-lung bypass machine is used during this procedure.

Robot-assisted technique. This type of procedure allows for even smaller, keyhole-sized incisions. A small video camera is inserted in one incision to show the heart, while the surgeon uses remote-controlled surgical instruments to do the surgery. A heart-lung bypass machine sometimes is used during this procedure.

Post Coronary Artery Bypass Grafting

Recovery in the Hospital

After surgery, you'll typically spend 1 or 2 days in an intensive care unit (ICU). Your heart rate, blood pressure, and oxygen levels will be checked regularly during this time.

An intravenous line (IV) will likely be inserted into a vein in your arm. Through the IV line, you may get medicines to control blood circulation and blood pressure. You also will likely have a tube in your bladder to drain urine and a tube to drain fluid from your chest.

You may receive oxygen therapy (oxygen given through nasal prongs or a mask) and a temporary pacemaker while in the ICU. A pacemaker is a small device that's placed in the chest or abdomen to help control abnormal heart rhythms.

Your doctor may recommend that you wear compression stockings on your legs as well. These stockings are tight at the ankle and become looser as they go up the leg. This creates gentle pressure up the leg. The pressure keeps blood from pooling and clotting.

While in the ICU, you'll also have bandages on your chest incision (cut) and on the areas where an artery or vein was removed for grafting.

After you leave the ICU, you'll be moved to a less intensive care area of the hospital for 3 to 5 days before going home.

Recovery at Home

Your doctor will give you specific instructions for recovering at home, especially concerning:

- How to care for your healing incisions
- How to recognize signs of infection or other complications
- When to call the doctor right away
- When to make follow-up appointments

You also may get instructions on how to deal with common side effects from surgery. Side effects often go away within 4 to 6 weeks after surgery, but may include:

- Discomfort or itching from healing incisions

- Swelling of the area where an artery or vein was removed for grafting

- Muscle pain or tightness in the shoulders and upper back

- Fatigue (tiredness), mood swings, or depression

- Problems sleeping or loss of appetite

- Constipation

- Chest pain around the site of the chest bone incision (more frequent with traditional CABG)

Full recovery from traditional CABG may take 6 to 12 weeks or more. Less recovery time is needed for nontraditional CABG.

Your doctor will tell you when you can start physical activity again. It varies from person to person, but there are some typical timeframes. Most people can resume sexual activity within about 4 weeks and driving after 3 to 8 weeks.

Returning to work after 6 weeks is common unless your job involves specific and demanding physical activity. Some people may need to find less physically demanding types of work or work a reduced schedule at first.

Ongoing Care

Care after surgery may include periodic checkups with doctors. During these visits, tests may be done to see how your heart is working. Tests may include EKG, stress testing, echocardiography, and cardiac CT.

CABG is not a cure for CHD. You and your doctor may develop a treatment plan that includes lifestyle changes to help you stay healthy and reduce the chance of CHD getting worse.

Lifestyle changes may include making changes to your diet, quitting smoking, doing physical activity regularly, and lowering and managing stress.

Your doctor also may refer you to cardiac rehabilitation (rehab). Cardiac rehab is a medically supervised program that helps improve the health and well-being of people who have heart problems.

Rehab programs include exercise training, education on heart healthy living, and counseling to reduce stress and help you return to an active life. Doctors supervise these programs, which may be offered in hospitals and other community facilities. Talk to your doctor about whether cardiac rehab might benefit you.

Taking medicines as prescribed also is an important part of care after surgery. Your doctor may prescribe medicines to manage pain during recovery; lower cholesterol and blood pressure; reduce the risk of blood clots forming; manage diabetes; or treat depression.

What Are the Risks of Coronary Artery Bypass Grafting?

As with any type of surgery, coronary artery bypass grafting (CABG) has risks. The risks of CABG include:

- wound infection and bleeding

- reactions to anesthesia

- fever

- pain

- stroke, heart attack, or even death

Some patients have a fever associated with chest pain, irritability, and decreased appetite. This is due to inflammation involving the lung and heart sac.

This complication sometimes occurs after surgeries that involve cutting through the pericardium (the outer covering of the heart). The problem usually is mild, but some patients may develop fluid buildup around the heart that requires treatment.

Memory loss and other issues, such as problems concentrating or thinking clearly, might occur in some people.

These problems are more likely to affect older patients and women. These issues often improve within 6–12 months of surgery.

In general, the risk of complications is higher if CABG is done in an emergency situation (for example, during a heart attack). The risk also is higher if you have other diseases or conditions, such as diabetes, kidney disease, lung disease, or peripheral arterial disease (P.A.D.).

Section 27.4

Valve Repair and Replacement

This section includes text excerpted from "How Is
Heart Valve Disease Treated?" National Heart, Lung, and
Blood Institute (NHLBI), June 22, 2015.

Treatment of Heart Valve Disease

Currently, no medicines can cure heart valve disease. However,
lifestyle changes and medicines often can treat symptoms successfully
and delay problems for many years. Eventually, though, you may need
surgery to repair or replace a faulty heart valve.

The goals of treating heart valve disease might include:

- Medicines

- Repairing or replacing faulty valves

- Heart-healthy lifestyle changes to treat other related heart
  conditions

Medicines

In addition to heart-healthy lifestyle changes, your doctor may
prescribe medicines to:

- Lower high blood pressure or high blood cholesterol.

- Prevent arrhythmias (irregular heartbeats).

- Thin the blood and prevent clots (if you have a man-made
  replacement valve). Doctors also prescribe these medicines for
  mitral stenosis or other valve defects that raise the risk of blood
  clots.

- Treat coronary heart disease. Medicines for coronary heart disease can reduce your heart's workload and relieve symptoms.

- Treat heart failure. Heart failure medicines widen blood vessels
  and rid the body of excess fluid.

Repairing or Replacing Heart Valves

Your doctor may recommend repairing or replacing your heart valve(s), even if your heart valve disease isn't causing symptoms. Repairing or replacing a valve can prevent lasting damage to your heart and sudden death.

The decision to repair or replace heart valves depends on many factors, including:

- The severity of your valve disease

- Whether you need heart surgery for other conditions, such as bypass surgery to treat coronary heart disease. Bypass surgery and valve surgery can be performed at the same time.

- Your age and general health

When possible, heart valve repair is preferred over heart valve replacement. Valve repair preserves the strength and function of the heart muscle. People who have valve repair also have a lower risk of infective endocarditis after the surgery, and they don't need to take blood-thinning medicines for the rest of their lives.

However, heart valve repair surgery is harder to do than valve replacement. Also, not all valves can be repaired. Mitral valves often can be repaired. Aortic and pulmonary valves often have to be replaced.

Repairing Heart Valves

Heart surgeons can repair heart valves by:

- Adding tissue to patch holes or tears or to increase the support at the base of the valve

- Removing or reshaping tissue so the valve can close tighter

- Separating fused valve flaps

Sometimes cardiologists repair heart valves using cardiac catheterization. Although catheter procedures are less invasive than surgery, they may not work as well for some patients. Work with your doctor to decide whether repair is appropriate. If so, your doctor can advise you on the best procedure.

Heart valves that cannot open fully (stenosis) can be repaired with surgery or with a less invasive catheter procedure called balloon valvuloplasty. This procedure also is called balloon valvotomy.

During the procedure, a catheter (thin tube) with a balloon at its tip is threaded through a blood vessel to the faulty valve in your heart. The balloon is inflated to help widen the opening of the valve. Your doctor then deflates the balloon and removes both it and the tube. You're awake during the procedure, which usually requires an overnight stay in a hospital.

Balloon valvuloplasty relieves many symptoms of heart valve disease, but may not cure it. The condition can worsen over time. You still may need medicines to treat symptoms or surgery to repair or replace the faulty valve. Balloon valvuloplasty has a shorter recovery time than surgery. The procedure may work as well as surgery for some patients who have mitral valve stenosis. For these people, balloon valvuloplasty often is preferred over surgical repair or replacement.

Balloon valvuloplasty doesn't work as well as surgery for adults who have aortic valve stenosis. Doctors often use balloon valvuloplasty to repair valve stenosis in infants and children.

Replacing Heart Valves

Sometimes heart valves can't be repaired and must be replaced. This surgery involves removing the faulty valve and replacing it with a man-made or biological valve.

Biological valves are made from pig, cow, or human heart tissue and may have man-made parts as well. These valves are specially treated, so you won't need medicines to stop your body from rejecting the valve.

Man-made valves last longer than biological valves and usually don't have to be replaced. Biological valves usually have to be replaced after about 10 years, although newer ones may last 15 years or longer. Unlike biological valves, however, man-made valves require you to take blood-thinning medicines for the rest of your life. These medicines prevent blood clots from forming on the valve. Blood clots can cause a heart attack or stroke. Man-made valves also raise your risk of infective endocarditis.

You and your doctor will decide together whether you should have a man-made or biological replacement valve.

If you're a woman of childbearing age or if you're athletic, you may prefer a biological valve so you don't have to take blood-thinning medicines. If you're elderly, you also may prefer a biological valve, as it will likely last for the rest of your life.

Ross Procedure

Doctors also can treat faulty aortic valves with the Ross procedure. During this surgery, your doctor removes your faulty aortic valve and replaces it with your pulmonary valve. Your pulmonary valve is then replaced with a pulmonary valve from a deceased human donor.

This is more involved surgery than typical valve replacement, and it has a greater risk of complications. The Ross procedure may be especially useful for children because the surgically replaced valves continue to grow with the child. Also, lifelong treatment with blood-thinning medicines isn't required. But in some patients, one or both valves fail to work well within a few years of the surgery. Researchers continue to study the use of this procedure.

Other Approaches for Repairing and Replacing Heart Valves

Some forms of heart valve repair and replacement surgery are less invasive than traditional surgery. These procedures use smaller incisions (cuts) to reach the heart valves. Hospital stays for these newer types of surgery usually are 3 to 5 days, compared with a 5-day stay for traditional heart valve surgery.

New surgeries tend to cause less pain and have a lower risk of infection. Recovery time also tends to be shorter—2 to 4 weeks versus 6 to 8 weeks for traditional surgery.

Transcatheter Valve Therapy. Interventional cardiologists perform procedures that involve threading clips or other devices to repair faulty heart valves using a catheter (tube) inserted through a large blood vessel. The clips or devices are used to reshape the valves and stop the backflow of blood. People who receive these clips recover more easily than people who have surgery. However, the clips may not treat backflow as well as surgery.

Doctors also may use a catheter to replace faulty aortic valves. This procedure is called transcatheter aortic valve replacement (TAVR). For this procedure, the catheter usually is inserted into an artery in the groin (upper thigh) and threaded to the heart. A deflated balloon with a folded replacement valve around it is at the end of the catheter.

Once the replacement valve is placed properly, the balloon is used to expand the new valve so it fits securely within the old valve. The balloon is then deflated, and the balloon and catheter are removed.

A replacement valve also can be inserted in an existing replacement valve that is failing. This is called a valve-in-valve procedure.

Heart-Healthy Lifestyle Changes to Treat Other Related
Heart Conditions

To help treat heart conditions related to heart valve disease, your doctor may advise you to make heart-healthy lifestyle changes, such as:

- Heart-healthy eating

- Aiming for a healthy weight

- Managing stress

- Physical activity

- Quitting smoking

Section 27.5

Arrhythmia Surgery

This section includes text excerpted from "Arrhythmia,"
National Heart, Lung, and Blood Institute (NHLBI), July 1, 2011.
Reviewed June 2017.

Arrhythmia

An arrhythmia is a problem with the rate or rhythm of the heartbeat. During an arrhythmia, the heart can beat too fast, too slow, or with an irregular rhythm.

A heartbeat that is too fast is called tachycardia. A heartbeat that is too slow is called bradycardia.

Most arrhythmias are harmless, but some can be serious or even life threatening. During an arrhythmia, the heart may not be able to pump enough blood to the body. Lack of blood flow can damage the brain, heart, and other organs.

Understanding the Heart's Electrical System

To understand arrhythmias, it helps to understand the heart's internal electrical system. The heart's electrical system controls the rate and rhythm of the heartbeat.

With each heartbeat, an electrical signal spreads from the top of the heart to the bottom. As the signal travels, it causes the heart to contract and pump blood.

Each electrical signal begins in a group of cells called the sinus node or sinoatrial (SA) node. The SA node is located in the heart's upper right chamber, the right atrium. In a healthy adult heart at rest, the SA node fires off an electrical signal to begin a new heartbeat 60 to 100 times a minute.

From the SA node, the electrical signal travels through special pathways in the right and left atria. This causes the atria to contract and pump blood into the heart's two lower chambers, the ventricles.

The electrical signal then moves down to a group of cells called the atrioventricular (AV) node, located between the atria and the ventricles. Here, the signal slows down just a little, allowing the ventricles time to finish filling with blood.

The electrical signal then leaves the AV node and travels along a pathway called the bundle of His. This pathway divides into a right bundle branch and a left bundle branch. The signal goes down these branches to the ventricles, causing them to contract and pump blood to the lungs and the rest of the body.

The ventricles then relax, and the heartbeat process starts all over again in the SA node.

A problem with any part of this process can cause an arrhythmia. For example, in atrial fibrillation, a common type of arrhythmia, electrical signals travel through the atria in a fast and disorganized way. This causes the atria to quiver instead of contract.

How Are Arrhythmias Treated?

Common arrhythmia treatments include medicines, medical procedures, and surgery. Your doctor may recommend treatment if your arrhythmia causes serious symptoms, such as dizziness, chest pain, or fainting.

Your doctor also may recommend treatment if the arrhythmia increases your risk for problems such as heart failure, stroke, or sudden cardiac arrest.

Medicines

Medicines can slow down a heart that's beating too fast. They also can change an abnormal heart rhythm to a normal, steady rhythm. Medicines that do this are called antiarrhythmics.

Some of the medicines used to slow a fast heart rate are beta blockers (such as metoprolol and atenolol), calcium channel blockers (such as diltiazem and verapamil), and digoxin (digitalis). These medicines often are used to treat atrial fibrillation (AF).

Some of the medicines used to restore a normal heart rhythm are amiodarone, sotalol, flecainide, propafenone, dofetilide, ibutilide, quinidine, procainamide, and disopyramide. These medicines often have side effects. Some side effects can make an arrhythmia worse or even cause a different kind of arrhythmia.

Currently, no medicine can reliably speed up a slow heart rate. Abnormally slow heart rates are treated with pacemakers.

People who have AF and some other arrhythmias may be treated with blood-thinning medicines. These medicines reduce the risk of blood clots forming. Warfarin (Coumadin®), dabigatran, heparin, and aspirin are examples of blood-thinning medicines.

Medicines also can control an underlying medical condition that might be causing an arrhythmia, such as heart disease or a thyroid condition.

Medical Procedures

Some arrhythmias are treated with pacemakers. A pacemaker is a small device that's placed under the skin of your chest or abdomen to help control abnormal heart rhythms.

Pacemakers have sensors that detect the heart's electrical activity. When the device senses an abnormal heart rhythm, it sends electrical pulses to prompt the heart to beat at a normal rate.

Some arrhythmias are treated with a jolt of electricity to the heart. This type of treatment is called cardioversion or defibrillation, depending on which type of arrhythmia is being treated.

Some people who are at risk for ventricular fibrillation are treated with a device called an implantable cardioverter defibrillator (ICD). Like a pacemaker, an ICD is a small device that's placed under the skin in the chest. This device uses electrical pulses or shocks to help control life-threatening arrhythmias.

An ICD continuously monitors the heartbeat. If it senses a dangerous ventricular arrhythmia, it sends an electric shock to the heart to restore a normal heartbeat.

A procedure called catheter ablation is used to treat some arrhythmias if medicines don't work. During this procedure, a thin, flexible tube is put into a blood vessel in your arm, groin (upper thigh), or neck. Then, the tube is guided to your heart.

A special machine sends energy through the tube to your heart. The energy finds and destroys small areas of heart tissue where abnormal heart rhythms may start. Catheter ablation usually is done in a hospital as part of an electrophysiology study.

Your doctor may recommend transesophageal echocardiography before catheter ablation to make sure no blood clots are present in the atria (the heart's upper chambers).

Surgery

Doctors treat some arrhythmias with surgery. This may occur if surgery is already being done for another reason, such as repair of a heart valve.

One type of surgery for AF is called maze surgery. During this surgery, a surgeon makes small cuts or burns in the atria. These cuts or burns prevent the spread of disorganized electrical signals.

If coronary heart disease is the cause of your arrhythmia, your doctor may recommend coronary artery bypass grafting. This surgery improves blood flow to the heart muscle.

Section 27.6

Carotid Endarterectomy

This section includes text excerpted from "Carotid
Endarterectomy," National Heart, Lung, and Blood
Institute (NHLBI), December 9, 2016.

Carotid endarterectomy, also known as carotid artery surgery, is surgery that removes plaque buildup from inside a carotid artery in your neck. This surgery is done to restore normal blood flow to the brain to prevent a stroke if you already have symptoms of reduced blood flow. Carotid endarterectomy also may be performed preventively if a diagnostic test such as carotid ultrasound shows significant blockage that is likely to trigger a stroke. Carotid endarterectomy is not a cure. Your arteries can become blocked again if your underlying condition, such as high blood cholesterol, is not controlled and causes new plaque buildup.

The Procedure

Carotid endarterectomy is done in a hospital. You may have general anesthesia and will not be awake or feel pain during the surgery. Your surgeon instead may decide to use local anesthesia to numb only the part of your body being worked on so that he or she can check your brain's reaction to the decreased blood flow during surgery. You also will be given medicine to relax you during the surgery. Your vital signs will be monitored during surgery. You will lie on your back on an operating table with your head turned to one side. Your surgeon will make an incision, or cut, on your neck to expose the blocked section of the carotid artery. Your surgeon will cut into the affected artery and remove the plaque through this cut. A temporary flexible tube may be inserted so blood can flow around the blocked area as the plaque is cleared. After removing the plaque from your artery, the surgeon will close the artery and neck incisions with stitches.

Recovering from Surgery

After surgery, you will recover in the hospital for one to two days. Your neck may hurt for a few days, and you may find it hard to swallow. Your doctor may prescribe medicine to prevent clots and suggest steps to keep your carotid arteries healthy.

Carotid endarterectomy is fairly safe when performed by experienced surgeons. However, serious complications such as clotting, stroke, or death may occur. Taking anticlotting medicines before and after surgery can reduce this risk. Other complications may include a reaction to anesthesia, short-term nerve injury that causes temporary numbness in your face or tongue, bleeding, infection, high blood pressure, heart attack, and seizure. The risk of complications is higher in women, older people, those with certain conditions such as chronic kidney disease or diabetes, and those with other serious medical conditions.

Section 27.7

Aneurysm Repair

This section contains text excerpted from the following
sources: Text beginning with the heading "Aortic Aneurysm"
is excerpted from "Aortic Aneurysm Fact Sheet," Centers for
Disease Control and Prevention (CDC), June 16, 2016; Text
under the heading "Treatment of Aneurysm" is excerpted from
"How Is an Aneurysm Treated?" National Heart, Lung, and Blood
Institute (NHLBI), April 1, 2011. Reviewed June 2017.

Aortic Aneurysm

An aortic aneurysm is a balloon-like bulge in the aorta, the large
artery that carries blood from the heart through the chest and torso.
Aortic aneurysms work in two ways:

- The force of blood pumping can split the layers of the artery
  wall, allowing blood to leak in between them. This process is
  called a **dissection**.

- The aneurysm can burst completely, causing bleeding inside the
  body. This is called a **rupture**.

- Dissections and ruptures are the cause of most deaths from aortic aneurysms.

Aortic Aneurysm in the United States

- Aortic aneurysms were the primary cause of **9,863 deaths in
  2014** and a contributing cause in more than **17,215 deaths** in
  the United States in 2009.

- About **two-thirds** of people who have an aortic dissection are
  male.

- The U.S. Preventive Services Task Force (USPSTF) recommends
  that men aged 65–75 years who have ever smoked should get an
  ultrasound screening for abdominal aortic aneurysms, even if
  they have no symptoms.

Types of Aortic Aneurysm

Thoracic Aortic Aneurysms

A thoracic aortic aneurysm occurs in the chest. Men and women are equally likely to get thoracic aortic aneurysms, which become more common with increasing age. Thoracic aortic aneurysms are usually caused by high blood pressure or sudden injury.

Signs and symptoms of thoracic aortic aneurysm can include:

- Sharp, sudden pain in the chest or upper back.

- Shortness of breath.

- Trouble breathing or swallowing.

Abdominal Aortic Aneurysms

An abdominal aortic aneurysm occurs below the chest. Abdominal aortic aneurysms happen more often than thoracic aortic aneurysms.

Abdominal aortic aneurysms are more common in men and among people aged 65 years and older. Abdominal aortic aneurysms are less common among blacks compared with whites.

Abdominal aortic aneurysms are usually caused by atherosclerosis (hardened arteries), but infection or injury can also cause them.

Abdominal aortic aneurysms often don't have any symptoms. If an individual does have symptoms, they can include:

- Throbbing or deep pain in your back or side.

- Pain in the buttocks, groin, or legs.

Other Types of Aneurysms

Aneurysms can occur in other parts of your body. A ruptured aneurysm in the brain can cause a stroke. Peripheral aneurysms—those found in arteries other than the aorta—can occur in the neck, in the groin, or behind the knees. These aneurysms are less likely to rupture or dissect than aortic aneurysms, but they can form blood clots. These clots can break away and block blood flow through the artery.

Risk Factors for Aortic Aneurysm

Diseases that damage your heart and blood vessels also increase your risk for aortic aneurysm. These diseases include:

- high blood pressure

340

- high cholesterol
- atherosclerosis (hardened arteries)
- smoking

Some inherited connective tissue disorders, such as Marfan syndrome and Ehlers-Danlos syndrome, can also increase your risk for aortic aneurysm. Your family may also have a history of aortic aneurysms that can increase your risk.

Unhealthy behaviors can also increase your risk for aortic aneurysm, especially for people who have one of the diseases listed above. Tobacco use is the most important behavior related to aortic aneurysm. People who have a history of smoking are 3 to 5 times more likely to develop an abdominal aortic aneurysm.

Treatment of Aneurysm

Aortic aneurysms are treated with medicines and surgery. Small aneurysms that are found early and aren't causing symptoms may not need treatment. Other aneurysms need to be treated.

The goals of treatment may include:

- Preventing the aneurysm from growing
- Preventing or reversing damage to other body structures
- Preventing or treating a rupture or dissection
- Allowing you to continue doing your normal daily activities

Treatment for an aortic aneurysm is based on its size. Your doctor may recommend routine testing to make sure an aneurysm isn't getting bigger. This method usually is used for aneurysms that are smaller than 5 centimeters (about 2 inches) across.

How often you need testing (for example, every few months or every year) is based on the size of the aneurysm and how fast it's growing. The larger it is and the faster it's growing, the more often you may need to be checked.

Medicines

If you have an aortic aneurysm, your doctor may prescribe medicines before surgery or instead of surgery. Medicines are used to lower blood pressure, relax blood vessels, and lower the risk that the aneurysm will rupture (burst). Beta blockers and calcium channel blockers are the medicines most commonly used.

Surgery

Your doctor may recommend surgery if your aneurysm is growing quickly or is at risk of rupture or dissection.

The two main types of surgery to repair aortic aneurysms are open abdominal or open chest repair and endovascular repair.

Open Abdominal or Open Chest Repair

The standard and most common type of surgery for aortic aneurysms is open abdominal or open chest repair. This surgery involves a major incision (cut) in the abdomen or chest.

General anesthesia is used during this procedure. The term "anesthesia" refers to a loss of feeling and awareness. General anesthesia temporarily puts you to sleep.

During the surgery, the aneurysm is removed. Then, the section of aorta is replaced with a graft made of material such as Dacron® or Teflon® The surgery takes 3 to 6 hours; you'll remain in the hospital for 5 to 8 days.

If needed, repair of the aortic heart valve also may be done during open abdominal or open chest surgery.

It often takes a month to recover from open abdominal or open chest surgery and return to full activity. Most patients make a full recovery.

Endovascular Repair

In endovascular repair, the aneurysm isn't removed. Instead, a graft is inserted into the aorta to strengthen it. Surgeons do this type of surgery using catheters (tubes) inserted into the arteries; it doesn't require surgically opening the chest or abdomen. General anesthesia is used during this procedure.

The surgeon first inserts a catheter into an artery in the groin (upper thigh) and threads it to the aneurysm. Then, using an X-ray to see the artery, the surgeon threads the graft (also called a stent graft) into the aorta to the aneurysm.

The graft is then expanded inside the aorta and fastened in place to form a stable channel for blood flow. The graft reinforces the weakened section of the aorta. This helps prevent the aneurysm from rupturing.

The recovery time for endovascular repair is less than the recovery time for open abdominal or open chest repair. However, doctors can't repair all aortic aneurysms with endovascular repair. The location or size of an aneurysm may prevent the use of a stent graft.

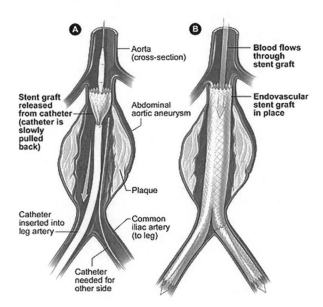

Figure 27.3. *Placement of a Stent Graft in an Aortic Aneurysm*

The illustration shows the placement of a stent graft in an aortic aneurysm. In figure A, a catheter is inserted into an artery in the groin (upper thigh). The catheter is threaded to the abdominal aorta, and the stent graft is released from the catheter. In figure B, the stent graft allows blood to flow through the aneurysm.

Section 27.8

Heart Transplant

This section includes text excerpted from "Heart Transplant," National Heart, Lung, and Blood Institute (NHLBI), December 9, 2016.

Heart transplant is surgery that removes a diseased heart and replaces it with a healthy heart from a deceased donor to improve your quality of life and increase your lifespan. Most heart transplants are done on patients who have end-stage heart failure, a condition in which your heart is severely damaged or weakened, and on people who have failed other treatment options. End-stage heart failure may be caused by conditions such as coronary heart disease, viral infections, or hereditary conditions. In rare instances, heart transplant may be performed at the same time as lung transplant in patients who have severe heart and lung disease.

Eligibility for Heart Transplant Surgery

You may be eligible for heart transplant surgery if you have severe heart disease that does not respond to other treatments. If you are otherwise healthy enough for surgery, you will be placed on the National Organ Procurement and Transplantation Network's (OPTN) waiting list. This national network handles the organ-sharing process for the United States. If a match is found, you will need to have your heart transplant surgery right away.

The Procedure

Heart transplant surgery will be done in a hospital. You will have general anesthesia and will not be awake during the surgery. You will receive medicine through an intravenous (IV) line in your arm. A breathing tube connected to a ventilator will help you breathe. A surgeon will open your chest, connect your heart's arteries and veins to a heart-lung bypass machine, and remove your diseased heart. The body's arteries and veins will be taken off the bypass machine and reconnected to the healthy donor heart. The heart transplant is complete after the surgeon closes your chest.

Recovering from Surgery

After the surgery, you will recover in the hospital's intensive care unit (ICU) and stay in the hospital for up to three weeks. During your recovery, you may start a cardiac rehabilitation program. Before leaving the hospital, you will learn how to keep track of your overall health; monitor your weight, blood pressure, pulse, and temperature; and learn the signs of heart transplant rejection and infection. For the first three months after leaving the hospital, you will return often for tests to check for infection or rejection of your new heart, to test your heart function, and to make sure that you are recovering well.

Practicing good hygiene, obtaining routine vaccines, and making healthy lifestyle choices are very important after a heart transplant to reduce your risk of infection. Regular dental care is also important. Your doctor or dentist may prescribe antibiotics before any dental work to prevent infection. Following your doctor's advice will help you recover and stay as healthy as possible.

Heart transplant has some serious risks. Primary graft dysfunction happens when the donor heart fails and cannot function. This is the most frequent cause of death for the first month after transplant. Your immune system also may reject your new heart. Rejection is most likely to occur within six months after the transplant. You will need to take medicines for the rest of your life to suppress your immune system and help prevent your body from rejecting your new heart. These medicines weaken your immune system and increase your chance for infection. Their long-term use also can increase your risk for cancer, cause diabetes and osteoporosis, and damage your kidneys. Cardiac allograft vasculopathy is a common and serious complication of heart transplant. Cardiac allograft vasculopathy is an aggressive form of atherosclerosis that over months or a few years can quickly block the heart's arteries and cause the donor heart to fail. Over time, your new heart may fail due to the same reasons that caused your original heart to fail. Some patients who have a heart transplant that fails may be eligible for another transplant.

Despite these risks, heart transplant has a good success rate that has improved over many decades of research. Recent survival rates are about 85 percent at one year after surgery, with survival rates decreasing by about three to four percent each additional year after surgery because of serious complications. Mechanical circulatory support, possibly from left ventricular assist devices, may be an alternative to heart transplant. But more research is needed to determine long-term survival rates for these new devices.

Risks in Heart Transplant Surgery

Heart transplant has some serious risks. Primary graft dysfunction happens when the donor heart fails and cannot function. This is the most frequent cause of death for the first month after transplant. Your immune system also may reject your new heart. Rejection is most likely to occur within six months after the transplant. You will need to take medicines for the rest of your life to suppress your immune system and help prevent your body from rejecting your new heart. These medicines weaken your immune system and increase your chance for infection. Their long-term use also can increase your risk for cancer, cause diabetes and osteoporosis, and damage your kidneys. Cardiac allograft vasculopathy is a common and serious complication of heart transplant. Cardiac allograft vasculopathy is an aggressive form of atherosclerosis that over months or a few years can quickly block the heart's arteries and cause the donor heart to fail. Over time, your new heart may fail due to the same reasons that caused your original heart to fail. Some patients who have a heart transplant that fails may be eligible for another transplant.

Despite these risks, heart transplant has a good success rate that has improved over many decades of research. Recent survival rates are about 85 percent at one year after surgery, with survival rates decreasing by about three to four percent each additional year after surgery because of serious complications. Mechanical circulatory support, possibly from left ventricular assist devices, may be an alternative to heart transplant. But more research is needed to determine long-term survival rates for these new devices.

Chapter 28

Implantable Devices for Heart Problems

Chapter Contents

347

Section 28.1

Cardioverter Defibrillator

This section includes text excerpted from "Implantable
Cardioverter Defibrillators," National Heart, Lung, and Blood
Institute (NHLBI), November 9, 2011. Reviewed June 2017.

Implantable Cardioverter Defibrillator

An implantable cardioverter defibrillator (ICD) is a small device
that's placed in the chest or abdomen. Doctors use the device to help
treat irregular heartbeats called arrhythmias.

An ICD uses electrical pulses or shocks to help control life-threatening arrhythmias, especially those that can cause sudden cardiac
arrest (SCA).

SCA is a condition in which the heart suddenly stops beating. If
the heart stops beating, blood stops flowing to the brain and other
vital organs. SCA usually causes death if it's not treated within
minutes.

Understanding the Heart's Electrical System

Your heart has its own internal electrical system that controls the
rate and rhythm of your heartbeat. With each heartbeat, an electrical
signal spreads from the top of your heart to the bottom. As the signal
travels, it causes the heart to contract and pump blood.

Each electrical signal normally begins in a group of cells called
the sinus node or sinoatrial (SA) node. As a signal spreads from the
top of the heart to the bottom, it coordinates the timing of heart cell
activity.

First, the heart's two upper chambers, the atria, contract. This
contraction pumps blood into the heart's two lower chambers, the
ventricles. The ventricles then contract and pump blood to the rest
of the body. The combined contraction of the atria and ventricles is a
heartbeat.

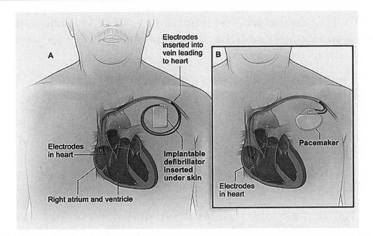

Figure 28.1. *Comparison of an Implantable Cardioverter Defibrillator and a Pacemaker*

The image compares an ICD with a pacemaker. Figure A shows the location and general size of an ICD in the upper chest. The wires with electrodes on the ends are inserted into the heart through a vein in the upper chest. Figure B shows the location and general size of a pacemaker in the upper chest. The wires with electrodes on the ends are inserted into the heart through a vein in the upper chest.

Who Needs an Implantable Cardioverter Defibrillator?

Implantable cardioverter defibrillators (ICDs) are used in children, teens, and adults. Your doctor may recommend an ICD if you're at risk for certain types of arrhythmia.

ICDs are used to treat life-threatening ventricular arrhythmias, such as those that cause the ventricles to beat too fast or quiver. You may be considered at high risk for a ventricular arrhythmia if you:

- Have had a ventricular arrhythmia before

- Have had a heart attack that has damaged your heart's electrical system

Doctors often recommend ICDs for people who have survived SCA. They also may recommend them for people who have certain heart conditions that put them at high risk for SCA.

For example, some people who have long QT syndrome, Brugada syndrome, or congenital heart disease may benefit from an ICD, even if they've never had ventricular arrhythmias before.

Some people who have heart failure may need a CRT-D device. This device combines a type of pacemaker called a cardiac resynchronization therapy (CRT) device with a defibrillator. CRT-D devices help both ventricles work together. This allows them to do a better job of pumping blood out of the heart.

Diagnostic Tests

Your doctor may recommend an ICD if he or she sees signs of a ventricular arrhythmia (or heart damage that would make one likely) on the following tests.

EKG (Electrocardiogram)

An EKG is a simple, painless test that detects and records the heart's electrical activity. The test shows how fast the heart is beating and its rhythm (steady or irregular). An EKG also records the strength and timing of electrical signals as they pass through the heart.

A standard EKG only records the heartbeat for a few seconds. It won't detect arrhythmias that don't happen during the test.

To diagnose arrhythmias that come and go, your doctor may have you wear a portable EKG monitor. The two most common types of portable EKGs are Holter and event monitors.

Holter and Event Monitors

A Holter monitor records the heart's electrical activity for a full 24- or 48-hour period. You wear one while you do your normal daily activities. This allows the monitor to record your heart for a longer time than a standard EKG.

An event monitor is similar to a Holter monitor. You wear an event monitor while doing your normal activities. However, an event monitor only records your heart's electrical activity at certain times while you're wearing it.

You may wear an event monitor for 1 to 2 months, or as long as it takes to get a recording of your heart during symptoms.

Echocardiography

Echocardiography (echo) uses sound waves to create a moving picture of your heart. The test shows the size and shape of your heart and how well your heart chambers and valves are working.

Echo also can identify areas of poor blood flow to the heart, areas of heart muscle that aren't contracting normally, and injury to the heart muscle caused by poor blood flow.

Electrophysiology Study

For this test, a thin, flexible wire is passed through a vein in your groin (upper thigh) or arm to your heart. The wire records the heart's electrical signals.

Your doctor uses the wire to electrically stimulate your heart. This allows him or her to see how your heart's electrical system responds. The electrical stimulation helps pinpoint where the heart's electrical system is damaged.

Stress Test

Some heart problems are easier to diagnose when your heart is working hard and beating fast. During stress testing, you exercise to make your heart work hard and beat fast while heart tests, such as an EKG or echo, are done. If you can't exercise, you may be given medicine to raise your heart rate.

How an Implantable Cardioverter Defibrillator Work

An ICD has wires with electrodes on the ends that connect to one or more of your heart's chambers. These wires carry the electrical signals from your heart to a small computer in the ICD. The computer monitors your heart rhythm.

If the ICD detects an irregular rhythm, it sends low-energy electrical pulses to prompt your heart to beat at a normal rate. If the low-energy pulses restore your heart's normal rhythm, you might avoid the high-energy pulses or shocks of the defibrillator (which can be painful).

Single-chamber ICDs have a wire that goes to either the right atrium or right ventricle. The wire senses electrical activity and corrects faulty electrical signaling within that chamber.

Dual-chamber ICDs have wires that go to both an atrium and a ventricle. These ICDs provide low-energy pulses to either or both chambers. Some dual-chamber ICDs have three wires. They go to an atrium and both ventricles.

The wires on an ICD connect to a small metal box implanted in your chest or abdomen. The box contains a battery, pulse generator, and small computer. When the computer detects irregular heartbeats, it triggers the ICD's pulse generator to send electrical pulses. Wires carry these pulses to the heart.

The ICD also can record the heart's electrical activity and heart rhythms. The recordings can help your doctor fine-tune the programming of your ICD so it works better to correct irregular heartbeats.

The type of ICD you get is based on your heart's pumping abilities, structural defects, and the type of irregular heartbeats you've had. Your ICD will be programmed to respond to the type of arrhythmia you're most likely to have.

During Implantable Cardioverter Defibrillator Surgery

Placing an ICD requires minor surgery, which usually is done in a hospital. You'll be given medicine right before the surgery that will help you relax and might make you fall asleep.

Your doctor will give you medicine to numb the area where he or she will put the ICD. He or she also may give you antibiotics to prevent infections.

First, your doctor will thread the ICD wires through a vein to the correct place in your heart. An X-ray "movie" of the wires as they pass through your vein and into your heart will help your doctor place them.

Once the wires are in place, your doctor will make a small cut into the skin of your chest or abdomen. He or she will then slip the ICD's small metal box through the cut and just under your skin. The box contains the battery, pulse generator, and computer.

Once the ICD is in place, your doctor will test it. You'll be given medicine to help you sleep during this testing so you don't feel any electrical pulses. Then your doctor will sew up the cut. The entire surgery takes a few hours.

Post Implantable Cardioverter Defibrillator Surgery

Expect to stay in the hospital 1–2 days after ICD surgery. This allows your healthcare team to check your heartbeat and make sure your ICD is working well.

You'll need to arrange for a ride home from the hospital because you won't be able to drive for at least a week while you recover from the surgery.

For a few days to weeks after the surgery, you may have pain, swelling, or tenderness in the area where your ICD was placed. The pain usually is mild, and over-the-counter medicines can help relieve it. Talk to your doctor before taking any pain medicines.

Your doctor may ask you to avoid high-impact activities and heavy lifting for about a month after ICD surgery. Most people return to their normal activities within a few days of having the surgery.

The Risks of Having an Implantable Cardioverter Defibrillator

Unnecessary Electrical Pulses

ICDs can sometimes give electrical pulses or shocks that aren't needed.

A damaged wire or a very fast heart rate due to extreme physical activity may trigger unnecessary pulses. These pulses also can occur if you forget to take your medicines.

Children tend to be more physically active than adults. Thus, younger people who have ICDs are more likely to receive unnecessary pulses than older people.

Pulses sent too often or at the wrong time can damage the heart or trigger an irregular, sometimes dangerous heartbeat. They also can be painful and upsetting.

If needed, your doctor can reprogram your ICD or prescribe medicine so unnecessary pulses occur less often.

Risks Related to Surgery

Although rare, some ICD risks are related to the surgery used to place the device. These risks include:

- swelling, bruising, or infection at the area where the ICD was placed

- bleeding from the site where the ICD was placed

- blood vessel, heart, or nerve damage

- a collapsed lung

- a bad reaction to the medicine used to make you relax or sleep during the surgery

Other Risks

People who have ICDs may be at higher risk for heart failure. Heart failure is a condition in which your heart can't pump enough blood to meet your body's needs. It's not clear whether an ICD increases the risk of heart failure, or whether heart failure is just more common in people who need ICDs.

Although rare, an ICD may not work properly. This will prevent the device from correcting irregular heartbeats. If this happens, your doctor may be able to reprogram the device. If that doesn't work, you doctor might have to replace the ICD.

The longer you have an ICD, the more likely it is that you'll have some of the related risks.

Impact of an Implantable Cardioverter Defibrillator on Lifestyle

The low-energy electrical pulses your ICD gives aren't painful. You may not notice them, or you may feel a fluttering in your chest.

The high-energy pulses or shocks your ICD gives last only a fraction of a second. They may feel like thumping or a painful kick in the chest, depending on their strength.

Your doctor may give you medicine to decrease the number of irregular heartbeats you have. This will reduce the number of high-energy pulses sent to your heart. Such medicines include amiodarone or sotalol and beta blockers.

Your doctor may want you to call his or her office or come in within 24 hours of getting a strong shock from your ICD. See your doctor or go to an emergency room right away if you get many strong shocks within a short time.

Devices That Can Disrupt Implantable Cardioverter Defibrillator Functions

Once you have an ICD, you have to avoid close or prolonged contact with electrical devices or devices that have strong magnetic fields. Devices that can interfere with an ICD include:

- cell phones and MP3 players (for example, iPods)
- household appliances, such as microwave ovens
- high-tension wires
- metal detectors
- industrial welders
- electrical generators

These devices can disrupt the electrical signaling of your ICD and prevent it from working well. You may not be able to tell whether your ICD has been affected.

How likely a device is to disrupt your ICD depends on how long you're exposed to it and how close it is to your ICD.

To be on the safe side, some experts recommend not putting your cell phone or MP3 player in a shirt pocket over your ICD (if they're turned on). You may want to hold your cell phone up to the ear that's opposite the site where your ICD was implanted. If you strap your MP3 player to your arm while listening to it, put it on the arm that's farther from your ICD.

You can still use household appliances, but avoid close and prolonged contact, as it may interfere with your ICD.

You can walk through security system metal detectors at your normal pace. Someone can check you with a metal detector wand as long as it isn't held for too long over your ICD site. You should avoid sitting or standing close to a security system metal detector. Notify airport screeners if you have an ICD.

Stay at least 2 feet away from industrial welders or electrical generators. Rarely, ICDs have caused unnecessary shocks during long, high-altitude flights.

Procedures That Can Disrupt Implantable Cardioverter Defibrillator Functions

Some medical procedures can disrupt your ICD. These procedures include:

- magnetic resonance imaging (MRI)

- shock-wave lithotripsy to treat kidney stones

- electrocauterization to stop bleeding during surgery

Let all of your doctors, dentists, and medical technicians know that you have an ICD. Your doctor can give you a card that states what kind of ICD you have. Carry this card in your wallet. You might want to wear a medical ID bracelet or necklace that states that you have an ICD.

Maintaining Daily Activities

Physical Activity

An ICD usually won't limit you from taking part in sports and exercise, including strenuous activities.

You may need to avoid full-contact sports, such as football. Such contact could damage your ICD or shake loose the wires in your heart. Ask your doctor how much and what kinds of physical activity are safe for you.

Driving

You'll have to avoid driving for at least a week while you recover from ICD surgery. If you've had sudden cardiac arrest, a ventricular arrhythmia, or certain symptoms of a ventricular arrhythmia (such as fainting), your doctor may ask you to not drive until you have gone 6 months without fainting. Some people may still faint even with an ICD.

Commercial driving isn't permitted with an ICD.

Ongoing Care

Your doctor will want to check your ICD regularly. Over time, your ICD may stop working well because:

- its wires get dislodged or broken

- its battery fails

- your heart disease progresses

- other devices have disrupted its electrical signaling

To check your ICD, your doctor may ask you to come in for an office visit several times a year. Some ICD functions can be checked over the phone or through a computer connection to the Internet.

Your doctor also may recommend an EKG (electrocardiogram) to check for changes in your heart's electrical activity.

Battery Replacement

ICD batteries last between 5 and 7 years. Your doctor will replace the generator along with the battery before the battery begins to run down.

Replacing the generator/battery is less involved surgery than the original surgery to implant the ICD. The wires of your ICD also may need to be replaced eventually. Your doctor can tell you whether you need to replace your ICD or its wires.

Benefits of Having an Implantable Cardioverter Defibrillator

An ICD works well at detecting and stopping certain life-threatening arrhythmias. An ICD can work better than drug therapy at preventing sudden cardiac arrest, depending on the cause of the arrest.

An ICD can't cure heart disease. However, it can lower the risk of dying from SCA.

Section 28.2

Pacemaker

This section includes text excerpted from "Pacemakers,"
National Heart, Lung, and Blood Institute (NHLBI),
February 28, 2012. Reviewed June 2017.

A pacemaker is a small device that's placed in the chest or abdomen to help control abnormal heart rhythms. This device uses electrical pulses to prompt the heart to beat at a normal rate.

Pacemakers are used to treat arrhythmias. Arrhythmias are problems with the rate or rhythm of the heartbeat. During an arrhythmia, the heart can beat too fast, too slow, or with an irregular rhythm.

A heartbeat that's too fast is called tachycardia. A heartbeat that's too slow is called bradycardia.

During an arrhythmia, the heart may not be able to pump enough blood to the body. This can cause symptoms such as fatigue (tiredness), shortness of breath, or fainting. Severe arrhythmias can damage the body's vital organs and may even cause loss of consciousness or death.

A pacemaker can relieve some arrhythmia symptoms, such as fatigue and fainting. A pacemaker also can help a person who has abnormal heart rhythms resume a more active lifestyle.

Understanding the Heart's Electrical System

Your heart has its own internal electrical system that controls the rate and rhythm of your heartbeat. With each heartbeat, an electrical signal spreads from the top of your heart to the bottom. As the signal travels, it causes the heart to contract and pump blood.

Each electrical signal normally begins in a group of cells called the sinus node or sinoatrial (SA) node. As the signal spreads from the top of the heart to the bottom, it coordinates the timing of heart cell activity.

First, the heart's two upper chambers, the atria, contract. This contraction pumps blood into the heart's two lower chambers, the ventricles. The ventricles then contract and pump blood to the rest of the body. The combined contraction of the atria and ventricles is a heartbeat.

Who Needs a Pacemaker?

Doctors recommend pacemakers for many reasons. The most common reasons are bradycardia and heart block.

Bradycardia is a heartbeat that is slower than normal. Heart block is a disorder that occurs if an electrical signal is slowed or disrupted as it moves through the heart.

Heart block can happen as a result of aging, damage to the heart from a heart attack, or other conditions that disrupt the heart's electrical activity. Some nerve and muscle disorders also can cause heart block, including muscular dystrophy.

Your doctor also may recommend a pacemaker if:

- Aging or heart disease damages your sinus node's ability to set the correct pace for your heartbeat. Such damage can cause slower than normal heartbeats or long pauses between heartbeats. The damage also can cause your heart to switch between slow and fast rhythms. This condition is called sick sinus syndrome.

- You've had a medical procedure to treat an arrhythmia called atrial fibrillation. A pacemaker can help regulate your heartbeat after the procedure.

- You need to take certain heart medicines, such as beta blockers. These medicines can slow your heartbeat too much.

- You faint or have other symptoms of a slow heartbeat. For example, this may happen if the main artery in your neck that supplies your brain with blood is sensitive to pressure. Just quickly turning your neck can cause your heart to beat slower than normal. As a result, your brain might not get enough blood flow, causing you to feel faint or collapse.

- You have heart muscle problems that cause electrical signals to travel too slowly through your heart muscle. Your pacemaker may provide cardiac resynchronization therapy (CRT) for this problem. CRT devices coordinate electrical signaling between the heart's lower chambers.

- You have long QT syndrome, which puts you at risk for dangerous arrhythmias.

Doctors also may recommend pacemakers for people who have certain types of congenital heart disease or for people who have had heart transplants. Children, teens, and adults can use pacemakers.

Before recommending a pacemaker, your doctor will consider any arrhythmia symptoms you have, such as dizziness, unexplained fainting, or shortness of breath. He or she also will consider whether you have a history of heart disease, what medicines you're currently taking, and the results of heart tests.

Diagnostic Tests

Many tests are used to detect arrhythmias. You may have one or more of the following tests.

EKG (Electrocardiogram)

An EKG is a simple, painless test that detects and records the heart's electrical activity. The test shows how fast your heart is beating and its rhythm (steady or irregular).

An EKG also records the strength and timing of electrical signals as they pass through your heart. The test can help diagnose bradycardia and heart block (the most common reasons for needing a pacemaker).

A standard EKG only records the heartbeat for a few seconds. It won't detect arrhythmias that don't happen during the test.

To diagnose heart rhythm problems that come and go, your doctor may have you wear a portable EKG monitor. The two most common types of portable EKGs are Holter and event monitors.

Holter and Event Monitors

A Holter monitor records the heart's electrical activity for a full 24- or 48-hour period. You wear one while you do your normal daily activities. This allows the monitor to record your heart for a longer time than a standard EKG.

An event monitor is similar to a Holter monitor. You wear an event monitor while doing your normal activities. However, an event monitor only records your heart's electrical activity at certain times while you're wearing it.

For many event monitors, you push a button to start the monitor when you feel symptoms. Other event monitors start automatically when they sense abnormal heart rhythms.

You can wear an event monitor for weeks or until symptoms occur.

Echocardiography

Echocardiography (echo) uses sound waves to create a moving picture of your heart. The test shows the size and shape of your heart and how well your heart chambers and valves are working.

Echo also can show areas of poor blood flow to the heart, areas of heart muscle that aren't contracting normally, and injury to the heart muscle caused by poor blood flow.

Electrophysiology Study

For this test, a thin, flexible wire is passed through a vein in your groin (upper thigh) or arm to your heart. The wire records the heart's electrical signals.

Your doctor uses the wire to electrically stimulate your heart. This allows him or her to see how your heart's electrical system responds. This test helps pinpoint where the heart's electrical system is damaged.

Stress Test

Some heart problems are easier to diagnose when your heart is working hard and beating fast.

During stress testing, you exercise to make your heart work hard and beat fast while heart tests, such as an EKG or echo, are done. If you can't exercise, you may be given medicine to raise your heart rate.

How a Pacemaker Works

A pacemaker consists of a battery, a computerized generator, and wires with sensors at their tips. (The sensors are called electrodes.) The battery powers the generator, and both are surrounded by a thin metal box. The wires connect the generator to the heart.

A pacemaker helps monitor and control your heartbeat. The electrodes detect your heart's electrical activity and send data through the wires to the computer in the generator.

If your heart rhythm is abnormal, the computer will direct the generator to send electrical pulses to your heart. The pulses travel through the wires to reach your heart.

Newer pacemakers can monitor your blood temperature, breathing, and other factors. They also can adjust your heart rate to changes in your activity.

The pacemaker's computer also records your heart's electrical activity and heart rhythm. Your doctor will use these recordings to adjust your pacemaker so it works better for you.

Your doctor can program the pacemaker's computer with an external device. He or she doesn't have to use needles or have direct contact with the pacemaker.

Pacemakers have one to three wires that are each placed in different chambers of the heart.

- The wires in a single-chamber pacemaker usually carry pulses from the generator to the right ventricle (the lower right chamber of your heart).

- The wires in a dual-chamber pacemaker carry pulses from the generator to the right atrium (the upper right chamber of your heart) and the right ventricle. The pulses help coordinate the timing of these two chambers' contractions.

- The wires in a biventricular pacemaker carry pulses from the generator to an atrium and both ventricles. The pulses help coordinate electrical signaling between the two ventricles. This type of pacemaker also is called a cardiac resynchronization therapy (CRT) device.

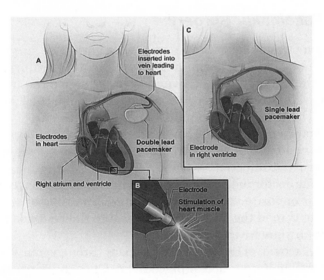

Figure 28.2. *Cross-Section of a Chest with a Pacemaker*

The image shows a cross-section of a chest with a pacemaker. Figure A shows the location and general size of a double-lead, or dual-chamber, pacemaker in the upper chest. The wires with electrodes are inserted into the heart's right atrium and ventricle through a vein in the upper chest. Figure B shows an electrode electrically stimulating the heart muscle. Figure C shows the location and general size of a single-lead, or single-chamber, pacemaker in the upper chest.

Types of Pacemaker Programming

The two main types of programming for pacemakers are demand pacing and rate-responsive pacing.

A demand pacemaker monitors your heart rhythm. It only sends electrical pulses to your heart if your heart is beating too slow or if it misses a beat.

A rate-responsive pacemaker will speed up or slow down your heart rate depending on how active you are. To do this, the device monitors your sinus node rate, breathing, blood temperature, and other factors to determine your activity level.

Your doctor will work with you to decide which type of pacemaker is best for you.

A rate-responsive pacemaker will speed up or slow down your heart rate depending on how active you are. To do this, the device monitors your sinus node rate, breathing, blood temperature, and other factors to determine your activity level.

Your doctor will work with you to decide which type of pacemaker is best for you.

During Pacemaker Surgery

Placing a pacemaker requires minor surgery. The surgery usually is done in a hospital or special heart treatment laboratory.

Before the surgery, an intravenous (IV) line will be inserted into one of your veins. You will receive medicine through the IV line to help you relax. The medicine also might make you sleepy.

Your doctor will numb the area where he or she will put the pacemaker so you don't feel any pain. Your doctor also may give you antibiotics to prevent infection.

First, your doctor will insert a needle into a large vein, usually near the shoulder opposite your dominant hand. Your doctor will then use the needle to thread the pacemaker wires into the vein and to correctly place them in your heart.

An X-ray "movie" of the wires as they pass through your vein and into your heart will help your doctor place them. Once the wires are in place, your doctor will make a small cut into the skin of your chest or abdomen.

He or she will slip the pacemaker's small metal box through the cut, place it just under your skin, and connect it to the wires that lead to your heart. The box contains the pacemaker's battery and generator.

Once the pacemaker is in place, your doctor will test it to make sure it works properly. He or she will then sew up the cut. The entire surgery takes a few hours.

After Pacemaker Surgery

Expect to stay in the hospital overnight so your healthcare team can check your heartbeat and make sure your pacemaker is working well. You'll likely have to arrange for a ride to and from the hospital because your doctor may not want you to drive yourself.

For a few days to weeks after surgery, you may have pain, swelling, or tenderness in the area where your pacemaker was placed. The pain usually is mild; over-the-counter medicines often can relieve it. Talk to your doctor before taking any pain medicines.

Your doctor may ask you to avoid vigorous activities and heavy lifting for about a month after pacemaker surgery. Most people return to their normal activities within a few days of having the surgery.

Risks of Pacemaker Surgery

Pacemaker surgery generally is safe. If problems do occur, they may include:

- swelling, bleeding, bruising, or infection in the area where the pacemaker was placed

- blood vessel or nerve damage

- a collapsed lung

- a bad reaction to the medicine used during the procedure

Talk with your doctor about the benefits and risks of pacemaker surgery.

Impact of a Pacemaker on Lifestyle

Once you have a pacemaker, you have to avoid close or prolonged contact with electrical devices or devices that have strong magnetic fields. Devices that can interfere with a pacemaker include:

- cell phones and MP3 players (for example, iPods)

- household appliances, such as microwave ovens

- high-tension wires

- metal detectors

- industrial welders

- electrical generators

These devices can disrupt the electrical signaling of your pacemaker and stop it from working properly. You may not be able to tell whether your pacemaker has been affected.

How likely a device is to disrupt your pacemaker depends on how long you're exposed to it and how close it is to your pacemaker.

To be safe, some experts recommend not putting your cell phone or MP3 player in a shirt pocket over your pacemaker (if the devices are turned on).

You may want to hold your cell phone up to the ear that's opposite the site where your pacemaker is implanted. If you strap your MP3 player to your arm while listening to it, put it on the arm that's farther from your pacemaker.

You can still use household appliances, but avoid close and prolonged exposure, as it may interfere with your pacemaker.

You can walk through security system metal detectors at your normal pace. Security staff can check you with a metal detector wand as long as it isn't held for too long over your pacemaker site. You should avoid sitting or standing close to a security system metal detector. Notify security staff if you have a pacemaker.

Also, stay at least 2 feet away from industrial welders and electrical generators.

Some medical procedures can disrupt your pacemaker. These procedures include:

- magnetic resonance imaging, or MRI

- shock-wave lithotripsy to get rid of kidney stones

- electrocauterization to stop bleeding during surgery

Let all of your doctors, dentists, and medical technicians know that you have a pacemaker. Your doctor can give you a card that states what kind of pacemaker you have. Carry this card in your wallet. You may want to wear a medical ID bracelet or necklace that states that you have a pacemaker.

Physical Activity

In most cases, having a pacemaker won't limit you from doing sports and exercise, including strenuous activities.

You may need to avoid full-contact sports, such as football. Such contact could damage your pacemaker or shake loose the wires in your heart. Ask your doctor how much and what kinds of physical activity are safe for you.

Ongoing Care

Your doctor will want to check your pacemaker regularly (about every 3 months). Over time, a pacemaker can stop working properly because:

- its wires get dislodged or broken
- its battery gets weak or fails
- your heart disease progresses
- other devices have disrupted its electrical signaling

To check your pacemaker, your doctor may ask you to come in for an office visit several times a year. Some pacemaker functions can be checked remotely using a phone or the Internet.

Your doctor also may ask you to have an EKG (electrocardiogram) to check for changes in your heart's electrical activity.

Battery Replacement

Pacemaker batteries last between 5 and 15 years (average 6 to 7 years), depending on how active the pacemaker is. Your doctor will replace the generator along with the battery before the battery starts to run down.

Replacing the generator and battery is less-involved surgery than the original surgery to implant the pacemaker. Your pacemaker wires also may need to be replaced eventually.

Your doctor can tell you whether your pacemaker or its wires need to be replaced when you see him or her for followup visits.

Chapter 29

Joint, Bone, and Spine Surgery

Chapter Contents

Section 29.1

Joint Replacement Surgery

This section includes text excerpted from "Joint Replacement Surgery: Health Information Basics for You and Your Family," National Institute of Arthritis and Musculoskeletal and Skin Diseases (NIAMS), August 2016.

What Is Joint Replacement Surgery?

Joint replacement surgery is removing a damaged joint and putting in a new one. A joint is where two or more bones come together, like the shoulder, knee, and hip. The surgery is usually done by a doctor called an orthopaedic surgeon. Sometimes, the surgeon will not remove the whole joint, but will only replace or fix the damaged parts.

The doctor may suggest a joint replacement to improve how you live. Replacing a joint can relieve pain and help you move and feel better. Hips and knees are replaced most often. Other joints that can be replaced include the shoulders, fingers, ankles, and elbows.

What Can Happen to My Joints?

Joints can be damaged by arthritis and other diseases, injuries, or other causes. Arthritis or simply years of use may cause the joint to wear away. This can cause pain, stiffness, and swelling. Diseases and damage inside a joint can limit blood flow, causing problems in the bones, which needs blood to be healthy, grow, and repair themselves.

What Is a New Joint Like?

A new joint, called a prosthesis, can be made of plastic, metal, or ceramic parts. It may be cemented into place or not cemented, so that your bone will grow into it. Both methods may be combined to keep the new joint in place.

A cemented joint is used more often in older people who do not move around as much and in people with "weak" bones. The cement holds the new joint to the bone. An uncemented joint is often recommended for younger, more active people and those with good bone quality. It may take longer to heal, because it takes longer for bone to grow and attach to it.

New joints generally last at least 10 to 15 years. Therefore, younger patients may need to have the same damaged joint replaced more than once.

Do Many People Have Joints Replaced?

Joint replacement is becoming more common. More than 1 million Americans have a hip or knee replaced each year. Research has shown that even if you are older, joint replacement can help you move around and feel better.

Any surgery has risks. Risks of joint surgery will depend on your health of your joints before surgery and the type of surgery done. Many hospitals and doctors have been replacing joints for several decades, and this experience results in better patient outcomes. For answers to their questions, some people talk with their doctor or someone who has had the surgery. A doctor specializing in joints will probably work with you before, during, and after surgery to make sure you heal quickly and recover successfully.

Do I Need to Have My Joint Replaced?

Only a doctor can tell if you need a joint replaced. He or she will look at your joint with an X-ray machine or another machine. The doctor may put a small, lighted tube (arthroscope) into your joint to look for damage. A small sample of your tissue could also be tested.

After looking at your joint, the doctor may say that you should consider exercise, walking aids such as braces or canes, physical therapy, or medicines and vitamin supplements. Medicines for arthritis include drugs that reduce inflammation. Depending on the type of arthritis, the doctor may prescribe corticosteroids or other drugs.

However, all drugs may cause side effects, including bone loss.

If these treatments do not work, the doctor may suggest an operation called an osteotomy, where the surgeon "aligns" the joint. Here, the surgeon cuts the bone or bones around the joint to improve alignment. This may be simpler than replacing a joint, but it may take longer to recover. However, this operation has become less common.

Joint replacement is often the answer if you have constant pain and can't move the joint well—for example, if you have trouble with things such as walking, climbing stairs, and taking a bath.

What Happens during Surgery?

First, the surgical team will give you medicine so you won't feel pain (anesthesia). The medicine may block the pain only in one part of the body (regional), or it may put your whole body to sleep (general). The team will then replace the damaged joint with a new man-made joint.

Each surgery is different. How long it takes depends on how badly the joint is damaged and how the surgery is done. To replace a knee or a hip takes about 2 hours or less, unless there are complicating factors. After surgery, you will be moved to a recovery room for 1 to 2 hours until you are fully awake or the numbness goes away.

What Happens after Surgery?

With knee or hip surgery, you will probably need to stay in the hospital for a few days. If you are elderly or have additional disabilities, you may then need to spend several weeks in an intermediate-care facility before going home. You and your team of doctors will determine how long you stay in the hospital.

After hip or knee replacement, you will often stand or begin walking the day of surgery. At first, you will walk with a walker or crutches. You may have some temporary pain in the new joint because your muscles are weak from not being used. Also, your body is healing. The pain can be helped with medicines and should end in a few weeks or months.

Physical therapy can begin the day after surgery to help strengthen the muscles around the new joint and help you regain motion in the joint. If you have your shoulder joint replaced, you can usually begin exercising the same day of your surgery! A physical therapist will help you with gentle, range-of-motion exercises. Before you leave the hospital, your therapist will show you how to use a pulley device to help bend and extend your arm.

Will My Surgery Be Successful?

The success of your surgery depends a lot on what you do when you go home. Follow your doctor's advice about what to eat, what medicines to take, and how to exercise. Talk with your doctor about any pain or trouble moving.

Joint replacement is usually a success in most people who have it. When problems do occur, most are treatable. Possible problems include:

- **Infection.** Areas in the wound or around the new joint may get infected. It may happen while you're still in the hospital or after you go home. It may even occur years later. Minor infections in the wound are usually treated with drugs. Deep infections may need a second operation to treat the infection or replace the joint.

- **Blood clots.** If your blood moves too slowly, it may begin to form lumps of blood parts called clots. If pain and swelling develop in your legs after hip or knee surgery, blood clots may be the cause. The doctor may suggest drugs to make your blood thin or special stockings, exercises, or boots to help your blood move faster. If swelling, redness, or pain occurs in your leg after you leave the hospital, contact your doctor right away.

- **Loosening.** The new joint may loosen, causing pain. If the loosening is bad, you may need another operation to reattach the joint to the bone.

- **Dislocation.** Sometimes after hip or other joint replacement, the ball of the prosthesis can come out of its socket. In most cases, the hip can be corrected without surgery. A brace may be worn for a while if a dislocation occurs.

- **Wear.** Some wear can be found in all joint replacements. Too much wear may help cause loosening. The doctor may need to operate again if the prosthesis comes loose. Sometimes, the plastic can wear thin, and the doctor may just replace the plastic and not the whole joint.

- **Nerve and blood vessel injury.** Nerves near the replaced joint may be damaged during surgery, but this does not happen often. Over time, the damage often improves and may disappear. Blood vessels may also be injured.

As you move your new joint and let your muscles grow strong again, pain will lessen, flexibility will increase, and movement will improve.

Section 29.2

Carpal Tunnel Surgery

This section includes text excerpted from "Carpal Tunnel Syndrome Fact Sheet," National Institute of Neurological Disorders and Stroke (NINDS), January 2017.

What Is Carpal Tunnel Syndrome (CTS)?

Carpal tunnel syndrome (CTS) occurs when the median nerve, which runs from the forearm into the palm of the hand, becomes pressed or squeezed at the wrist. The carpal tunnel—a narrow, rigid passageway of ligament and bones at the base of the hand—houses the median nerve and the tendons that bend the fingers. The median nerve provides feeling to the palm side of the thumb and to the index, middle, and part of the ring fingers (although not the little finger). It also controls some small muscles at the base of the thumb.

Sometimes, thickening from the lining of irritated tendons or other swelling narrows the tunnel and causes the median nerve to be compressed. The result may be numbness, weakness, or sometimes pain in the hand and wrist, or occasionally in the forearm and arm. CTS is the most common and widely known of the entrapment neuropathies, in which one of the body's peripheral nerves is pressed upon.

What Are the Symptoms of CTS?

Symptoms usually start gradually, with frequent burning, tingling, or itching numbness in the palm of the hand and the fingers, especially the thumb and the index and middle fingers. Some carpal tunnel sufferers say their fingers feel useless and swollen, even though little or no swelling is apparent. The symptoms often first appear in one or both hands during the night, since many people sleep with flexed wrists. A person with carpal tunnel syndrome may wake up feeling the need to "shake out" the hand or wrist. As symptoms worsen, people might feel tingling during the day. Decreased grip strength may make it difficult to form a fist, grasp small objects, or perform other manual tasks. In chronic and/or untreated cases, the muscles at the base of the thumb may waste away. Some people are unable to tell between hot and cold by touch.

What Are the Causes of CTS?

Carpal tunnel syndrome is often the result of a combination of factors that reduce the available space for the median nerve within the carpal tunnel, rather than a problem with the nerve itself. Contributing factors include trauma or injury to the wrist that cause swelling, such as sprain or fracture; an overactive pituitary gland; an underactive thyroid gland; and rheumatoid arthritis. Mechanical problems in the wrist joint, work stress, repeated use of vibrating hand tools, fluid retention during pregnancy or menopause, or the development of a cyst or tumor in the canal also may contribute to the compression. Often, no single cause can be identified.

Who Is at Risk of Developing CTS?

Women are three times more likely than men to develop carpal tunnel syndrome, perhaps because the carpal tunnel itself may be smaller in women than in men. The dominant hand is usually affected first and produces the most severe pain. Persons with diabetes or other metabolic disorders that directly affect the body's nerves and make them more susceptible to compression are also at high risk. Carpal tunnel syndrome usually occurs only in adults.

The risk of developing carpal tunnel syndrome is not confined to people in a single industry or job, but is especially common in those performing assembly line work—manufacturing, sewing, finishing, cleaning, and meat, poultry, or fish packing. In fact, carpal tunnel syndrome is three times more common among assemblers than among data-entry personnel.

How Is CTS Diagnosed?

Early diagnosis and treatment are important to avoid permanent damage to the median nerve.

- A medical history and physical examination of the hands, arms, shoulders, and neck can help determine if the person's discomfort is related to daily activities or to an underlying disorder, and can rule out other conditions that cause similar symptoms. The wrist is examined for tenderness, swelling, warmth, and discoloration. Each finger should be tested for sensation and the

373

muscles at the base of the hand should be examined for strength and signs of atrophy.

- Routine laboratory tests and X-rays can reveal fractures, arthritis, and detect diseases that can damage the nerves, such as diabetes.

- Specific tests may reproduce the symptoms of CTS. In the Tinel test, the doctor taps on or presses over the median nerve in the person's wrist. The test is positive when tingling occurs in the affected fingers. Phalen maneuver (or wrist-flexion test) involves the person pressing the backs of the hands and fingers together with their wrists flexed as far as possible. This test is positive if tingling or numbness occur in the affected fingers within 1–2 minutes. Doctors may also ask individuals to try to make a movement that brings on symptoms.

- Electrodiagnostic tests may help confirm the diagnosis of CTS. A nerve conduction study measures electrical activity of the nerves and muscles by assessing the nerve's ability to send a signal along the nerve or to the muscle. Electromyography is a special recording technique that detects electrical activity of muscle fibers and can determine the severity of damage to the median nerve.

- Ultrasound imaging can show abnormal size of the median nerve. Magnetic resonance imaging (MRI) can show the anatomy of the wrist but to date has not been especially useful in diagnosing carpal tunnel syndrome.

How Is CTS Treated?

Treatments for carpal tunnel syndrome should begin as early as possible, under a doctor's direction. Underlying causes such as diabetes or arthritis should be treated first.

Nonsurgical Treatments

- **Splinting.** Initial treatment is usually a splint worn at night.

- **Avoiding daytime activities that may provoke symptoms.** Some people with slight discomfort may wish to take frequent breaks from tasks, to rest the hand. If the wrist is red, warm and swollen, applying cool packs can help.

- **Over-the-counter drugs.** In special circumstances, drugs can ease the pain and swelling associated with carpal tunnel syndrome. Nonsteroidal anti-inflammatory drugs, such as aspirin, ibuprofen, and other nonprescription pain relievers, may provide some short-term relief from discomfort but haven't been shown to treat CTS itself.

- **Prescription medicines.** Corticosteroids (such as prednisone) or the drug lidocaine can be injected directly into the wrist or taken by mouth (in the case of prednisone) to relieve pressure on the median nerve in people with mild or intermittent symptoms. (Caution: Individuals with diabetes and those who may be predisposed to diabetes should note that prolonged use of corticosteroids can make it difficult to regulate insulin levels.)

- **Alternative therapies.** Yoga has been shown to reduce pain and improve grip strength among those with CTS. Some people report relief using acupuncture and chiropractic care but the effectiveness of these therapies remains unproved.

Surgery

Carpal tunnel release is one of the most common surgical procedures in the United States. Generally, surgery involves severing a ligament around the wrist to reduce pressure on the median nerve. Surgery is usually done under local or regional anesthesia (involving some sedation) and does not require an overnight hospital stay. Many people require surgery on both hands. While all carpal tunnel surgery involves cutting the ligament to relieve the pressure on the nerve, there are two different methods used by surgeons to accomplish this.

- **Open release surgery,** the traditional procedure used to correct carpal tunnel syndrome, consists of making an incision up to 2 inches in the wrist and then cutting the carpal ligament to enlarge the carpal tunnel. The procedure is generally done under local anesthesia on an outpatient basis, unless there are unusual medical conditions.

- **Endoscopic surgery** may allow somewhat faster functional recovery and less postoperative discomfort than traditional open release surgery but it may also have a higher risk of complications and the need for additional surgery. The surgeon makes one or two incisions (about ½ inch each) in the wrist and palm, inserts a camera attached to a tube, observes the nerve, ligament, and tendons on a monitor, and cuts the carpal ligament (the tissue that holds joints together) with a small knife that is inserted through the tube.

Following surgery, the ligaments usually grow back together and allow more space than before. Although symptoms may be relieved immediately after surgery, full recovery from carpal tunnel surgery can take months. Almost always there is a decrease in grip strength, which improves over time. Some individuals may develop infections, nerve damage, stiffness, and pain at the scar. Most people need to modify work activity for several weeks following surgery, and some people may need to adjust job duties or even change jobs after recovery from surgery.

Although recurrence of carpal tunnel syndrome following treatment is rare, fewer than half of individuals report their hand(s) feeling completely normal following surgery. Some residual numbness or weakness is common.

How Can CTS Be Prevented?

At the workplace, workers can do on-the-job conditioning, perform stretching exercises, take frequent rest breaks, and ensure correct posture and wrist position. Wearing fingerless gloves can help keep hands warm and flexible. Workstations, tools and tool handles, and tasks can be redesigned to enable the worker's wrist to maintain a natural position during work. Jobs can be rotated among workers. Employers can develop programs in ergonomics, the process of adapting workplace conditions and job demands to the capabilities of workers. However, research has not conclusively shown that these workplace changes prevent the occurrence of carpal tunnel syndrome.

Section 29.3

Hip Replacement Surgery

This section includes text excerpted from "Hip Replacement," NIHSeniorHealth, National Institute on Aging (NIA), February 2015.

Who Needs a Hip Replacement?

Hip replacement is an operation in which a damaged hip joint is removed and replaced with an artificial joint. There are many medical conditions that can damage the hip joint.

Reasons for Hip Replacement

The most common reason for hip replacement is osteoarthritis. Osteoarthritis occurs when the cartilage covering the ends of the bones where they meet to form joints breaks down. This causes the bones of the joint to rub together. Growths of bone, called spurs, may form around the joint. These changes lead to pain and stiffness.

Other possible causes of hip damage include injuries, fractures, bone tumors, rheumatoid arthritis, and osteonecrosis.

Rheumatoid arthritis is a condition in which the body's immune system attacks the membrane that lines the joint. This can lead to pain, inflammation, and destruction of the joint. Osteonecrosis is a condition in which the blood supply to the bone is cut off, causing the bone to die.

Doctors often recommend hip replacement if pain and stiffness interfere with your ability to do everyday activities—particularly if other treatments have not helped.

Before Choosing Hip Replacement

Treatments your doctor will likely recommend first include exercises to strengthen the muscles around the hip, walking aids such as canes to reduce stress on the joint, and medicines to relieve pain.

Medicines for Hip Pain

Several different medicines can be useful for hip pain. For pain without inflammation, doctors usually recommend the analgesic acetaminophen.

For pain with inflammation, your doctor may prescribe a nonsteroidal anti-inflammatory drug (NSAID) such as ibuprofen or naproxen. For additional pain relief, your doctor may recommend acetaminophen and an NSAID, but you shouldn't combine the two without first speaking with your doctor.

In some cases, stronger medicines may be needed. These include the analgesic tramadol or a product containing both acetaminophen and a narcotic codeine to control pain. For inflammation, doctors may prescribe corticosteroids; however, they should not be used any longer than necessary because of their harmful side effects.

Hip Replacement Isn't for Everyone

For example, people with Parkinson disease or conditions causing severe muscle weakness are more likely to damage or dislocate an artificial hip. People who are in poor health or at high risk for infection are less likely to recover successfully.

If You Are Considering Surgery

The decision to have hip replacement surgery is one you must make with your doctor and your family. If you would like to consider hip replacement, ask your doctor to refer you for an evaluation to an orthopaedic surgeon, a doctor specially trained to treat problems with the bones and joints.

The surgeon must consider many factors before recommending hip replacement. Although most people who have hip replacement are between 60 and 80 years old, age is less of an issue than factors such as pain, disability, and general health. In fact, more and more people under the age of 60 are turning to hip replacement as a way to maintain function and quality of life.

People who are generally healthy are the best candidates for the surgery. Recent studies also suggest that people who choose to have surgery before advanced joint damage occurs tend to recover more easily and have better outcomes.

Types of Surgeries

There are two major types of hip replacement surgery: traditional and minimally invasive, also called mini-incision hip replacement.

Traditional Surgery

In a traditional surgery, the surgeon makes a 10- to 12-inch incision through some of the muscles around the hip to expose the joint. Then the surgeon removes the damaged bone and cartilage and replaces them with an artificial joint, or prosthesis.

Minimally Invasive Surgery

In minimally invasive surgery, the surgeon makes one or two much smaller incisions between the muscles. These incisions may be in the back, side, or front of the hip. The recovery time for the mini-incision surgery is shorter than for traditional surgery.

Doctors tend to recommend minimally invasive surgery for younger patients and those who are of normal weight and healthier than those who are candidates for traditional hip replacement surgery.

The Artificial Joint

Regardless of which type of surgery you have, the artificial joint will consist of two basic parts: a ball made of highly polished strong metal or ceramic material and a socket made of plastic, ceramic, or metal. The ball attaches to the top of the thighbone, or femur; the new socket attaches to your pelvis.

Cemented and Uncemented Parts

These components come in two basic varieties: cemented and uncemented, which refers to the way the parts are attached to your existing bone.

Surgeons fasten cemented parts to existing, healthy bone with a special glue or cement. Uncemented parts rely on a process called biologic fixation to hold them in place. This means that the parts are made with a porous surface. Over time, your own bone grows into the holes in the joint surface to secure them.

Sometimes surgeons use an uncemented part for the socket and a cemented part for the femur. This combination is called a hybrid replacement.

Studies show that cemented and uncemented joints are similarly successful; however, doctors usually use cemented joints for older, less active people and people with weak bones.

Uncemented joints are often reserved for younger, more active people. The main disadvantage of uncemented joints is a longer recovery time because it takes time for bone to grow into the surface of the replacement part(s). Also, recovery may be more painful as bone grows into the prosthesis.

Preparing for Surgery

Have a Medical Evaluation

Preparing for surgery will likely begin with a medical evaluation. During the evaluation, your doctor will assess your general health, looking for any problems that could complicate surgery or your recovery.

During the evaluation, your doctor may order tests on blood and urine samples as well as tests like an electrocardiogram or chest X-rays.

If you are taking any medications, it's important to tell your doctor the specific medications and doses you are taking. You may need to stop taking some of your medicines for a while before surgery, while you can continue others. Be certain you report all over-the-counter and herbal supplements you are taking. You may be asked to stop taking some of these before the surgery.

What Your Doctor May Recommend

If you are overweight, your doctor may recommend that you lose some weight before surgery to minimize the stress on your new hip and possibly decrease the risks of surgery. Your doctor may also recommend exercise to strengthen your muscles and improve your general health and recovery.

In case you might need blood during surgery, your doctor may recommend autologous blood donation. This means you have your own blood drawn several weeks before surgery and stored in case you need it.

Because dental procedures can allow bacteria to enter the body and these bacteria can potentially lodge in the joint, your doctor may recommend that you have any needed dental work before your surgery.

Before any future procedures, tell the healthcare provider about your artificial joint. You may need to take antibiotics for some dental, eye, and certain other procedures to prevent the possibility of infection in and around the artificial joint.

Learn about the Procedure

It's also important to know as much as you can about the procedure and what to expect before you have it. Your doctor should be able to give you written information or recommend other sources.

Many people find it helpful to speak with someone who has already had the surgery. If you think you like might to speak with someone, ask your doctor to recommend someone.

Also, some hospitals have classes for prospective hip replacement patients. Ask if the hospital where you will be having your surgery has one and sign up to learn more about the surgery itself and recovery afterwards.

Having Surgery

Having hip replacement usually requires a hospital stay of 3 to 5 days. During that time you will have the surgery and begin recovery and rehabilitation. You will also learn about possible complications, including how to prevent them and recognize them if they occur.

Before Surgery

You will most likely be admitted to the hospital on the day of your surgery. Before you are admitted, however, you will see an anesthesiologist, who will evaluate your general health and talk with you about the types of anesthesia, or pain relief, during surgery.

Two common types of anesthesia for hip replacement are general anesthesia and spinal or epidural anesthesia. With general anesthesia, you are asleep during surgery and a machine helps you breathe. With spinal or epidural anesthesia, you are numbed from the waist down during the operation. Regardless of the method used, the surgery itself will not be painful.

After Surgery

Hip replacement surgery usually takes 1 to 2 hours. After surgery, you will be taken to the recovery room where you will be monitored for an hour or two. Once you are fully awake and alert, you will be moved to a hospital room for the rest of your stay.

In the first hours after your surgery, you will be allowed to move very little. Your hospital bed will have special pillows or devices to hold your hip in the correct position.

You may have an IV tube inserted to replace any fluids you lost during surgery. You may also have a tube near the incision to drain fluid and a tube called a catheter to drain urine until you are able to go to the bathroom. You will also receive medicine to relieve pain.

The surgery site will be closed with staples or stitches, which will be removed about two weeks after surgery. In the meantime, it will be important to avoid getting the wound wet until it heals. A bandage can help prevent clothing or stockings from irritating the wound.

Shortly after surgery, a respiratory therapist may visit you and ask you to breathe deeply, cough, or blow into a device to increase your lung capacity. Doing these things will help reduce the risk of infection in your lungs.

Physical Therapy

Later in the day after your surgery or the following day, physical therapists will begin to teach you exercises to help your recovery. A day or two after surgery, you will be allowed to sit on the edge of the bed and stand and walk with help.

A physical therapist will teach you exercises to strengthen the hip muscles and help you safely do daily activities. Because your new hip's range of motion is more limited than that of a natural hip, it is important to use proper techniques for activities such as sitting and bending, to avoid injuring your new hip.

Possible Complications

While new technology and advances in surgical techniques have greatly reduced the risks involved with hip replacements, there are still some risks you should be aware of. Two of the most common possible problems that might occur in the short-term (just after surgery or up to 3 months after) are dislocation and blood clots.

Dislocation

Because the artificial ball and socket are smaller than natural ones, the ball can come out of the socket if you put the hip in certain positions. Positions to avoid include pulling your knees up to your chest, crossing your legs, or bending your hips farther than a right angle.

Blood Clots

Blood clots can occur in the veins of your legs or pelvis after hip replacement surgery. To reduce the risk of clots your doctor will prescribe some combination of special exercises, support hose, and/or blood thinners.

Other Complications

Other complications such as new or ongoing pain, stiffness, fracture, bleeding, or injury to the blood vessels can occur. Sometimes infections elsewhere in the body can travel to your prosthesis, but this is not common. Serious medical complications, such as heart attack or stroke, are even rarer, and if they happened, would most likely occur just after the surgery.

Reducing Your Risk for Complications

To minimize the risk of complications, it's important to know how to prevent problems and to recognize signs of potential problems early and contact your doctor. For example tenderness, redness and swelling of your calf, or swelling of your thigh, ankle, or foot. could be warning signs of a possible blood clot. Warning signs of infection include fever, chills, tenderness and swelling, or drainage from the wound. You should call your doctor if you experience any of these symptoms.

It is important to get instructions from your doctor before leaving the hospital and follow them carefully once you get home. Doing so will you give you the greatest chance of a successful surgery.

Section 29.4

Knee Replacement Surgery

This section includes text excerpted from "Knee Replacement," NIHSeniorHealth, National Institute on Aging (NIA), August 2014.

Who Needs a Knee Replacement?

Knee replacement is an operation that involves removing parts of one's natural knee joint and replacing them with artificial ones. Knee replacement is the most common joint replacement surgery.

The main reason to have knee replacement surgery is to ease pain and disability caused by arthritis or other joint problems, while preserving movement. Less commonly, it is used to correct some kinds of knee deformity.

Arthritis and Other Joint Problems

Several forms of arthritis can damage knees to the point that they need to be replaced. They include:

- **osteoarthritis,** which occurs when the cartilage covering the ends of the bones where they meet to form joints breaks down. This causes the bones of the joint to rub together. Growths of bone, called spurs, may form around the joint. These changes lead to pain and stiffness.

- **rheumatoid arthritis,** a condition in which the body's immune system attacks the membrane that lines the joint. This can lead to pain, inflammation and destruction of the joint.

- **posttraumatic arthritis,** a form of osteoarthritis that may occur after a knee injury such as a fracture or ligament tear. These kinds of injuries can cause inflammation and affect the alignment of the knee, leading to cartilage damage over time. Because of this, an injury that you suffered earlier in life can cause you to have arthritis at middle age or later.

Knee damage can also result from a problem called avascular necrosis, or osteonecrosis, in which the bones lose their blood supply, die, and eventually collapse. Although the cause of avascular necrosis is not well understood, in many people it appears to result from trauma to the knee.

Knee Deformities

Knee deformities—such as bowed legs or knock knees—occur when the knees are not formed or aligned properly. Over time, this creates stress on the joints that can wear down cartilage and lead to pain and disability. In these cases, knee replacement can restore the normal alignment of the knee and correct disability.

Other Treatments

Your doctor may recommend knee replacement if pain and stiffness interfere with your ability to do everyday activities—particularly if other treatments have not helped.

Treatments your doctor will likely recommend before knee replacement include:

- **exercises** to strengthen the muscles around the knee and improve flexibility

- **weight loss,** if needed, to reduce the load the knee must bear

- **walking aids** such as canes to reduce stress on the joint

- **shoe inserts** to improve the knee's alignment

- **medicines** to relieve pain.

Medicines to Relieve Knee Pain

Several different medicines can be useful for knee pain. Some medicines are taken by mouth. These include analgesic medications such as acetaminophen and tramadol, and nonsteroidal anti-inflammatory drugs (NSAIDs) such as ibuprofen or naproxen. Some, referred to as topical analgesics, are rubbed into the skin directly over the knee. Others are injected into the knee joint. These include corticosteroids, which are strong inflammation-fighting drugs, and hyaluronic acid substitutes, also called viscosupplements, which are designed to replace a substance that gives joint fluid its "slipperiness."

Who Shouldn't Have Knee Replacement Surgery

Although knee replacement is a common surgery, it is not for everyone. For example, you should not have a knee replacement if you have an infection of the knee, a severe nerve disorder, or severe blood vessel disease. Your doctor may also advise against surgery if you are severely overweight, have heart or lung disorders that could complicate surgery or anesthesia, or have a skin condition such as psoriasis where the incisions would be made.

The Decision to Have Surgery

The decision to have knee replacement surgery is one you must make with your doctor and your family. If you would like to consider knee replacement surgery, ask your doctor to refer you for evaluation to an orthopaedic surgeon, a doctor specially trained to treat problems with the bones and joints.

The surgeon must consider many factors before recommending knee replacement. People who are generally healthy are the best candidates for the surgery, and those who have surgery before advanced joint damage occurs tend to recover more quickly and have better outcomes.

Types of Knee Replacement

There are many different types and designs of artificial knees. Most consist of three components:

- the femoral component, which is the part that attaches to the thigh bone

- the tibial component, the part that attaches to the shin bone

- the patellar component, the knee cap.

Total and Partial Knee Replacement

Knee replacement may be either total or partial/unicompartmental.

In total knee replacement, as the name suggests, the entire knee joint is replaced. You will likely need a total knee replacement if you have damage to several parts of your knee.

In partial/unicompartmental knee replacement, the surgeon replaces just the damaged part of the knee. You may be able to have a partial knee replacement if only one section of your knee is damaged. However, when one part is replaced, there is a chance that another part will develop arthritis, requiring further surgery.

Cemented and Uncemented Joint Components

Joint components may also be attached to your own bone in different ways. Most are cemented with a special joint glue into your existing bone; others rely on a process called biologic fixation to hold them in place. This means that the parts are made with a porous surface, and over time your own bone grows into the joint surface to secure them. In some cases, surgeons use a combination of cemented and uncemented parts. This is referred to as a hybrid implant.

Minimally Invasive Surgery

While some knee replacement surgery requires an 8- to 12-inch incision in the front of the knee, surgeons at many medical centers are now performing what is called minimally invasive surgery using incisions of 3 to 5 inches or even smaller. Because the incision is smaller, there may be less pain and a shorter recovery time. If you think you might be interested in minimally invasive surgery, speak with your surgeon.

Preparing for Surgery

One of the most important factors in successful surgery is preparation. As a patient, part of preparation is learning what to expect of surgery itself as well as during the recovery—both in the hospital and at home. This includes knowing the warning signs of complications that warrant a call to your doctor.

Your first step in preparing for surgery will likely be a medical evaluation. During the evaluation, your doctor will evaluate not only the knee to be replaced, but also the ankle and hip on the same leg. If either of these joints is severely damaged, replacing the damaged knee may do little to improve function.

Your doctor will also assess your general health, looking for any problems that could complicate surgery or your recovery. This may involve blood and urine tests as well as tests like an electrocardiogram (ECG) or chest X-ray.

If you are taking medications of any kind—prescription or over-the-counter medications, or herbal or alternative therapies—it is important to tell your doctor about all the medications and doses you are taking. You may need to stop taking some of your medicines for a while before surgery, while you can continue others.

Weight Loss and Exercise

If you are overweight, your doctor may recommend that you lose some weight before surgery to minimize the stress on your new knee and possibly decrease the risks of surgery. Your doctor may also recommend exercise to strengthen your muscles and improve your general health and recovery.

Storing Blood

In the event that you need blood during surgery, your doctor may recommend autologous blood donation—particularly if you are anemic. Autologous blood donation means you have your own blood drawn several weeks before surgery and stored in case you need it.

Because dental procedures can allow bacteria to enter the body, and bacteria that enter the body can potentially get into the joint, your doctor may recommend that you have any needed dental work before your surgery. Your doctor may also prescribe an antibiotic before surgery to reduce your risk of infection.

Learning About the Procedure

It is important to know as much as you can about the procedure and what to expect before you have it. Your doctor should also be able to give you written information or recommend other sources.

Many people find it helpful to speak with someone who has already had the surgery. If you think you might like to speak with someone, ask your doctor to recommend someone.

Also, some hospitals have classes for patients who will be getting knee replacement. Ask if the hospital where you will be having your surgery has one, and sign up to learn more about the surgery itself and recovery afterward.

Having Surgery

Having knee replacement usually requires a hospital stay of three to five days. During that time, you will have the surgery and begin recovery and rehabilitation. You will also learn about possible complications, including how to prevent them and recognize them if they occur.

You will most likely be admitted to the hospital on the day of your surgery. Before you are admitted, however, you will see an anesthesiologist, who will evaluate your general health and talk with you about the types of anesthesia, or pain relief, that will be used during surgery.

Two Types of Anesthesia

Two common types of anesthesia for knee replacement are:

- **general anesthesia**, which keeps you asleep during surgery while a machine helps you breathe

- **spinal anesthesia**, which numbs you only from the waist down.

Regardless of the method used, the surgery itself will not be painful.

What to Expect after Surgery

Knee replacement surgery usually takes one to two hours. After surgery, you will be taken to the recovery room where you will be monitored for an hour or two. Once you are fully awake and alert, you will be moved to a hospital room for the rest of your stay.

You may have an intravenous (IV) tube inserted to replace any fluids you lost during surgery. You may also have a tube near the incision to drain fluid and a tube called a catheter to drain urine until you are able to go to the bathroom. In addition, you will receive medicine to relieve pain.

The surgery site will be closed with staples or stitches, which will be removed a few weeks after surgery. In the meantime, it will be important to avoid getting the wound wet as it heals. A bandage can help prevent clothing or stockings from irritating the wound.

Shortly after surgery, a respiratory therapist may visit you and ask you to breathe deeply, cough, or blow into a device to measure your lung capacity. Doing these things will help reduce fluid in your lungs.

Physical Therapy

The day after surgery, a physical therapist will begin to teach you exercises to help your recovery. You can expect some pain, discomfort, and stiffness as you begin therapy, but to get the best results from your new knee, it is important to do all of the exercises your physical therapist recommends.

Your physical therapist may also use a device called a continuous passive motion (CPM) machine to help speed your recovery. This machine cradles your leg and slowly bends and straightens your knee while you relax. For some people, this may keep the knee from getting stiff and increase its range of motion.

A day or two after surgery, you will be allowed to sit on the edge of the bed and stand and walk. You will begin walking with help, using a walker or crutches. Eventually you will be able to walk on flat surfaces, climb stairs, and return to normal activities without help.

Possible Complications

While new technology and advances in surgical techniques have greatly reduced the risks involved with knee replacements, there are still some risks you should be aware of. Two of the most common possible problems are blood clots and infection.

Preventing Blood Clots

Blood clots can occur in the veins of your legs after knee replacement surgery. To reduce the risk of clots, your doctor may have you elevate your leg periodically and prescribe special exercises, support hose, or blood thinners.

Preventing Infections

Infection can occur when bacteria enter the bloodstream from skin or urinary tract infections. To reduce the risk of infection, your doctors may prescribe antibiotics for you to take prior to your surgery and for a short time afterward.

Other Complications

Other complications, such as new or ongoing pain, stiffness, fracture, bleeding, or injury to the blood vessels can occur. Serious medical complications, such as heart attack or stroke, are very rare.

Warning Signs to Watch For

To minimize the risk of complications, it is important to recognize signs of potential problems early and contact your doctor. For example, tenderness, redness, and swelling of your calf or swelling of your thigh, ankle, calf, or foot could be warning signs of a possible blood clot.

Warning signs of infection include fever or chills, tenderness and swelling of the wound, and drainage from the wound. You should call your doctor if you experience any of these symptoms.

It is important to get instructions from your doctor before leaving the hospital and follow them carefully once you get home. Doing so will give you the greatest chance of a successful surgery.

What to Expect in Recovery

Recovery from knee replacement extends long after you leave the hospital. Preparing for recovery requires learning what to expect in the days and weeks following surgery. It requires understanding what you will and won't be able to do—and when. It also means arranging for social support and arranging your house to make everyday tasks easier and to help speed your recovery.

Find Someone to Stay with You

Because you will not be able to drive for several weeks after surgery, you will need someone to take you home from the hospital and be on hand to run errands or take you to appointments until you can drive yourself.

If you live with someone, you should have them plan to stay home with you or at least stay close by, in case you need help. If you don't live with a family member or have one close by, a friend or neighbor may be able to help. Other options include staying in an extended-care facility during your recovery or hiring someone to come to your home and help you. Your hospital social worker should be able to help you make arrangements.

Prepare Your Home for Your Recovery

To prepare your home for your recovery, stock up on needed items before you leave for the hospital. Make sure you have plenty of non-perishable foods on hand. Prepare meals and freeze them to put in the microwave when you need an easy meal.

In the first weeks after surgery, you should avoid going up and down stairs. If your bedroom is on the second floor of your home, consider moving to a downstairs bedroom temporarily or sleeping on the sofa.

Set Up a "Recovery Station"

Set up a "recovery station" at home. Place a sturdy chair where you plan to spend most of your time sitting during the first weeks after surgery. The chair should be 18 to 20 inches high and should have two arms and a firm seat and back. Place a foot stool in front of the chair so you can elevate your legs, and place items you will need—such as the television remote control, telephone, medicine, and tissues—where you can reach them easily from the chair.

Place items you use every day at arm's level to avoid reaching up or bending down. Ask your doctor or physical therapist about devices and tips that may make daily activities easier once you get home.

Devices you may find helpful include long-handled reachers to retrieve items placed on high shelves or dropped on the floor, aprons with pockets that allow you to carry items while leaving your hands free for crutches, shower benches that let you sit while you shower, and dressing sticks to help you get dressed without bending your new knee excessively.

Safeguard Against Falls

Because a fall can damage your new knee, making your home a safe place is crucial. Before your surgery, look for and correct hazards, including cluttered floors, loose electrical cords, unsecured rugs, and dark hallways.

Bathrooms are likely places to fall, so particular attention is needed there. A raised toilet seat can make it easier to get up and down. Grab bars in the tub can keep you steady. Textured shapes on the shower floor can minimize slipping.

Gradually Increase Activity

It is also important to exercise to get stronger while avoiding any activities that can damage or dislocate your new joint. Activity should include a graduated walking program (where you slowly increase the time, distance, and pace that you walk) and specific exercises several times a day to prevent scarring, restore movement, and stabilize and strengthen your new knee.

Remember Follow-Ups

Your surgeon will let you know about follow-up visits. Even after you have healed from surgery, you will need to see your surgeon periodically for examinations and X-rays to detect any potential problems with your knee.

By preparing for surgery and recovery and following your doctor's advice, you can get the greatest benefits from your new knee with the least risk of complications for many years to come.

Section 29.5

Spinal Stenosis Surgery

This section includes text excerpted from "Spinal Stenosis—Questions and Answers about Spinal Stenosis," National Institute of Arthritis and Musculoskeletal and Skin Diseases (NIAMS), August 2016.

What Is Spinal Stenosis?

Spinal stenosis is a narrowing of spaces in the spine (backbone) that results in pressure on the spinal cord and/or nerve roots. This disorder usually involves the narrowing of one or more of three areas of the spine:

1. the canal in the center of the column of bones (vertebral or spinal column) through which the spinal cord and nerve roots run,

2. the canals at the base or roots of nerves branching out from the spinal cord, or

3. the openings between vertebrae (bones of the spine) through which nerves leave the spine and go to other parts of the body.

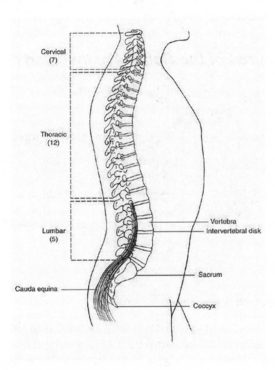

Figure 29.1. *Side View of Spine*

Who Gets Spinal Stenosis?

This disorder is most common in men and women over 50 years of age. However, it may occur in younger people who are born with a narrowing of the spinal canal or who suffer an injury to the spine.

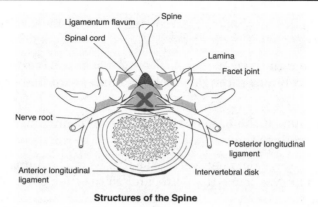

Structures of the Spine

Figure 29.2. *Structures of the Spine*

What Structures of the Spine Are Involved?

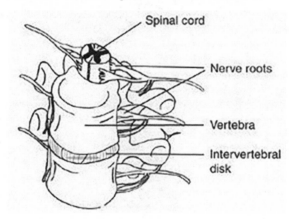

Figure 29.3. *Section of the Spine*

The spine is a column of 26 bones that extend in a line from the base of the skull to the pelvis (see Figure 29.1). Twenty-four of the bones are called vertebrae. The bones of the spine include 7 cervical vertebrae in the neck; 12 thoracic vertebrae at the back wall of the chest; 5 lumbar vertebrae at the inward curve (small) of the lower back; the sacrum, composed of 5 fused vertebrae between the hip bones; and the coccyx, composed of 3 to 5 fused bones at the lower tip of the vertebral column.

The vertebrae link to each other and are cushioned by shock-absorbing disks that lie between them. Other structures of the spine include:

- **Facet joints.** Joints located on the back of the main part of the vertebra. They are formed by a portion of one vertebra and the vertebra above it. They connect the vertebrae to each other and permit backward motion.

- **Ligaments.** Elastic bands of tissue that support the spine by preventing the vertebrae from slipping out of line as the spine moves.

- **Spinal cord/nerve roots.** A major part of the central nervous system that extends from the base of the brain down to the lower back and that is encased by the vertebral column. It consists of nerve cells and bundles of nerves. The cord connects the brain to all parts of the body via 31 pairs of nerves that branch out from the cord and leave the spine between vertebrae.

- **Cauda equina.** A sack of nerve roots that continues from the lumbar region, where the spinal cord ends, and continues down to provide neurologic function to the lower part of the body. It resembles a "horse's tail" (*cauda equina* in Latin).

What Causes Spinal Stenosis?

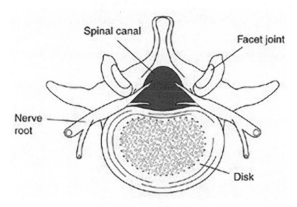

Figure 29.4. *Normal Vertebra (Cross Section)*

The normal vertebral canal (see Figure 29.4) provides adequate room for the spinal cord and cauda equina. Narrowing of the canal, which occurs in spinal stenosis, may be inherited or acquired. Some people inherit a small spinal canal (see Figure 29.5) or have a curvature of the spine (scoliosis) that produces pressure on nerves and soft tissue and compresses or stretches ligaments. In an inherited condition called achondroplasia, defective bone formation results in changes that reduce the diameter (distance across) of the spinal canal.

Acquired conditions that can cause spinal stenosis are explained in more detail in the sections that follow.

Degenerative Conditions

Spinal stenosis most often results from a gradual, degenerative aging process. Either structural changes or inflammation can begin the process. As people age, the ligaments of the spine may thicken and calcify (harden from deposits of calcium salts). Bones and joints may also enlarge; when surfaces of the bone begin to project out from the body, these projections are called osteophytes (bone spurs).

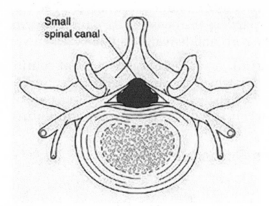

Figure 29.5. *Small Spinal Canal*

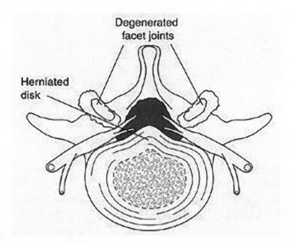

Figure 29.6. *Herniated Disk*

When the health of one part of the spine fails, it usually places increased stress on other parts of the spine. For example, a herniated (bulging) disk may place pressure on the spinal cord or nerve root (see

Figure 29.6). When a segment of the spine becomes too mobile, the capsules (enclosing membranes) of the facet joints thicken in an effort to stabilize the segment, and bone spurs may occur. This decreases the space available for nerve roots leaving the spinal cord.

Spondylolisthesis, a condition in which one vertebra slips forward on another, may result from a degenerative condition or an accident, or, very rarely, may be acquired at birth. Poor alignment of the spinal column when a vertebra slips forward onto the one below it can place pressure on the spinal cord or nerve roots at that place.

Aging with secondary changes is the most common cause of spinal stenosis. Two forms of arthritis that may affect the spine are osteoarthritis and rheumatoid arthritis.

- **Osteoarthritis.** Osteoarthritis is the most common form of arthritis and is more likely to occur in middle-aged and older people. It is a chronic, degenerative process that may involve multiple joints of the body. It wears away the surface cartilage layer of joints, and is often accompanied by overgrowth of bone, formation of bone spurs, and impaired function. If the degenerative process of osteoarthritis affects the facet joint(s) and the disk, the condition is sometimes referred to as spondylosis. This condition may be accompanied by disk degeneration, and an enlargement or overgrowth of bone that narrows the central and nerve root canals.

- **Rheumatoid Arthritis.** Rheumatoid arthritis usually affects people at an earlier age than osteoarthritis does and is associated with inflammation and enlargement of the soft tissues (the synovium) of the joints. Although not a common cause of spinal stenosis, damage to ligaments, bones, and joints that begins as synovitis (inflammation of the synovial membrane that lines the inside of the joint) has a severe and disrupting effect on joint function. The portions of the vertebral column with the greatest mobility (for example, the neck area) are often the ones most affected in people with rheumatoid arthritis.

Other Acquired Conditions

The following conditions that are not related to degenerative disease are causes of acquired spinal stenosis:

- **Tumors of the spine** are abnormal growths of soft tissue that may affect the spinal canal directly by inflammation or by growth of tissue into the canal. Tissue growth may lead to bone resorption (bone loss due to overactivity of certain bone cells) or displacement of bone.

- **Trauma** (accidents) may either dislocate the spine and the spinal canal or cause burst fractures that produce fragments of bone that penetrate the canal.

- **Paget disease of bone** is a chronic (long-term) disorder that typically results in enlarged and abnormal bones. Excessive bone breakdown and formation cause thick and fragile bone. As a result, bone pain, arthritis, noticeable bone structure changes, and fractures can occur. The disease can affect any bone of the body, but is often found in the spine. The blood supply that feeds healthy nerve tissue may be diverted to the area of involved bone. Also, structural problems of the involved vertebrae can cause narrowing of the spinal canal, producing a variety of neurological symptoms. Other developmental conditions may also result in spinal stenosis.

- **Ossification of the posterior longitudinal ligament** occurs when calcium deposits form on the ligament that runs up and down behind the spine and inside the spinal canal (see Figure 29.7). These deposits turn the fibrous tissue of the ligament into bone. (Ossification means "forming bone.") These deposits may press on the nerves in the spinal canal.

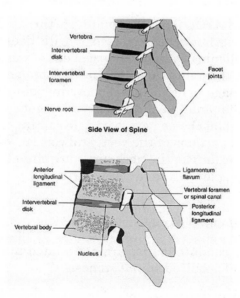

Figure 29.7. *Side View of Spine (Cross Section)*

What Are the Symptoms of Spinal Stenosis?

The space within the spinal canal may narrow without producing any symptoms. However, if narrowing places pressure on the spinal cord, cauda equina, or nerve roots, there may be a slow onset and progression of symptoms. The neck or back may or may not hurt. More often, people experience numbness, weakness, cramping, or general pain in the arms or legs. If the narrowed space within the spine is pushing on a nerve root, people may feel pain radiating down the leg (sciatica). Sitting or flexing the lower back should relieve symptoms. (The flexed position "opens up" the spinal column, enlarging the spaces between vertebrae at the back of the spine.) Flexing exercises are often advised, along with stretching and strengthening exercises.

People with more severe stenosis may have problems with bowel and bladder function and foot disorders. For example, cauda equina syndrome is a severe, and very rare, form of spinal stenosis. It occurs because of compression of the cauda equina, and symptoms may include loss of control of the bowel, bladder, or sexual function and/ or pain, weakness, or loss of feeling in one or both legs. Cauda equina syndrome is a serious condition requiring urgent medical attention.

How Is Spinal Stenosis Diagnosed?

The doctor may use a variety of approaches to diagnose spinal stenosis and rule out other conditions.

- **Medical history.** The patient tells the doctor details about symptoms and about any injury, condition, or general health problem that might be causing the symptoms.

- **Physical examination.** The doctor (1) examines the patient to determine the extent of limitation of movement, (2) checks for pain or symptoms when the patient hyper-extends the spine (bends backwards), and (3) checks for normal neurologic function (for instance, sensation, muscle strength, and reflexes) in the arms and legs.

- **X-ray.** An X-ray beam is passed through the back to produce a two-dimensional picture. An X-ray may be done before other tests to look for signs of an injury, tumor, or inherited problem. This test can show the structure of the vertebrae and the outlines of joints, and can detect calcification.

- **Magnetic resonance imaging (MRI).** Energy from a powerful magnet (rather than X-rays) produces signals that are detected by a scanner and analyzed by computer. This produces a series of cross-sectional images ("slices") and/or a three-dimensional view of parts of the back. An MRI is particularly sensitive for detecting damage or disease of soft tissues, such as the disks between vertebrae or ligaments. It shows the spinal cord, nerve roots, and surrounding spaces, as well as enlargement, degeneration, or tumors.

- **Computerized axial tomography (CAT).** X-rays are passed through the back at different angles, detected by a scanner, and analyzed by a computer. This produces a series of cross-sectional images and/or three-dimensional views of the parts of the back. The scan shows the shape and size of the spinal canal, its contents, and structures surrounding it.

- **Myelogram.** A liquid dye that X-rays cannot penetrate is injected into the spinal column. The dye circulates around the spinal cord and spinal nerves, which appear as white objects against bone on an X-ray film. A myelogram can show pressure on the spinal cord or nerves from herniated disks, bone spurs, or tumors.

Who Treats Spinal Stenosis?

Nonsurgical treatment of spinal stenosis may be provided by internists or general practitioners. The disorder is also treated by specialists such as rheumatologists, who treat arthritis and related disorders; and neurologists, who treat nerve diseases. Orthopaedic surgeons and neurosurgeons also provide nonsurgical treatment and perform spinal surgery if it is required. Allied health professionals such as physical therapists may also help treat patients.

What Are the Major Risks of Surgery?

All surgery, particularly that involving general anesthesia and older patients, carries risks. The most common complications of surgery for spinal stenosis are a tear in the membrane covering the spinal cord at the site of the operation, infection, or a blood clot that forms in the veins. These conditions can be treated but may prolong recovery. The presence of other diseases and the physical condition of the patient are also significant factors to consider when making decisions about surgery.

When Should Surgery Be Considered and What Is Involved?

In many cases, the conditions causing spinal stenosis cannot be permanently altered by nonsurgical treatment, even though these measures may relieve pain for a period of time. To determine how much nonsurgical treatment will help, a doctor may recommend such treatment first. However, surgery might be considered immediately if a patient has numbness or weakness that interferes with walking, impaired bowel or bladder function, or other neurological involvement. The effectiveness of nonsurgical treatments, the extent of the patient's pain, and the patient's preferences may all factor into whether or not to have surgery.

The purpose of surgery is to relieve pressure on the spinal cord or nerves and restore and maintain alignment and strength of the spine. This can be done by removing, trimming, or adjusting diseased parts that are causing the pressure or loss of alignment. The most common surgery is called decompressive laminectomy: removal of the lamina (roof) of one or more vertebrae to create more space for the nerves. A surgeon may perform a laminectomy with or without fusing vertebrae or removing part of a disk. Various devices may be used to enhance fusion and strengthen unstable segments of the spine following decompression surgery.

Patients with spinal stenosis caused by spinal trauma or achondroplasia may need surgery at a young age. When surgery is required in patients with achondroplasia, laminectomy (removal of the roof) without fusion is usually sufficient.

What Are the Long-Term Outcomes of Surgical Treatment for Spinal Stenosis?

Removal of the obstruction that has caused the symptoms usually gives patients some relief; most patients have less leg pain and are able to walk better following surgery. However, if nerves were badly damaged before surgery, there may be some remaining pain or numbness or no improvement. Also, the degenerative process will likely continue, and pain or limitation of activity may reappear after surgery. National Institute of Arthritis and Musculoskeletal and Skin Diseases (NIAMS)-supported researchers have published results from the Spine Patient Outcomes Research Trial (SPORT), the largest trial to date comparing surgical and nonsurgical interventions for the treatment of low back and associated leg pain caused by spinal stenosis. The study found that for patients with spinal stenosis, surgical treatment was more effective than nonsurgical treatment in relieving symptoms and improving function. However, the functional status of patients who received nonsurgical therapies also improved somewhat during the study.

Section 29.6

Low Back Surgery

This section includes text excerpted from "Low Back Pain Fact Sheet," National Institute of Neurological Disorders and Stroke (NINDS), December 2014.

If you have lower back pain, you are not alone. About 80 percent of adults experience low back pain at some point in their lifetimes. It is the most common cause of job-related disability and a leading contributor to missed work days. In a large survey, more than a quarter of adults reported experiencing low back pain during the past 3 months.

Men and women are equally affected by low back pain, which can range in intensity from a dull, constant ache to a sudden, sharp sensation that leaves the person incapacitated. Pain can begin abruptly as a result of an accident or by lifting something heavy, or it can develop over time due to age-related changes of the spine. Sedentary lifestyles also can set the stage for low back pain, especially when a weekday routine of getting too little exercise is punctuated by strenuous weekend workout.

Most low back pain is acute, or short-term, and lasts a few days to a few weeks. It tends to resolve on its own with self-care and there is no residual loss of function. The majority of acute low back pain is mechanical in nature, meaning that there is a disruption in the way the components of the back (the spine, muscle, intervertebral discs, and nerves) fit together and move.

Subacute low back pain is defined as pain that lasts between 4 and 12 weeks.

Chronic back pain is defined as pain that persists for 12 weeks or longer, even after an initial injury or underlying cause of acute low back pain has been treated. About 20 percent of people affected by acute low back pain develop chronic low back pain with persistent symptoms at one year. In some cases, treatment successfully relieves chronic low back pain, but in other cases pain persists despite medical and surgical treatment.

The magnitude of the burden from low back pain has grown worse in recent years. In 1990, a study ranking the most burdensome conditions in the United States in terms of mortality or poor health as a result of disease put low back pain in sixth place; in 2010, low back pain jumped to third place, with only ischemic heart disease and chronic obstructive pulmonary disease ranking higher.

What Structures Make up the Back?

The lower back where most back pain occurs includes the five vertebrae (referred to as L1-L5) in the lumbar region, which supports much of the weight of the upper body. The spaces between the vertebrae are maintained by round, rubbery pads called intervertebral discs that act like shock absorbers throughout the spinal column to cushion the bones as the body moves. Bands of tissue known as ligaments hold the vertebrae in place, and tendons attach the muscles to the spinal column. Thirty-one pairs of nerves are rooted to the spinal cord and they control body movements and transmit signals from the body to the brain.

What Causes Lower Back Pain?

The vast majority of low back pain is mechanical in nature. In many cases, low back pain is associated with spondylosis, a term that refers to the general degeneration of the spine associated with normal wear and tear that occurs in the joints, discs, and bones of the spine as people get older. Some examples of mechanical causes of low back pain include:

- **Sprains and strains** account for most acute back pain. Sprains are caused by overstretching or tearing ligaments, and strains are tears in tendon or muscle. Both can occur from twisting or lifting something improperly, lifting something too heavy, or overstretching. Such movements may also trigger spasms in back muscles, which can also be painful.

403

- **Intervertebral disc degeneration** is one of the most common mechanical causes of low back pain, and it occurs when the usually rubbery discs lose integrity as a normal process of aging. In a healthy back, intervertebral discs provide height and allow bending, flexion, and torsion of the lower back. As the discs deteriorate, they lose their cushioning ability.

- **Herniated or ruptured discs** can occur when the intervertebral discs become compressed and bulge outward (herniation) or rupture, causing low back pain.

- **Radiculopathy** is a condition caused by compression, inflammation and/or injury to a spinal nerve root. Pressure on the nerve root results in pain, numbness, or a tingling sensation that travels or radiates to other areas of the body that are served by that nerve. Radiculopathy may occur when spinal stenosis or a herniated or ruptured disc compresses the nerve root.

- **Sciatica** is a form of radiculopathy caused by compression of the sciatic nerve, the large nerve that travels through the buttocks and extends down the back of the leg. This compression causes shock-like or burning low back pain combined with pain through the buttocks and down one leg, occasionally reaching the foot. In the most extreme cases, when the nerve is pinched between the disc and the adjacent bone, the symptoms may involve not only pain, but numbness and muscle weakness in the leg because of interrupted nerve signaling. The condition may also be caused by a tumor or cyst that presses on the sciatic nerve or its roots.

- **Spondylolisthesis** is a condition in which a vertebra of the lower spine slips out of place, pinching the nerves exiting the spinal column.

- **A traumatic injury,** such as from playing sports, car accidents, or a fall can injure tendons, ligaments or muscle resulting in low back pain. Traumatic injury may also cause the spine to become overly compressed, which in turn can cause an intervertebral disc to rupture or herniate, exerting pressure on any of the nerves rooted to the spinal cord. When spinal nerves become compressed and irritated, back pain and sciatica may result.

- **Spinal stenosis** is a narrowing of the spinal column that puts pressure on the spinal cord and nerves that can cause pain or numbness with walking and over time leads to leg weakness and sensory loss.

- **Skeletal irregularities** include scoliosis, a curvature of the spine that does not usually cause pain until middle age; lordosis, an abnormally accentuated arch in the lower back; and other congenital anomalies of the spine.

Low back pain is rarely related to serious underlying conditions, but when these conditions do occur, they require immediate medical attention. Serious underlying conditions include:

- **Infections** are not a common cause of back pain. However, infections can cause pain when they involve the vertebrae, a condition called osteomyelitis; the intervertebral discs, called discitis; or the sacroiliac joints connecting the lower spine to the pelvis, called sacroiliitis.

- **Tumors** are a relatively rare cause of back pain. Occasionally, tumors begin in the back, but more often they appear in the back as a result of cancer that has spread from elsewhere in the body.

- **Cauda equina syndrome** is a serious but rare complication of a ruptured disc. It occurs when disc material is pushed into the spinal canal and compresses the bundle of lumbar and sacral nerve roots, causing loss of bladder and bowel control. Permanent neurological damage may result if this syndrome is left untreated.

- **Abdominal aortic aneurysms** occur when the large blood vessel that supplies blood to the abdomen, pelvis, and legs becomes abnormally enlarged. Back pain can be a sign that the aneurysm is becoming larger and that the risk of rupture should be assessed.

- **Kidney stones** can cause sharp pain in the lower back, usually on one side.

Other underlying conditions that predispose people to low back pain include:

- **Inflammatory diseases of the joints** such as arthritis, including osteoarthritis and rheumatoid arthritis as well as spondylitis, an inflammation of the vertebrae, can also cause low back pain. Spondylitis is also called spondyloarthritis or spondyloarthropathy.

- **Osteoporosis** is a metabolic bone disease marked by a progressive decrease in bone density and strength, which can lead to painful fractures of the vertebrae.

- **Endometriosis** is the buildup of uterine tissue in places outside the uterus.

- **Fibromyalgia,** a chronic pain syndrome involving widespread muscle pain and fatigue.

What Are the Risk Factors for Developing Low Back Pain?

Beyond underlying diseases, certain other risk factors may elevate one's risk for low back pain, including:

- **Age.** The first attack of low back pain typically occurs between the ages of 30 and 50, and back pain becomes more common with advancing age. As people grow older, loss of bone strength from osteoporosis can lead to fractures, and at the same time, muscle elasticity and tone decrease. The intervertebral discs begin to lose fluid and flexibility with age, which decreases their ability to cushion the vertebrae. The risk of spinal stenosis also increases with age.

- **Fitness level.** Back pain is more common among people who are not physically fit. Weak back and abdominal muscles may not properly support the spine. "Weekend warriors"—people who go out and exercise a lot after being inactive all week—are more likely to suffer painful back injuries than people who make moderate physical activity a daily habit. Studies show that low-impact aerobic exercise is beneficial for the maintaining the integrity of intervertebral discs.

- **Pregnancy.** Pregnancy is commonly accompanied by low back pain, which results from pelvic changes and alterations in weight loading. Back symptoms almost always resolve postpartum.

- **Weight gain.** Being overweight, obese, or quickly gaining significant amounts of weight can put stress on the back and lead to low back pain.

- **Genetics.** Some causes of back pain, such as ankylosing spondylitis, a form of arthritis that involves fusion of the spinal joints leading to some immobility of the spine, have a genetic component.

- **Occupational risk factors.** Having a job that requires heavy lifting, pushing, or pulling, particularly when it involves twisting or vibrating the spine, can lead to injury and back pain. An inactive job or a desk job may also lead to or contribute to pain, especially if you have poor posture or sit all day in a chair with inadequate back support.

- **Mental health factors.** Preexisting mental health issues such as anxiety and depression can influence how closely one focuses on their pain as well as their perception of its severity. Pain that becomes chronic also can contribute to the development of such psychological factors. Stress can affect the body in numerous ways, including causing muscle tension.

- **Backpack overload in children.** Low back pain unrelated to injury or other known cause is unusual in preteen children. However, a backpack overloaded with schoolbooks and supplies can strain the back and cause muscle fatigue. The American Academy of Orthopaedic Surgeons recommends that a child's backpack should weigh no more than 15 to 20 percent of the child's body weight.

How Is Low Back Pain Diagnosed?

A complete medical history and physical exam can usually identify any serious conditions that may be causing the pain. During the exam, a healthcare provider will ask about the onset, site, and severity of the pain; duration of symptoms and any limitations in movement; and history of previous episodes or any health conditions that might be related to the pain. Along with a thorough back examination, neurologic tests are conducted to determine the cause of pain and appropriate treatment. The cause of chronic lower back pain is often difficult to determine even after a thorough examination.

Imaging tests are not warranted in most cases. Under certain circumstances, however, imaging may be ordered to rule out specific causes of pain, including tumors and spinal stenosis. Imaging and other types of tests include:

X-ray is often the first imaging technique used to look for broken bones or an injured vertebra. X-rays show the bony structures and any vertebral misalignment or fractures. Soft tissues such as muscles, ligaments, or bulging discs are not visible on conventional X-rays.

Computerized tomography (CT) is used to see spinal structures that cannot be seen on conventional X-rays, such as disc rupture, spinal stenosis, or tumors. Using a computer, the CT scan creates a three-dimensional image from a series of two dimensional pictures.

Myelograms enhance the diagnostic imaging of X-rays and CT scans. In this procedure, a contrast dye is injected into the spinal canal, allowing spinal cord and nerve compression caused by herniated discs or fractures to be seen on an X-ray or CT scans.

Discography may be used when other diagnostic procedures fail to identify the cause of pain. This procedure involves the injection of a contrast dye into a spinal disc thought to be causing low back pain. The fluid's pressure in the disc will reproduce the person's symptoms if the disc is the cause. The dye helps to show the damaged areas on CT scans taken following the injection. Discography may provide useful information in cases where people are considering lumbar surgery or when their pain has not responded to conventional treatments.

Magnetic resonance imaging (MRI) uses a magnetic force instead of radiation to create a computer-generated image. Unlike X-ray, which shows only bony structures, MRI scans also produce images of soft tissues such as muscles, ligaments, tendons, and blood vessels. An MRI may be ordered if a problem such as infection, tumor, inflammation, disc herniation or rupture, or pressure on a nerve is suspected. MRI is a noninvasive way to identify a condition requiring prompt surgical treatment. However, in most instances, unless there are "red flags" in the history or physical exam, an MRI scan is not necessary during the early phases of low back pain.

Electrodiagnostics are procedures that, in the setting of low back pain, are primarily used to confirm whether a person has lumbar radiculopathy. The procedures include electromyography (EMG), nerve conduction studies (NCS), and evoked potential (EP) studies. EMG assesses the electrical activity in a muscle and can detect if muscle weakness results from a problem with the nerves that control the muscles. Very fine needles are inserted in muscles to measure electrical activity transmitted from the brain or spinal cord to a particular area of the body. NCSs are often performed along with EMG to exclude conditions that can mimic radiculopathy. In NCSs, two sets of electrodes are placed on the skin over the muscles. The first set provides a mild shock to stimulate the nerve that runs to a particular muscle. The second set records the nerve's electrical signals, and from this information nerve damage that slows conduction of the nerve signal can be detected. EP tests also involve two sets of electrodes—one set to stimulate a sensory nerve, and the other placed on the scalp to record the speed of nerve signal transmissions to the brain.

Bone scans are used to detect and monitor infection, fracture, or disorders in the bone. A small amount of radioactive material is injected into the bloodstream and will collect in the bones, particularly in areas with some abnormality. Scanner-generated images can be used to identify specific areas of irregular bone metabolism or abnormal blood flow, as well as to measure levels of joint disease.

Ultrasound imaging, also called ultrasound scanning or sonography, uses high-frequency sound waves to obtain images inside the body. The sound wave echoes are recorded and displayed as a real-time visual image. Ultrasound imaging can show tears in ligaments, muscles, tendons, and other soft tissue masses in the back.

Blood tests are not routinely used to diagnose the cause of back pain; however in some cases they may be ordered to look for indications of inflammation, infection, and/or the presence of arthritis. Potential tests include complete blood count, erythrocyte sedimentation rate, and C-reactive protein. Blood tests may also detect HLA-B27, a genetic marker in the blood that is more common in people with ankylosing spondylitis or reactive arthritis (a form of arthritis that occurs following infection in another part of the body, usually the genitourinary tract).

How Is Back Pain Treated?

Treatment for low back pain generally depends on whether the pain is acute or chronic. In general, surgery is recommended only if there is evidence of worsening nerve damage and when diagnostic tests indicate structural changes for which corrective surgical procedures have been developed.

Conventionally used treatments and their level of supportive evidence include:

Hot or cold packs have never been proven to quickly resolve low back injury; however, they may help ease pain and reduce inflammation for people with acute, subacute, or chronic pain, allowing for greater mobility among some individuals.

Activity. Bed rest should be limited. Individuals should begin stretching exercises and resume normal daily activities as soon as possible, while avoiding movements that aggravate pain. Strong evidence shows that persons who continue their activities without bed rest following onset of low back pain appeared to have better back flexibility than those who rested in bed for a week. Other studies suggest that bed rest alone may make back pain worse and can lead to secondary complications such as depression, decreased muscle tone, and blood clots in the legs.

Strengthening exercises, beyond general daily activities, are not advised for acute low back pain, but may be an effective way to speed recovery from chronic or subacute low back pain. Maintaining and building muscle strength is particularly important for persons with skeletal irregularities. Healthcare providers can provide a list of beneficial exercises that will help improve coordination and develop proper posture and muscle balance. Evidence supports short- and long-term benefits of yoga to ease chronic low back pain.

Physical therapy programs to strengthen core muscle groups that support the low back, improve mobility and flexibility, and promote proper positioning and posture are often used in combinations with other interventions.

Medications. A wide range of medications are used to treat acute and chronic low back pain. Some are available over the counter (OTC); others require a physician's prescription. Certain drugs, even those available OTC, may be unsafe during pregnancy, may interact with other medications, cause side effects, or lead to serious adverse effects such as liver damage or gastrointestinal ulcers and bleeding. Consultation with a healthcare provider is advised before use. The following are the main types of medications used for low back pain:

- **Analgesic medications** are those specifically designed to relieve pain. They include OTC acetaminophen and aspirin, as well as prescription opioids such as codeine, oxycodone, hydrocodone, and morphine. Opioids should be used only for a short period of time and under a physician's supervision. People can develop a tolerance to opioids and require increasingly higher dosages to achieve the same effect. Opioids can also be addictive. Their side effects can include drowsiness, constipation, decreased reaction time, and impaired judgment. Some specialists are concerned that chronic use of opioids is detrimental to people with back pain because they can aggravate depression, leading to a worsening of the pain.

- **Nonsteroidal anti-inflammatory drugs (NSAIDS)** relieve pain and inflammation and include OTC formulations (ibuprofen, ketoprofen, and naproxen sodium). Several others, including a type of NSAID called COX-2 inhibitors, are available only by prescription. Long-term use of NSAIDs has been associated with stomach irritation, ulcers, heartburn, diarrhea, fluid retention, and in rare cases, kidney dysfunction and cardiovascular disease. The longer a person uses NSAIDs the more likely they are to develop side effects. Many other drugs cannot be taken at the same time a person is treated with NSAIDs because they alter the way the body processes or eliminates other medications.

- **Anticonvulsants**—drugs primarily used to treat seizures—may be useful in treating people with radiculopathy and radicular pain.

- **Antidepressants** such as tricyclics and serotonin and norepinephrine reuptake inhibitors have been commonly prescribed for chronic low back pain, but their benefit for nonspecific low back pain is unproven, according to a review of studies assessing their benefit.

- **Counter-irritants** such as creams or sprays applied topically stimulate the nerves in the skin to provide feelings of warmth or cold in order to dull the sensation of pain. Topical analgesics reduce inflammation and stimulate blood flow.

Spinal manipulation and spinal mobilization are approaches in which professionally licensed specialists (doctors of chiropractic care) use their hands to mobilize, adjust, massage, or stimulate the spine and the surrounding tissues. Manipulation involves a rapid movement over which the individual has no control; mobilization involves slower adjustment movements. The techniques have been shown to provide small to moderate short-term benefits in people with chronic low back pain. Evidence supporting their use for acute or subacute low back pain is generally of low quality. Neither technique is appropriate when a person has an underlying medical cause for the back pain such as osteoporosis, spinal cord compression, or arthritis.

Traction involves the use of weights and pulleys to apply constant or intermittent force to gradually "pull" the skeletal structure into better alignment. Some people experience pain relief while in traction, but that relief is usually temporary. Once traction is released the back pain tends to return. There is no evidence that traction provides any long-term benefits for people with low back pain.

Acupuncture is moderately effective for chronic low back pain. It involves the insertion of thin needles into precise points throughout the body. Some practitioners believe this process helps clear away blockages in the body's life force known as Qi. Others who may not believe in the concept of Qi theorize that when the needles are inserted and then stimulated (by twisting or passing a low-voltage electrical current through them) naturally occurring painkilling chemicals such as endorphins, serotonin, and acetylcholine are released. Evidence of acupuncture's benefit for acute low back pain is conflicting and clinical studies continue to investigate its benefits.

Biofeedback is used to treat many acute pain problems, most notably back pain and headache. The therapy involves the attachment of electrodes to the skin and the use of an electromyography machine that allows people to become aware of and self-regulate their breathing, muscle tension, heart rate, and skin temperature. People regulate their response to pain by using relaxation techniques. Biofeedback is often used in combination with other treatment methods, generally without side effects. Evidence is lacking that biofeedback provides a clear benefit for low back pain.

Nerve block therapies aim to relieve chronic pain by blocking nerve conduction from specific areas of the body. Nerve block approaches range from injections of local anesthetics, botulinum toxin, or steroids into affected soft tissues or joints to more complex nerve root blocks and spinal cord stimulation. When extreme pain is involved, low doses of drugs may be administered by catheter directly into the spinal cord. The success of a nerve block approach depends on the ability of a practitioner to locate and inject precisely the correct nerve. Chronic use of steroid injections may lead to increased functional impairment.

Epidural steroid injections are a commonly used short-term option for treating low back pain and sciatica associated with inflammation. Pain relief associated with the injections, however, tends to be temporary and the injections are not advised for long-term use. An NIH-funded randomized controlled trial assessing the benefit of epidural steroid injections for the treatment of chronic low back pain associated with spinal stenosis showed that long-term outcomes were worse among those people who received the injections compared with those who did not.

Transcutaneous electrical nerve stimulation (TENS) involves wearing a battery-powered device consisting of electrodes placed on the skin over the painful area that generate electrical impulses designed to block incoming pain signals from the peripheral nerves. The theory is that stimulating the nervous system can modify the perception of pain. Early studies of TENS suggested that it elevated levels of endorphins, the body's natural pain-numbing chemicals. More recent studies, however, have produced mixed results on its effectiveness for providing relief from low back pain.

Surgery

When other therapies fail, surgery may be considered an option to relieve pain caused by serious musculoskeletal injuries or nerve compression. It may be months following surgery before the patient is fully healed, and he or she may suffer permanent loss of flexibility.

Surgical procedures are not always successful, and there is little evidence to show which procedures work best for their particular indications. Patients considering surgical approaches should be fully informed of all related risks. Surgical options include:

- **Vertebroplasty and kyphoplasty** are minimally invasive treatments to repair compression fractures of the vertebrae caused by osteoporosis. Vertebroplasty uses three-dimensional imaging to assist in guiding a fine needle through the skin into the vertebral body, the largest part of the vertebrae. A glue-like bone cement is then injected into the vertebral body space, which quickly hardens to stabilize and strengthen the bone and provide pain relief. In kyphoplasty, prior to injecting the bone cement, a special balloon is inserted and gently inflated to restore height to the vertebral structure and reduce spinal deformity.

- **Spinal laminectomy** (also known as spinal decompression) is performed when spinal stenosis causes a narrowing of the spinal canal that causes pain, numbness, or weakness. During the procedure, the lamina or bony walls of the vertebrae, along with any bone spurs, are removed. The aim of the procedure is to open up the spinal column to remove pressure on the nerves.

- **Discectomy or microdiscectomy** may be recommended to remove a disc, in cases where it has herniated and presses on a nerve root or the spinal cord, which may cause intense and enduring pain. Microdiscectomy is similar to a conventional

413

discectomy; however, this procedure involves removing the herniated disc through a much smaller incision in the back and a more rapid recovery. Laminectomy and discectomy are frequently performed together and the combination is one of the more common ways to remove pressure on a nerve root from a herniated disc or bone spur.

- **Foraminotomy** is an operation that "cleans out" or enlarges the bony hole (foramen) where a nerve root exits the spinal canal. Bulging discs or joints thickened with age can cause narrowing of the space through which the spinal nerve exits and can press on the nerve, resulting in pain, numbness, and weakness in an arm or leg. Small pieces of bone over the nerve are removed through a small slit, allowing the surgeon to cut away the blockage and relieve pressure on the nerve.

- **Intradiscal electrothermal therapy (IDET)** is a treatment for discs that are cracked or bulging as a result of degenerative disc disease. The procedure involves inserting a catheter through a small incision at the site of the disc in the back. A special wire is passed through the catheter and an electrical current is applied to heat the disc, which helps strengthen the collagen fibers of the disc wall, reducing the bulging and the related irritation of the spinal nerve. IDET is of questionable benefit.

- **Nucleoplasty, also called plasma disc decompression (PDD),** is a type of laser surgery that uses radiofrequency energy to treat people with low back pain associated with mildly herniated discs. Under X-ray guidance, a needle is inserted into the disc. A plasma laser device is then inserted into the needle and the tip is heated to 40–70 degrees Celsius, creating a field that vaporizes the tissue in the disc, reducing its size and relieving pressure on the nerves. Several channels may be made depending on how tissue needs to be removed to decompress the disc and nerve root.

- **Radiofrequency denervation** is a procedure using electrical impulses to interrupt nerve conduction (including the conduction of pain signals). Using X-ray guidance, a needle is inserted into a target area of nerves and a local anesthetic is introduced as a way of confirming the involvement of the nerves in the person's back pain. Next, the region is heated, resulting in localized destruction of the target nerves. Pain relief associated with the technique is temporary and the evidence supporting this technique is limited.

- **Spinal fusion** is used to strengthen the spine and prevent pain-ful movements in people with degenerative disc disease or spon-dylolisthesis (following laminectomy). The spinal disc between two or more vertebrae is removed and the adjacent vertebrae are "fused" by bone grafts and/or metal devices secured by screws. The fusion can be performed through the abdomen, a procedure known as an anterior lumbar interbody fusion, or through the back, called posterior fusion. Spinal fusion may result in some loss of flexibility in the spine and requires a long recovery period to allow the bone grafts to grow and fuse the vertebrae together. Spinal fusion has been associated with an acceleration of disc degeneration at adjacent levels of the spine.

- **Artificial disc replacement** is considered an alternative to spinal fusion for the treatment of people with severely damaged discs. The procedure involves removal of the disc and its replace-ment by a synthetic disc that helps restore height and move-ment between the vertebrae.

Can Back Pain Be Prevented?

Recurring back pain resulting from improper body mechanics is often preventable by avoiding movements that jolt or strain the back, maintaining correct posture, and lifting objects properly. Many work-related injuries are caused or aggravated by stressors such as heavy lifting, contact stress (repeated or constant contact between soft body tissue and a hard or sharp object), vibration, repetitive motion, and awkward posture. Using ergonomically designed furniture and equipment to protect the body from injury at home and in the work-place may reduce the risk of back injury.

The use of lumbar supports in the form of wide elastic bands that can be tightened to provide support to the lower back and abdominal muscles to prevent low back pain remains controversial. Such supports are widely used despite a lack of evidence showing that they actually prevent pain. Multiple studies have determined that the use of lumbar supports provides no benefit in terms of the prevention and treatment of back pain. Although there have been anecdotal case reports of injury reduction among workers using lumbar support belts, many companies that have back belt programs also have training and ergonomic aware-ness programs. The reported injury reduction may be related to a com-bination of these or other factors. Furthermore, some caution is advised given that wearing supportive belts may actually lead to or aggravate back pain by causing back muscles to weaken from lack of use.

415

Recommendations for Keeping One's Back Healthy

Following any period of prolonged inactivity, a regimen of low-impact exercises is advised. Speed walking, swimming, or stationary bike riding 30 minutes daily can increase muscle strength and flexibility. Yoga also can help stretch and strengthen muscles and improve posture. Consult a physician for a list of low-impact, age-appropriate exercises that are specifically targeted to strengthening lower back and abdominal muscles.

- Always stretch before exercise or other strenuous physical activity.

- Don't slouch when standing or sitting. The lower back can support a person's weight most easily when the curvature is reduced. When standing, keep your weight balanced on your feet.

- At home or work, make sure work surfaces are at a comfortable height.

- Sit in a chair with good lumbar support and proper position and height for the task. Keep shoulders back. Switch sitting positions often and periodically walk around the office or gently stretch muscles to relieve tension. A pillow or rolled-up towel placed behind the small of the back can provide some lumbar support. During prolonged periods of sitting, elevate feet on a low stool or a stack of books.

- Wear comfortable, low-heeled shoes.

- Sleeping on one's side with the knees drawn up in a fetal position can help open up the joints in the spine and relieve pressure by reducing the curvature of the spine. Always sleep on a firm surface.

- Don't try to lift objects that are too heavy. Lift from the knees, pull the stomach muscles in, and keep the head down and in line with a straight back. When lifting, keep objects close to the body. Do not twist when lifting.

- Maintain proper nutrition and diet to reduce and prevent excessive weight gain, especially weight around the waistline that taxes lower back muscles. A diet with sufficient daily intake of calcium, phosphorus, and vitamin D helps to promote new bone growth.

- Quit smoking. Smoking reduces blood flow to the lower spine, which can contribute to spinal disc degeneration. Smoking also increases the risk of osteoporosis and impedes healing. Coughing due to heavy smoking also may cause back pain.

Chapter 30

Gastrointestinal Surgery

Chapter Contents

Section 30.1

Appendectomy

This section includes text excerpted from "Appendicitis,"
National Institute of Diabetes and Digestive and Kidney
Diseases (NIDDK), November 2014.

About Appendicitis

Appendicitis is inflammation of your appendix. In the United States, appendicitis is the most common cause of acute abdominal pain requiring surgery. Over 5 percent of the population develops appendicitis at some point. Appendicitis most commonly occurs in the teens and twenties but may occur at any age.

If appendicitis is not treated, it may lead to complications. The complications of a ruptured appendix are:

- peritonitis, which can be a dangerous condition. Peritonitis happens if your appendix bursts and infection spreads in your abdomen. If you have peritonitis, you may be very ill and have:

  - fever

  - nausea

  - severe tenderness in your abdomen

  - vomiting

- an abscess of the appendix called an appendiceal abscess.

Symptoms of Appendicitis

The most common symptom of appendicitis is pain in your abdomen.

If you have appendicitis, you'll most often have pain in your abdomen that:

- begins near your belly button and then moves lower and to your right

420

- gets worse in a matter of hours

- gets worse when you move around, take deep breaths, cough, or sneeze

- is severe and often described as different from any pain you've felt before

- occurs suddenly and may even wake you up if you're sleeping

- occurs before other symptoms

Other symptoms of appendicitis may include:

- loss of appetite

- nausea

- vomiting

- constipation or diarrhea

- an inability to pass gas

- a low-grade fever

- swelling in your abdomen

- the feeling that having a bowel movement will relieve discomfort

Symptoms can be different for each person and can seem like the following conditions that also cause pain in the abdomen:

- abdominal adhesions

- constipation

- inflammatory bowel disease, which includes Crohn's disease and ulcerative colitis, long-lasting disorders that cause irritation and ulcers in the gastrointestinal (GI) tract

- intestinal obstruction

- pelvic inflammatory disease

Causes of Appendicitis

Appendicitis can have more than one cause, and in many cases the cause is not clear. Possible causes include:

- Blockage of the opening inside the appendix

- enlarged tissue in the wall of your appendix, caused by infection in the GI tract or elsewhere in your body

- inflammatory bowel disease

- stool, parasites, or growths that can clog your appendiceal lumen

- trauma to your abdomen

Diagnosis of Appendicitis

Most often, healthcare professionals suspect the diagnosis of appendicitis based on your symptoms, your medical history, and a physical exam. A doctor can confirm the diagnosis with an ultrasound, X-ray, or magnetic resonance imaging (MRI) exam.

Medical History

A healthcare professional will ask specific questions about your symptoms and health history to help rule out other health problems. The healthcare professional will want to know:

- when your abdominal pain began

- the exact location and severity of your pain

- when your other symptoms appeared

- your other medical conditions, previous illnesses, and surgical procedures

- whether you use medicines, alcohol, or illegal drugs

Physical Exam

Healthcare professionals need specific details about the pain in your abdomen to diagnose appendicitis correctly. A healthcare professional will assess your pain by touching or applying pressure to specific areas of your abdomen.

The following responses to touch or pressure may indicate that you have appendicitis:

- Rovsing sign

- Psoas sign

- Obturator sign
- Guarding
- Rebound tenderness
- Digital rectal exam
- Pelvic exam

Lab Tests

Doctors use lab tests to help confirm the diagnosis of appendicitis or find other causes of abdominal pain.

- Blood tests
- Urinalysis
- Pregnancy test

Imaging Tests

Doctors use imaging tests to confirm the diagnosis of appendicitis or find other causes of pain in the abdomen.

- Abdominal ultrasound
- Magnetic resonance imaging (MRI)
- CT scan

Treatment for Appendicitis

Doctors typically treat appendicitis with surgery to remove the appendix. Surgeons perform the surgery in a hospital with general anesthesia. Your doctor will recommend surgery if you have continuous abdominal pain and fever, or signs of a burst appendix and infection. Prompt surgery decreases the chance that your appendix will burst.

Healthcare professionals call the surgery to remove the appendix an appendectomy. A surgeon performs the surgery using one of the following methods:

- **Laparoscopic surgery.** During laparoscopic surgery, surgeons use several smaller incisions and special surgical tools that they feed through the incisions to remove your appendix.

Laparoscopic surgery leads to fewer complications, such as hospital-related infections, and has a shorter recovery time.

• **Laparotomy.** Surgeons use laparotomy to remove the appendix through a single incision in the lower right area of your abdomen.

After surgery, most patients completely recover from appendicitis and don't need to make changes to their diet, exercise, or lifestyle. Surgeons recommend that you limit physical activity for the first 10 to 14 days after a laparotomy and for the first 3 to 5 days after laparoscopic surgery.

What If the Surgeon Finds a Normal Appendix?

In some cases, a surgeon finds a normal appendix during surgery. In this case, many surgeons will remove it to eliminate the future possibility of appendicitis. Sometimes surgeons find a different problem, which they may correct during surgery.

Can Doctors Treat Appendicitis without Surgery?

Some cases of mild appendicitis may be cured with antibiotics alone. All patients suspected of having appendicitis are treated with antibiotics before surgery, and some patients may improve completely before surgery is performed.

Section 30.2

Bowel Diversion Surgeries

This section includes text excerpted from "Ostomy Surgery of the Bowel," National Institute of Diabetes and Digestive and Kidney Diseases (NIDDK), August 2014.

About Ostomy Surgery of the Bowel

Ostomy surgery of the bowel, also known as bowel diversion, refers to surgical procedures that reroute the normal movement of intestinal contents out of the body when part of the bowel is diseased or removed. Creating an ostomy means bringing part of the intestine through the abdominal wall so that waste exits through the abdominal wall instead of passing through the anus.

Ostomy surgery of the bowel may be temporary or permanent, depending on the reason for the surgery. A surgeon specially trained in intestinal surgery performs the procedure in a hospital. During the surgery, the person receives general anesthesia.

Ostomy surgeries of the bowel include:

- ileostomy

- colostomy

- ileoanal reservoir

- continent ileostomy

Bowel

The bowel is another word for the small and large intestines. The bowel forms the largest part of the gastrointestinal (GI) tract—a series of hollow organs joined in a long, twisting tube from the mouth to the anus. The anus is a 1-inch-long opening through which stool leaves the body. Organs that make up the GI tract include the mouth, esophagus, stomach, small intestine, large intestine, and anus. The small intestine measures about 20 feet long in adults and includes:

- the duodenum—the first part of the small intestine nearest the stomach

- the jejunum—the middle section of the small intestine between the duodenum and ileum

- the ileum—the lower end of the small intestine

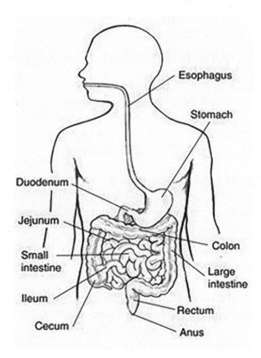

Figure 30.1. *Gastrointestinal (GI) Tract*

Peristalsis—a wavelike movement of muscles in the GI tract—moves food and liquid through the GI tract. Peristalsis, along with the release of hormones and enzymes, helps food digest. The small intestine absorbs nutrients from foods and liquids passed from the stomach. Most food digestion and nutrient absorption take place in the small intestine.

The large intestine consists of the cecum, colon, and rectum. The cecum connects to the last part of the ileum and contains the appendix. The large intestine measures about 5 feet in adults and absorbs water and any remaining nutrients from partially digested food passed from the small intestine. The large intestine then changes waste from liquid to semisolid or solid feces, or stool. Stool passes from the colon to the rectum. The rectum measures 6 to 8 inches in adults and is located between the last part of the colon and the anus. The rectum stores stool prior to a bowel movement. During a bowel movement, stool moves from the rectum, through the anus, and out of the body.

Need of Ostomy Surgery of the Bowel

A person may need ostomy surgery of the bowel if he or she has:

- cancer of the colon or rectum

- an injury to the small or large intestine

- inflammatory bowel disease—long lasting disorders, such as Crohn's disease and ulcerative colitis, that cause irritation or sores in the GI tract

- obstruction—a blockage in the bowel that prevents the flow of fluids or solids

- diverticulitis—a condition that occurs when small pouches in the colon called diverticula become inflamed, or irritated and swollen, and infected

Stoma

During ostomy surgery of the bowel, a surgeon creates a stoma by bringing the end of the intestine through an opening in the abdomen

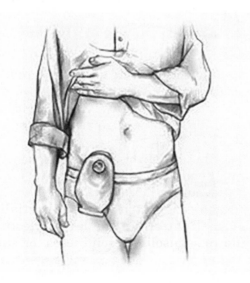

Figure 30.2. *Ostomy Pouch*

and attaching it to the skin to create an opening outside the body. A stoma may be three-fourths of an inch to a little less than 2 inches wide. The stoma is usually located in the lower part of the abdomen, just below the beltline. However, sometimes the stoma is located in the upper abdomen. The surgeon and a wound, ostomy, and continence (WOC) nurse or an enterostomal therapist will work together to select the best location for the stoma. A removable external collection pouch, called an ostomy pouch or ostomy appliance, is attached to the stoma and worn outside the body to collect intestinal contents or stool. Intestinal contents or stool passes through the stoma instead of passing through the anus. The stoma has no muscle, so it cannot control the flow of stool, and the flow occurs whenever peristalsis occurs. Ileostomy and colostomy are the two main types of ostomy surgery of the bowel during which a surgeon creates a stoma.

Ileostomy

An ileostomy is a stoma created from a part of the ileum. For this surgery, the surgeon brings the ileum through the abdominal wall to make a stoma. An ileostomy may be permanent or temporary. An

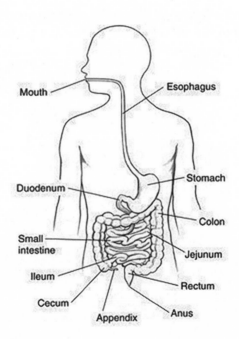

Figure 30.3. *Ileostomy*

ileostomy is permanent when the surgeon removes or bypasses the entire colon, rectum, and anus. A surgeon may perform a temporary ileostomy for a damaged or an inflamed colon or rectum that only needs time to rest or heal from injury or surgery. After the colon or rectum heals, the surgeon repairs the opening in the abdominal wall and reconnects the ileum so stool will pass into the colon normally. An ileostomy is the most common temporary bowel diversion. A surgeon performs an ileostomy most often to treat inflammatory bowel disease or rectal cancer.

Colostomy

A colostomy is a stoma created from a part of the colon. For this surgery, the surgeon brings the colon through the abdominal wall and makes a stoma. A colostomy may be temporary or permanent. The colostomy is permanent when the surgeon removes or bypasses the lower end of the colon or rectum. A surgeon may perform a temporary colostomy for a damaged or an inflamed lower part of the colon or rectum that only needs time to rest or heal from injury or surgery. Once the colon or rectum heals, the surgeon repairs the opening in the

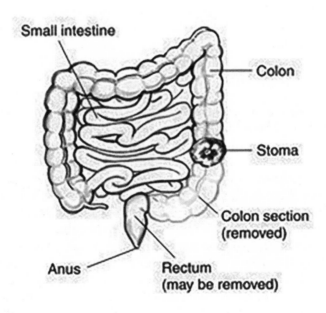

Figure 30.4. *Colostomy*

abdominal wall and reconnects the colon so stool will pass normally. A surgeon performs a colostomy most often to treat rectal cancer, diverticulitis, or fecal incontinence—the accidental loss of stool.

Ileoanal Reservoir

An ileoanal reservoir is an internal pouch made from the ileum. This surgery is a common alternative to an ileostomy and does not have a permanent stoma. Also known as a J-pouch or pelvic pouch, the ileoanal reservoir connects to the anus after a surgeon removes the colon and rectum. Stool collects in the ileoanal reservoir and then exits the body through the anus during a bowel movement. An ileoanal reservoir is an option after removal of the entire large intestine when the anus remains intact and disease-free. The surgeon often makes a temporary ileostomy before or at the time of making an ileoanal reservoir. Once the ileoanal reservoir heals from surgery, the surgeon reconnects the ileum to the ileoanal pouch and closes the temporary ileostomy. A person does not need a permanent external ostomy pouch for an ileoanal reservoir.

A surgeon creates an ileoanal reservoir most often to treat ulcerative colitis or familial adenomatous polyposis. Familial adenomatous polyposis is an inherited disease characterized by the presence of 100 or more polyps in the colon. The polyps may lead to colorectal cancer if not treated. People with Crohn's disease usually are not candidates for this procedure.

Continent Ileostomy

A continent ileostomy is an internal pouch, sometimes called a Kock pouch, fashioned from the end of the ileum just before it exits the abdominal wall as an ileostomy. The surgeon makes a valve inside the pouch so that intestinal contents do not flow out. The person drains the pouch each day by inserting a thin, flexible tube, called a catheter, through the stoma. The person covers the stoma with a simple patch or dressing. A continent ileostomy is an option for people who are not good candidates for an ileoanal reservoir because of damage to the rectum or anus and who do not want to wear an ostomy pouch.

Creating the Kock pouch is a delicate surgical procedure that requires a healthy bowel for proper healing. Therefore, a surgeon usually does not perform Kock pouch surgery during an acute attack of bowel disease. A continent ileostomy is now uncommon, and most hospitals do not have a specialist who knows how to perform this type of surgery. As with ileoanal reservoir surgery, the surgeon usually removes the colon and rectum to treat the original bowel disease, such as ulcerative colitis or familial adenomatous polyposis. People with Crohn's disease are not usually candidates for this procedure.

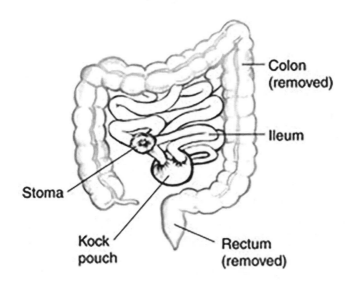

Figure 30.5. *Continent Ileostomy*

Complications of Ostomy Surgery of the Bowel

Complications of ostomy surgery of the bowel may include:

Skin Irritation

Skin irritation is the most common complication for people with an ostomy. If the external ostomy pouch does not fit properly, stool or stool contents can leak out around the stoma and under the pouch. When irritated, a person's skin will become itchy, red, and uncomfortable. When changing the pouch, a person can use an ostomy powder on the skin around the stoma to treat skin irritation. If the skin irritation does not improve, the person should talk with a WOC nurse or an enterostomal therapist—who are specially trained in ostomy care and rehabilitation—or another healthcare provider about the symptoms. Skin irritation may occur around the stoma for people who have an ileostomy or a colostomy. People who have ileoanal reservoir surgery may have skin irritation around the anus. Sometimes, using a barrier ointment to protect the skin around the anus can help treat and prevent irritation.

431

Stoma Problems

Stoma problems include the following:

- **Hernia.** A stoma hernia, seen as a bulge in the skin around the stoma, is a weakening of the abdominal wall around the stoma site. As with all hernias, a stoma hernia continues to increase in size and may eventually need surgical repair when it becomes too large. Rarely, the intestine gets trapped or kinked within the hernia and becomes blocked. A blocked intestine that loses its blood supply requires emergency surgery.

- **Prolapse.** A stoma prolapse occurs when the bowel pushes itself through the stoma. A person may be able to push the bowel back through the stoma and keep it in place with a stoma shield. If not, the stoma prolapse may require special care and a larger ostomy pouch. A stoma prolapse that becomes blocked or loses its blood supply requires surgical repair.

- **Narrowing of the stoma.** Narrowing of the stoma makes it difficult for stool to pass through the stoma. A narrowed stoma may need surgical repair.

Blockage

Occasionally, an ileostomy or a colostomy does not function for a short time. If the stoma has not passed intestinal content or stool for 4 to 6 hours and the person is experiencing cramping or nausea, the ileum or colon may be blocked. Blockage may occur when foods that are hard to digest get stuck in the ileum or colon.

Abdominal adhesions in the ileum or colon may cause blockage as well. Abdominal adhesions are bands of fibrous tissue that form between abdominal tissues and organs, causing them to kink or narrow. Most blockages get better without additional surgery by not eating food and drinking only clear liquids to rest the bowel for a short time.

Diarrhea

Diarrhea is loose, watery stools. A person has diarrhea if he or she passes loose stools three or more times a day. Diarrhea occurs when intestinal contents pass through the small intestine too quickly for fluid and mineral absorption. When fluids and minerals such as sodium and potassium are not absorbed, they leave the body. Diarrhea can lead to dehydration, malnutrition, and weight loss. Diarrhea is common, even normal, with an ileostomy or ileoanal reservoir. In most

432

cases of diarrhea, the only treatment necessary is replacing lost fluids and electrolytes to prevent dehydration. Electrolytes are minerals in body fluids that are part of salts, including sodium, potassium, magnesium, and chloride. People should maintain good daily hydration by drinking plenty of water and liquids, such as fruit juices, sports drinks, caffeine-free soft drinks, and broths. In some cases of diarrhea, a healthcare provider may recommend changes in diet and may prescribe medications to treat diarrhea.

Bleeding

As with any major surgery, ostomy surgery may cause internal bleeding. If too much blood is lost, the person may require a blood transfusion. Bleeding may also occur through the stoma or through the anus after surgery.

Electrolyte Imbalance

The main function of the large intestine is to absorb water, nutrients, and electrolytes from partially digested food that enters from the ileum. When a surgeon removes the large intestine, absorption of electrolytes does not occur to the same extent, making electrolyte imbalance more likely. Diarrhea, excessive sweating, and vomiting can increase the chance of developing electrolyte imbalance. Symptoms of electrolyte imbalance may include:

- fatigue, or feeling tired
- weakness
- nausea
- muscle problems such as spasms, weakness, uncontrolled twitching, and cramps
- dizziness and confusion

People with these symptoms require medical care and should contact a healthcare provider.

People who have had their large intestine removed should talk with a healthcare provider or dietitian about diets that help maintain electrolyte balance.

Infection

The GI tract is filled with bacteria that can leak out during ostomy surgery and infect areas inside the abdomen. Bacteria entering the body through the stoma or anus can also cause an infection. The person's skin around the stoma may also become infected with bacteria or skin fungus. Healthcare providers treat infections with antibiotics. Symptoms of infection may include:

- fever
- back pain
- poor appetite
- nausea and vomiting

Irritation of the Internal Pouch, or Pouchitis

Pouchitis is an irritation or inflammation of the lining of an ileoanal reservoir or a continent ileostomy pouch. A healthcare provider treats pouchitis with antibiotics. For severe or chronic pouchitis, a healthcare provider may prescribe immunosuppressive medications, such as corticosteroids. Symptoms of pouchitis include:

- frequent bowel movements with diarrhea
- an urgent need to have a bowel movement
- a feeling of pressure in the pouch
- abdominal pain
- cramping or bleeding
- dehydration
- low-grade fever
- a general unwell feeling

Vitamin B12 Deficiency

Ostomy surgery of the bowel may affect vitamin B12 absorption from food and result in a gradual drop in vitamin B12 levels in the body. Low levels of vitamin B12 can affect the body's ability to use nutrients and may cause anemia. Anemia is a condition in which red blood cells are fewer or smaller than normal, which prevents the body's cells from getting enough oxygen. Healthcare providers treat vitamin B12 deficiency with vitamin B12 supplements.

Phantom Rectum

Phantom rectum is the feeling of needing to have a bowel movement even though the rectum is not present. Phantom rectum is relatively common. Symptoms are usually mild and often go away without treatment. However, for some people, phantom rectum may occur for years after a surgeon removes the rectum. Some people with phantom rectum may feel pain. Healthcare providers treat rectal pain with medications such as pain relievers and sometimes antidepressants. To help control phantom rectum, a healthcare provider may recommend complementary therapies such as guided imagery and other relaxation techniques.

Short Bowel Syndrome

Short bowel syndrome is a group of problems related to inadequate absorption of nutrients after removal of part of the small intestine. People with short bowel syndrome cannot absorb enough water, vitamins, and other nutrients from food to sustain life. Diarrhea is the main symptom of short bowel syndrome. Other symptoms may include:

- cramping
- bloating
- heartburn
- weakness and fatigue
- vomiting
- excessive gas
- foul-smelling stool

Short bowel syndrome is uncommon and can occur with Crohn's disease, trauma, or other conditions that lead to removal of a large amount of the small intestine.

A healthcare provider will recommend a treatment for short bowel syndrome based on a person's nutritional needs. Treatment may include nutritional support, medications, and surgery.

Rectal Discharge

People with an ileostomy or a colostomy whose lower colon, rectum, and anus are still present may experience a discharge of mucus from their rectum. Mucus is a clear fluid made by the GI tract that coats and protects the lining of the bowel. Mucus within the bypassed part of the colon may leak out of the rectum from time to time or gradually buildup, forming a small, stool like ball that passes out of the rectum. A person cannot control mucus production and rectal discharge.

However, people who have rectal discharge can learn how to manage and cope with this problem.

Seek Immediate Care

People should seek immediate medical care if they have any of the following symptoms, as complications of ostomy surgery can become a medical emergency:

- continuous nausea and vomiting
- dramatic change in stoma size, shape, or color
- continuous bleeding at the junction between the stoma and the skin that does not stop by applying pressure
- obstruction, prolapse, or narrowing of the stoma
- a deep cut in the stoma
- no output of intestinal content or stool from the stoma for 4 to 6 hours, with cramping and nausea
- severe diarrhea with risk of dehydration
- excessive bleeding from the stoma opening

After Ostomy Surgery

Once the person is home from the hospital, the first week or two are considered an extension of the hospital stay. Most people will tire quite easily when they first come home. Getting enough rest is important. Gradually, stamina and strength will improve. Most people can return to work about 6 to 8 weeks after surgery. People may have certain GI issues—such as gas, diarrhea, and constipation—as the bowel heals, depending on the type of bowel diversion.

- **Ileostomy and colostomy.** During the early weeks and months after surgery, people with an ileostomy or a colostomy may have excessive gas. This extra gas will decrease once the bowel has had time to heal and the person resumes a regular diet.

- **Ileoanal reservoir.** People with an ileoanal reservoir initially have about six to 10 bowel movements a day. The newly formed ileoanal reservoir takes several months to stretch and adjust to its new function. After the adjustment period, bowel movements decrease to as few as four to six a day. People with an ileoanal reservoir may have mild fecal incontinence and may have to get up during periods of sleep to pass stool.

- **Continent ileostomy.** Similar to people with an ileostomy or a colostomy, people with a continent ileostomy may have excessive gas during the early weeks and months after surgery.

Resuming Normal Activities after Ostomy Surgery

After ostomy surgery, people should be able to resume their normal activities after healing completes and their strength returns. However, they may need to restrict activities, including driving and heavy lifting, during the first 2 to 3 weeks after surgery. Strenuous activities, such as heavy lifting, increase the chance of a stoma hernia. A person who has recovered from the ostomy surgery should be able to do most of the activities he or she enjoyed before the ostomy surgery, even swimming and other water sports. The only exceptions may be contact sports such as football or karate. People whose jobs include strenuous physical activities should talk with their healthcare provider and employer about making adjustments to job responsibilities.

People should avoid extreme physical exercise and sports activities for the first 3 months. Walking, biking, and swimming are fine and should be encouraged as long as they are not overly strenuous.

People with an ostomy should talk with their healthcare provider about when they can resume normal activities.

Section 30.3

Colectomy

What Is a Colectomy?

A colectomy is the surgical removal of all or a part of the colon, or large intestine, from the digestive system. The esophagus, stomach, small intestine and large intestine (colon) are part of the human digestive system. Digestion involves processing vitamins, minerals, carbohydrates, fats, proteins, and water from food and removing waste from the body. When a colectomy is performed, the severed portions of the colon may be reattached to facilitate bowel movement. Otherwise, a surgical procedure known as a colostomy becomes necessary. In this procedure, an opening known as a stoma is made to the outside the body to excrete stool.

When Is a Colectomy Recommended?

A colectomy is recommended for conditions like bowel obstruction, colon cancer, diverticulitis, inflammatory disease, such as Crohn's disease and ulcerative colitis, infection, and bleeding.

What Is the Surgical Procedure Used in a Colectomy?

Surgeons use one of two methods to perform a colectomy:

Open Surgery. The colon is accessed by making a long vertical incision on the abdomen and the surgeon operates on the infected/damaged part. This is termed an open colectomy.

Laparoscopic Surgery. The surgeon makes a few small incisions using specialized surgical tools. A video camera is then inserted into one of the incisions so that the surgeon can operate by looking at a screen. This is termed a laparoscopic-assisted colectomy and is the procedure of choice for certain types of cancerous conditions. There is less pain and blood loss and recovery is usually faster than after an open surgery.

What Are the Categories of Colectomy?

Depending on whether all or part of the colon is removed, a colectomy is categorized into the following types:

- **Total colectomy:** The entire colon is surgically removed.

- **Segmental resection:** Removal is confined to only the affected part of the colon.

- **Partial colectomy:** Part of the colon is removed. This is also known as a subtotal colectomy.

- **Sigmoidectomy:** The lower section of the colon is removed in this procedure.

- **Hemicolectomy:** Only the right or left quadrants of the colon is removed.

- **Total proctocolectomy:** The entire colon and the rectum are removed and the small intestine is attached to the anus for excretion of stool.

- **Abdominal perineal resection:** This involves the removal of the sigmoid colon, rectum and anus and replaced with a permanent colostomy.

- **Low anterior resection:** The top section of the rectum is removed.

How Do I Prepare before Surgery?

A few days before surgery you need to take care of a few things as listed below.

- Follow the diet advised by the surgeon.

- Stay hydrated with at least eight glasses of water daily.

- Cleanse your colon by following the instructions given by your surgeon. This could include laxatives, enemas, and special liquid preparations and diets.

- Take medicines as prescribed by your surgeon.

- Shower with an antibacterial soap the night before the procedure.

- Make arrangements for help at home and have someone drive you to hospital.

- Wear comfortable clothing.

- Stop taking regular medication as instructed by your surgeon.

What Happens in a Colectomy?

During a laparoscopic colectomy, the surgeon makes an incision that is less than half an inch in the abdomen and inserts a tube-like instrument known as a cannula or port into the abdomen. Carbon dioxide (CO_2) gas is pumped into the abdomen through the cannula to create enough space to carry out the procedure. A laparoscope is then inserted through the cannula. The laparoscope is a device with a camera and light source on it. It illuminates the surgical site and relays images of it to a high definition monitor for the surgeon to view. Up to four ports are used to insert specialized surgical instruments for the surgeon to perform the surgery. One of the incisions is made slightly bigger and the portion of the colon targeted for removal is pulled out of the abdomen. Depending on the type of surgery, the ends of the intestines are then joined together and inserted back into the abdomen.

An open surgery happens more or less the same way, except that the surgeon uses handheld instruments through a large incision made in the abdomen.

If most of the colon is removed, reattachment may not be possible and an ileostomy or a colostomy may be required. A stoma, or opening, is made in the abdominal wall and the open end of the intestine is attached to it. This allows waste to exit from the stoma. The patient will need to wear an ostomy bag which collects the waste material. Depending on the patient, the stoma could be temporary or permanent. People are able to lead a healthy and active life even with a permanent stoma.

What Are the Complications and Side Effects Associated with a Colectomy?

A colectomy is a generally safe procedure. But as with any operation, there are risks. If you are concerned, discuss them with your healthcare provider.

Some of the risks include:

- Bleeding

- Difficulty breathing

- Heart attack

- Injury to nearby organs during surgery

- Blood clots in the legs and lungs

- Obstruction caused by scar tissue after surgery

- Infection

- Tearing of sutures

- Anastomotic leaks in the colon because of failure of sutures

- Hematoma (accumulation of blood in the wound)

What Happens after the Procedure?

You may need to spend up to a week in the hospital after surgery to recover. You will be administered pain medication and put on a limited liquid diet. After a few days, solid food may be advised. Your surgeon as well as other doctors (such as your oncologist or general practitioner) will schedule a series of follow-up appointments. Make sure you attend all of them. You will also be given instructions on specific things to watch out for in order to spot complications that may arise when you are at home. Make sure you remain alert to them. You will also be given information on how to take care of the stoma.

How Should I Take Care of Myself at Home after Surgery?

Keep the following things in mind for a normal recovery and to identify complications at home:

- Watch for problems such as swelling, redness, bleeding, or discharge at the site of surgery. Intimate your healthcare provider immediately if you find something.

- If you experience pain, chills, or fever, contact your healthcare provider immediately.

- Do not lift heavy weights and do not engage in demanding activities at home for up to 6 weeks.

- Seek help at home for your daily activities until you can take care of yourself again.

- Follow a diet as per instructions from your healthcare provider.

- Do not expose the surgical site to water.

- Drink plenty of water to stay hydrated.

- Do not drive while on narcotic medication for pain.

- Follow instructions on showering, sexual activity, and taking care of your stoma.

- Use a thermometer to check for fever.

- Wear loose fitting clothes.

- Remain on medication as directed for pain, infection, and constipation. Call your healthcare provider if in doubt.

- Engage in deep breathing and relaxation techniques if you find yourself getting anxious.

What Is the Outcome of a Colectomy?

The outcome of a colectomy depends on why exactly you needed the procedure. For cancerous conditions, if the diseased section has been removed entirely, the possibility of a good outcome is greater. For precancerous conditions, such as polyps and ulcerative colitis, the outcome is similar. Most people go on to lead a healthy and productive life postsurgery.

References

1. "Frequently Asked Questions About Colectomy (Colon Resection)," The University of Chicago Medical Center, n.d.

2. Tresca, Amber J. "Types of Colectomy Surgery," VeryWell, January 4, 2017.

3. "Surgical Procedures: Colectomy," Trustees of the University of Pennsylvania, September 19, 2016.

4. "Colectomy," EBSCO Publishing, n.d.

5. "Colectomy," The Regents of the University of California, n.d.

6. "Colectomy," The Johns Hopkins University, The Johns Hopkins Hospital, and Johns Hopkins Health System, n.d.

7. Mayo Clinic Staff, "Colectomy," Mayo Foundation for Medical Education and Research (MFMER), November 17, 2015.

Section 30.4

Colon and Rectal Cancer Surgery

This section contains text excerpted from the following sources:
Text under the heading "Colon Cancer" is excerpted from "Colon
Cancer Treatment (PDQ®)—Patient Version," National Cancer
Institute (NCI), February 27, 2017; Text under the heading "Rectal
Cancer" is excerpted from "Rectal Cancer Treatment (PDQ®)—
Patient Version," National Cancer Institute (NCI), May 19, 2017.

Colon Cancer

Colon cancer is a disease in which malignant (cancer) cells form in
the tissues of the colon. The colon is part of the body's digestive system.
The digestive system removes and processes nutrients (vitamins, minerals, carbohydrates, fats, proteins, and water) from foods and helps
pass waste material out of the body. The digestive system is made up
of the esophagus, stomach, and the small and large intestines. The
colon (large bowel) is the first part of the large intestine and is about
five feet long. Together, the rectum and anal canal make up the last
part of the large intestine and are about 6–8 inches long. The anal
canal ends at the anus (the opening of the large intestine to the outside
of the body). Gastrointestinal stromal tumors can occur in the colon.

Colon Cancer Surgery

Surgery (removing the cancer in an operation) is the most common
treatment for all stages of colon cancer. A doctor may remove the cancer using one of the following types of surgery:

- **Local excision.** If the cancer is found at a very early stage,
  the doctor may remove it without cutting through the abdominal wall. Instead, the doctor may put a tube with a cutting tool
  through the rectum into the colon and cut the cancer out. This is
  called a local excision. If the cancer is found in a polyp (a small
  bulging area of tissue), the operation is called a polypectomy.

- **Resection of the colon with anastomosis.** If the cancer is
  larger, the doctor will perform a partial colectomy (removing the

443

cancer and a small amount of healthy tissue around it). The doctor may then perform an anastomosis (sewing the healthy parts of the colon together). The doctor will also usually remove lymph nodes near the colon and examine them under a microscope to see whether they contain cancer.

- **Resection of the colon with colostomy.** If the doctor is not able to sew the 2 ends of the colon back together, a stoma (an opening) is made on the outside of the body for waste to pass through. This procedure is called a colostomy. A bag is placed around the stoma to collect the waste. Sometimes the colostomy is needed only until the lower colon has healed, and then it can be reversed. If the doctor needs to remove the entire lower colon, however, the colostomy may be permanent.

Even if the doctor removes all the cancer that can be seen at the time of the operation, some patients may be given chemotherapy or radiation therapy after surgery to kill any cancer cells that are left. Treatment given after the surgery, to lower the risk that the cancer will come back, is called adjuvant therapy.

Rectal Cancer

Rectal cancer is a disease in which malignant (cancer) cells form in the tissues of the rectum. The rectum is part of the body's digestive system. The digestive system takes in nutrients (vitamins, minerals, carbohydrates, fats, proteins, and water) from foods and helps pass waste material out of the body. The digestive system is made up of the esophagus, stomach, and the small and large intestines. The colon (large bowel) is the first part of the large intestine and is about 5 feet long. Together, the rectum and anal canal make up the last part of the large intestine and are 6–8 inches long. The anal canal ends at the anus (the opening of the large intestine to the outside of the body).

Rectal Cancer Surgery

Surgery is the most common treatment for all stages of rectal cancer. The cancer is removed using one of the following types of surgery:

- **Polypectomy.** If the cancer is found in a polyp (a small piece of bulging tissue), the polyp is often removed during a colonoscopy.
- **Local excision.** If the cancer is found on the inside surface of the rectum and has not spread into the wall of the rectum, the

cancer and a small amount of surrounding healthy tissue is removed.

- **Resection.** If the cancer has spread into the wall of the rectum, the section of the rectum with cancer and nearby healthy tissue is removed. Sometimes the tissue between the rectum and the abdominal wall is also removed. The lymph nodes near the rectum are removed and checked under a microscope for signs of cancer.

- **Radiofrequency ablation.** The use of a special probe with tiny electrodes that kill cancer cells. Sometimes the probe is inserted directly through the skin and only local anesthesia is needed. In other cases, the probe is inserted through an incision in the abdomen. This is done in the hospital with general anesthesia.

- **Cryosurgery.** A treatment that uses an instrument to freeze and destroy abnormal tissue. This type of treatment is also called cryotherapy.

- **Pelvic exenteration.** If the cancer has spread to other organs near the rectum, the lower colon, rectum, and bladder are removed. In women, the cervix, vagina, ovaries, and nearby lymph nodes may be removed. In men, the prostate may be removed. Artificial openings (stoma) are made for urine and stool to flow from the body to a collection bag.

After the cancer is removed, the surgeon will either:

- do an anastomosis (sew the healthy parts of the rectum together, sew the remaining rectum to the colon, or sew the colon to the anus); or

- make a stoma (an opening) from the rectum to the outside of the body for waste to pass through. This procedure is done if the cancer is too close to the anus and is called a colostomy. A bag is placed around the stoma to collect the waste. Sometimes the colostomy is needed only until the rectum has healed, and then it can be reversed. If the entire rectum is removed, however, the colostomy may be permanent.

Radiation therapy and/or chemotherapy may be given before surgery to shrink the tumor, make it easier to remove the cancer, and help with bowel control after surgery. Treatment given before surgery is called neoadjuvant therapy. Even if all the cancer that can be seen at the time of the operation is removed, some patients may be given radiation therapy and/or chemotherapy after surgery to kill any cancer cells that are left. Treatment given after the surgery, to lower the risk that the cancer will come back, is called adjuvant therapy.

Section 30.5

Gallbladder Removal Surgery (Cholecystectomy)

This section includes text excerpted from "Gallstones," National Institute of Diabetes and Digestive and Kidney Diseases (NIDDK), November 2013. Reviewed June 2017.

Gallstones

Gallstones are hard particles that develop in the gallbladder. The gallbladder is a small, pear-shaped organ located in the upper right abdomen—the area between the chest and hips—below the liver.

Gallstones can range in size from a grain of sand to a golf ball. The gallbladder can develop a single large gallstone, hundreds of tiny stones, or both small and large stones. Gallstones can cause sudden pain in the upper right abdomen. This pain, called a gallbladder attack or biliary colic, occurs when gallstones block the ducts of the biliary tract.

Biliary Tract

The biliary tract consists of the gallbladder and the bile ducts. The bile ducts carry bile and other digestive enzymes from the liver and pancreas to the duodenum—the first part of the small intestine.

The liver produces bile—a fluid that carries toxins and waste products out of the body and helps the body digest fats and the fat-soluble vitamins A, D, E, and K. Bile mostly consists of cholesterol, bile salts, and bilirubin. Bilirubin, a reddish-yellow substance, forms when hemoglobin from red blood cells breaks down. Most bilirubin is excreted through bile.

The bile ducts of the biliary tract include the hepatic ducts, the common bile duct, the pancreatic duct, and the cystic duct. The gallbladder stores bile. Eating signals the gallbladder to contract and empty bile through the cystic duct and common bile duct into the duodenum to mix with food.

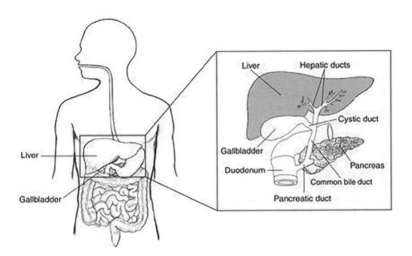

Figure 30.6. *The Biliary Tract*

Causes of Gallstones

Imbalances in the substances that make up bile cause gallstones. Gallstones may form if bile contains too much cholesterol, too much bilirubin, or not enough bile salts. Scientists do not fully understand why these imbalances occur. Gallstones also may form if the gallbladder does not empty completely or often enough.

The two types of gallstones are cholesterol and pigment stones:

- Cholesterol stones, usually yellow-green in color, consist primarily of hardened cholesterol. In the United States, more than 80 percent of gallstones are cholesterol stones.

- Pigment stones, dark in color, are made of bilirubin.

Risk Factors of Gallstones

Certain people have a higher risk of developing gallstones than others:

- Women are more likely to develop gallstones than men. Extra estrogen can increase cholesterol levels in bile and decrease gallbladder contractions, which may cause gallstones to form. Women may have extra estrogen due to pregnancy, hormone replacement therapy, or birth control pills.

- People over age 40 are more likely to develop gallstones than younger people.

- People with a family history of gallstones have a higher risk.

- American Indians have genetic factors that increase the amount of cholesterol in their bile. In fact, American Indians have the highest rate of gallstones in the United States— almost 65 percent of women and 30 percent of men have gallstones.

- Mexican Americans are at higher risk of developing gallstones.

Other factors that affect a person's risk of gallstones include:

- Obesity

- Rapid weight loss

- Diet

- Certain intestinal diseases

- Metabolic syndrome, diabetes, and insulin resistance

Pigment stones tend to develop in people who have:

- cirrhosis—a condition in which the liver slowly deteriorates and malfunctions due to chronic, or long lasting, injury

- infections in the bile ducts

- severe hemolytic anemias—conditions in which red blood cells are continuously broken down, such as sickle cell anemia

Symptoms and Complications of Gallstones

Many people with gallstones do not have symptoms. Gallstones that do not cause symptoms are called asymptomatic, or silent, gallstones. Silent gallstones do not interfere with the function of the gallbladder, liver, or pancreas.

If gallstones block the bile ducts, pressure increases in the gallbladder, causing a gallbladder attack. The pain usually lasts from 1 to several hours. Gallbladder attacks often follow heavy meals, and they usually occur in the evening or during the night.

Gallbladder attacks usually stop when gallstones move and no longer block the bile ducts. However, if any of the bile ducts remain blocked for more than a few hours, complications can occur. Complications include inflammation, or swelling, of the gallbladder and severe damage or infection of the gallbladder, bile ducts, or liver.

A gallstone that becomes lodged in the common bile duct near the duodenum and blocks the pancreatic duct can cause gallstone pancreatitis—inflammation of the pancreas.

Left untreated, blockages of the bile ducts or pancreatic duct can be fatal.

Consulting a Healthcare Provider about Gallstones

People who think they have had a gallbladder attack should notify their healthcare provider. Although these attacks usually resolve as gallstones move, complications can develop if the bile ducts remain blocked.

People with any of the following symptoms during or after a gallbladder attack should see a healthcare provider immediately:

- abdominal pain lasting more than five hours

- nausea and vomiting

- fever—even a low-grade fever—or chills

- yellowish color of the skin or whites of the eyes, called jaundice

- tea-colored urine and light-colored stools

These symptoms may be signs of serious infection or inflammation of the gallbladder, liver, or pancreas.

Diagnosis of Gallstones

A healthcare provider will usually order an ultrasound exam to diagnose gallstones. Other imaging tests may also be used.

- Ultrasound exam

- Computerized tomography (CT) scan

- Magnetic resonance imaging (MRI)

- Cholescintigraphy

- Endoscopic retrograde cholangiopancreatography (ERCP)

Healthcare providers also use blood tests to look for signs of infection or inflammation of the bile ducts, gallbladder, pancreas, or liver. A blood test involves drawing blood at a healthcare provider's office or commercial facility and sending the sample to a lab for analysis.

Gallstone symptoms may be similar to those of other conditions, such as appendicitis, ulcers, pancreatitis, and gastroesophageal reflux disease.

Sometimes, silent gallstones are found when a person does not have any symptoms. For example, a healthcare provider may notice gallstones when performing ultrasound for a different reason.

Treatment of Gallstones

If gallstones are not causing symptoms, treatment is usually not needed. However, if a person has a gallbladder attack or other symptoms, a healthcare provider will usually recommend treatment. A person may be referred to a gastroenterologist—a doctor who specializes in digestive diseases—for treatment. If a person has had one gallbladder attack, more episodes will likely follow.

The usual treatment for gallstones is surgery to remove the gallbladder. If a person cannot undergo surgery, nonsurgical treatments may be used to dissolve cholesterol gallstones. A healthcare provider may use ERCP to remove stones in people who cannot undergo surgery or to remove stones from the common bile duct in people who are about to have gallbladder removal surgery.

Surgery

Surgery to remove the gallbladder, called cholecystectomy, is one of the most common operations performed on adults in the United States.

The gallbladder is not an essential organ, which means a person can live normally without a gallbladder. Once the gallbladder is removed, bile flows out of the liver through the hepatic and common bile ducts and directly into the duodenum, instead of being stored in the gallbladder.

Surgeons perform two types of cholecystectomy:

- **Laparoscopic cholecystectomy.** In a laparoscopic cholecystectomy, the surgeon makes several tiny incisions in the abdomen and inserts a laparoscope—a thin tube with a tiny video camera attached. The camera sends a magnified image from inside the body to a video monitor, giving the surgeon a close-up view of organs and tissues. While watching the monitor, the surgeon uses instruments to carefully separate the gallbladder from the liver, bile ducts, and other structures. Then the surgeon removes the gallbladder through one of the small incisions. Patients usually receive general anesthesia.

Most cholecystectomies are performed with laparoscopy. Many laparoscopic cholecystectomies are performed on an outpatient basis, meaning the person is able to go home the same day. Normal physical activity can usually be resumed in about a week.

- **Open cholecystectomy.** An open cholecystectomy is performed when the gallbladder is severely inflamed, infected, or scarred from other operations. In most of these cases, open cholecystectomy is planned from the start. However, a surgeon may perform an open cholecystectomy when problems occur during a laparoscopic cholecystectomy. In these cases, the surgeon must switch to open cholecystectomy as a safety measure for the patient.

To perform an open cholecystectomy, the surgeon creates an incision about 4 to 6 inches long in the abdomen to remove the gallbladder. Patients usually receive general anesthesia. Recovery from open cholecystectomy may require some people to stay in the hospital for up to a week. Normal physical activity can usually be resumed after about a month.

A small number of people have softer and more frequent stools after gallbladder removal because bile flows into the duodenum more often. Changes in bowel habits are usually temporary; however, they should be discussed with a healthcare provider.

Though complications from gallbladder surgery are rare, the most common complication is injury to the bile ducts. An injured common bile duct can leak bile and cause a painful and possibly dangerous infection. One or more additional operations may be needed to repair the bile ducts. Bile duct injuries occur in less than 1 percent of cholecystectomies.

Nonsurgical Treatments for Cholesterol Gallstones

Nonsurgical treatments are used only in special situations, such as when a person with cholesterol stones has a serious medical condition that prevents surgery. Gallstones often recur within five years after nonsurgical treatment.

451

Two types of nonsurgical treatments can be used to dissolve cholesterol gallstones:

- **Oral dissolution therapy.** Ursodiol (Actigall) and chenodiol (Chenix) are medications that contain bile acids that can dissolve gallstones. These medications are most effective in dissolving small cholesterol stones. Months or years of treatment may be needed to dissolve all stones.

- **Shock wave lithotripsy.** A machine called a lithotripter is used to crush the gallstone. The lithotripter generates shock waves that pass through the person's body to break the gallstone into smaller pieces. This procedure is used only rarely and may be used along with ursodiol.

Eating, Diet, and Nutrition

Factors related to eating, diet, and nutrition that increase the risk of gallstones include:

- obesity

- rapid weight loss

- diets high in calories and refined carbohydrates and low in fiber

People can decrease their risk of gallstones by maintaining a healthy weight through proper diet and nutrition.

Ursodiol can help prevent gallstones in people who rapidly lose weight through low-calorie diets or bariatric surgery. People should talk with their healthcare provider or dietitian about what diet is right for them.

Section 30.6

Hemorrhoid Surgery

This section includes text excerpted from "Hemorrhoids,"
National Institute of Diabetes and Digestive and Kidney
Diseases (NIDDK), October 1, 2016.

About Hemorrhoids

Hemorrhoids, also called piles, are swollen and inflamed veins around your anus or in your lower rectum.

The two types of hemorrhoids are:

- external hemorrhoids, which form under the skin around the anus

- internal hemorrhoids, which form in the lining of the anus and lower rectum

Hemorrhoids are common in both men and women and affect about 1 in 20 Americans. About half of adults older than age 50 have hemorrhoids.

What Are the Complications of Hemorrhoids?

Complications of hemorrhoids can include the following:

- blood clots in an external hemorrhoid

- skin tags—extra skin left behind when a blood clot in an external hemorrhoid dissolves

- infection of a sore on an external hemorrhoid

- strangulated hemorrhoid—when the muscles around your anus cut off the blood supply to an internal hemorrhoid that has fallen through your anal opening

- anemia

Symptoms of Hemorrhoids

The symptoms of hemorrhoids depend on the type you have.

453

If you have external hemorrhoids, you may have:

- anal itching

- one or more hard, tender lumps near your anus

- anal ache or pain, especially when sitting

Too much straining, rubbing, or cleaning around your anus may make your symptoms worse. For many people, the symptoms of external hemorrhoids go away within a few days.

If you have internal hemorrhoids, you may have:

- bleeding from your rectum—bright red blood on stool, on toilet paper, or in the toilet bowl after a bowel movement

- a hemorrhoid that has fallen through your anal opening, called prolapse

Internal hemorrhoids that are not prolapsed most often are not painful. Prolapsed internal hemorrhoids may cause pain and discomfort.

Although hemorrhoids are the most common cause of anal symptoms, not every anal symptom is caused by a hemorrhoid. Some hemorrhoid symptoms are similar to those of other digestive tract problems. For example, bleeding from your rectum may be a sign of bowel diseases such as Crohn's disease, ulcerative colitis, or cancer of the colon or rectum.

Seeking a Doctor's Help

You should seek a doctor's help if you:

- still have symptoms after 1 week of at-home treatment

- have bleeding from your rectum

What Causes Hemorrhoids?

The causes of hemorrhoids include:

- straining during bowel movements

- sitting on the toilet for long periods of time

- chronic constipation or diarrhea

- a low-fiber diet

- weakening of the supporting tissues in your anus and rectum that happens with aging

- pregnancy
- often lifting heavy objects

Diagnosis of Hemorrhoids

Your doctor can often diagnose hemorrhoids based on your medical history and a physical exam. He or she can diagnose external hemorrhoids by checking the area around your anus. To diagnose internal hemorrhoids, your doctor will perform a digital rectal exam and may perform procedures to look inside your anus and rectum.

Medical History

Your doctor will ask you to provide your medical history and describe your symptoms. He or she will ask you about your eating habits, toilet habits, enema and laxative use, and current medical conditions.

Physical Exam

Your doctor will check the area around your anus for:

- lumps or swelling
- internal hemorrhoids that have fallen through your anal opening, called prolapse
- external hemorrhoids with a blood clot in a vein
- leakage of stool or mucus
- skin irritation
- skin tags—extra skin that is left behind when a blood clot in an external hemorrhoid dissolves
- anal fissures—a small tear in the anus that may cause itching, pain, or bleeding

Your doctor will perform a digital rectal exam to:

- check the tone of the muscles in your anus
- check for tenderness, blood, internal hemorrhoids, and lumps or masses

Procedures

Your doctor may use the following procedures to diagnose internal hemorrhoids:

- Anoscopy

- Rigid proctosigmoidoscopy

Your doctor may diagnose internal hemorrhoids while performing procedures for other digestive tract problems or during routine examination of your rectum and colon. These procedures include colonoscopy and flexible sigmoidoscopy.

Treatment of Hemorrhoids

You can most often treat your hemorrhoids at home by:

- eating foods that are high in fiber

- taking a stool softener or a fiber supplement such as psyllium (Metamucil) or methylcellulose (Citrucel)

- drinking water or other nonalcoholic liquids each day as recommended by your healthcare professional

- not straining during bowel movements

- not sitting on the toilet for long periods of time

- taking over-the-counter pain relievers such as acetaminophen, ibuprofen, naproxen, or aspirin

- sitting in a tub of warm water, called a sitz bath, several times a day to help relieve pain

Applying over-the-counter hemorrhoid creams or ointments or using suppositories—a medicine you insert into your rectum—may relieve mild pain, swelling, and itching of external hemorrhoids. Most often, doctors recommend using over-the-counter products for 1 week. You should follow up with your doctor if the products:

- do not relieve your symptoms after 1 week

- cause side effects such dry skin around your anus or a rash

Most prolapsed internal hemorrhoids go away without at-home treatment. However, severely prolapsed or bleeding internal hemorrhoids may need medical treatment.

How Do Doctors Treat Hemorrhoids?

Doctors treat hemorrhoids with procedures during an office visit or in an outpatient center or a hospital.

Office treatments include the following:

- Rubber band ligation
- Sclerotherapy
- Infrared photocoagulation
- Electrocoagulation

Outpatient center or hospital treatments include the following:

- **Hemorrhoidectomy.** A doctor, most often a surgeon, may perform a hemorrhoidectomy to remove large external hemorrhoids and prolapsing internal hemorrhoids that do not respond to other treatments. Your doctor will give you anesthesia for this treatment.

- **Hemorrhoid stapling.** A doctor, most often a surgeon, may use a special stapling tool to remove internal hemorrhoid tissue and pull a prolapsing internal hemorrhoid back into the anus. Your doctor will give you anesthesia for this treatment.

Sometimes complications of hemorrhoids also require treatment.

Eating, Diet, and Nutrition

Your doctor may recommend that you eat more foods that are high in fiber. Eating foods that are high in fiber can make stools softer and easier to pass and can help treat and prevent hemorrhoids. Drinking water and other liquids, such as fruit juices and clear soups, can help the fiber in your diet work better. Ask your doctor about how much you should drink each day based on your health and activity level and where you live.

The 2015–2020 *Dietary Guidelines for Americans* recommends a dietary fiber intake of 14 grams per 1,000 calories consumed. For example, for a 2,000-calorie diet, the fiber recommendation is 28 grams per day.

A doctor or dietitian can help you learn how to add more high-fiber foods to your diet.

What Should I Avoid Eating If I Have Hemorrhoids?

If your hemorrhoids are caused by chronic constipation, try not to eat too many foods with little or no fiber, such as:

- cheese

- chips

- fast food

- ice cream

- meat

- prepared foods, such as some frozen and snack foods

- processed foods, such as hot dogs and some microwavable dinners

Section 30.7

Hernia Surgery

This section includes text excerpted from "Hernia Surgical Mesh Implants," U.S. Food and Drug Administration (FDA), April 4, 2017.

About Hernia

A hernia occurs when an organ, intestine or fatty tissue squeezes through a hole or a weak spot in the surrounding muscle or connective tissue. Hernias often occur at the abdominal wall. Sometimes a hernia can be visible as an external bulge particularly when straining or bearing down.

Types of Hernias

The most common types of hernias are:

- **Inguinal.** occurs in the inner groin

- **Femoral.** occurs in the upper thigh/outer groin

- **Incisional.** occurs through an incision or scar in the abdomen

- **Ventral.** occurs in the general abdominal/ventral wall

- **Umbilical.** occurs at the belly button

- **Hiatal.** occurs inside the abdomen, along the upper stomach/ diaphragm

Causes of Hernias

Most hernias are caused by a combination of pressure and an opening or weakness of muscle or connective tissue. The pressure pushes an organ or tissue through the opening or weak spot. Sometimes the muscle weakness is present at birth but more often it occurs later in life. Anything that causes an increase in abdominal pressure can cause a hernia, including obesity, lifting heavy objects, diarrhea or constipation, or persistent coughing or sneezing. Poor nutrition, smoking, and overexertion can weaken muscles and contribute to the likelihood of a hernia.

Treatment Options for Hernias

Hernia repairs are common—more than one million hernia repairs are performed each year in the United States. Approximately 800,000 are to repair inguinal hernias and the rest are for other types of hernias.

- **Nonsurgical**
    - **Watchful Waiting**. Your surgeon will watch the hernia and make sure that it is not getting larger or causing problems. Although surgery is the only treatment that can repair hernias, many surgical procedures are elective for adult inguinal hernias. Watchful waiting is an option for people who do not have complications or symptoms with their hernias, and if recommended by their surgeon.

- **Surgical**
    - **Laparoscopic.** The surgeon makes several small incisions in the abdomen that allow surgical tools into the openings to repair the hernia. Laparoscopic surgery can be performed with or without surgical mesh.

    - **Open Repair.** The surgeon makes an incision near the hernia and the weak muscle area is repaired. Open repair can be done with or without surgical mesh. Open repair that uses sutures without mesh is referred to as primary closure. Primary closure is used to repair inguinal hernias in infants, small hernias, strangulated or infected hernias.

Hernias have a high rate of recurrence, and surgeons often use surgical mesh to strengthen the hernia repair and reduce the rate of recurrence. Since the 1980s, there has been an increase in mesh-based hernia repairs—by 2000, nonmesh repairs represented less than 10 percent of groin hernia repair techniques.

The use of surgical mesh may also improve patient outcomes through decreased operative time and minimized recovery time. However, recovery time depends on the type of hernia, the surgical approach, and the patient's condition both before and after surgery.

Information found in medical literature has consistently demonstrated a reduced hernia recurrence rate when surgical mesh is used to repair the hernia compared to hernia repair without surgical mesh. For example, inguinal hernia recurrence is higher with open repair using sutures (primary closure) than with mesh repair.

Despite reduced rates of recurrence, there are situations where the use of surgical mesh for hernia repair may not be recommended. Patients should talk to their surgeons about their specific circumstances and their best options and alternatives for hernia repair.

Surgical Mesh

Surgical mesh is a medical device that is used to provide additional support to weakened or damaged tissue. The majority of surgical mesh devices currently available for use are constructed from synthetic materials or animal tissue.

Surgical mesh made of synthetic materials can be found in knitted mesh or nonknitted sheet forms. The synthetic materials used can be absorbable, nonabsorbable or a combination of absorbable and nonabsorbable materials.

Animal-derived mesh are made of animal tissue, such as intestine or skin, that has been processed and disinfected to be suitable for use as an implanted device. These animal-derived mesh are absorbable. The majority of tissue used to produce these mesh implants are from a pig (porcine) or cow (bovine) source.

Nonabsorbable mesh will remain in the body indefinitely and is considered a permanent implant. It is used to provide permanent reinforcement to the repaired hernia. Absorbable mesh will degrade and lose strength over time. It is not intended to provide long-term reinforcement to the repair site. As the material degrades, new tissue growth is intended to provide strength to the repair.

Hernia Repair Surgery Complications

Based on U.S. Food and Drug Administration (FDA)'s analysis of medical device adverse event reports and of peer-reviewed, scientific literature, the most common adverse events for all surgical repair of hernias—with or without mesh—are pain, infection, hernia recurrence, scar-like tissue that sticks tissues together (adhesion), blockage of the large or small intestine (obstruction), bleeding, abnormal connection between organs, vessels, or intestines (fistula), fluid buildup at the surgical site (seroma), and a hole in neighboring tissues or organs (perforation).

The most common adverse events following hernia repair with mesh are pain, infection, hernia recurrence, adhesion, and bowel obstruction. Some other potential adverse events that can occur following hernia repair with mesh are mesh migration and mesh shrinkage (contraction).

Many complications related to hernia repair with surgical mesh that have been reported to the FDA have been associated with recalled mesh products that are no longer on the market. Pain, infection, recurrence, adhesion, obstruction, and perforation are the most common complications associated with recalled mesh. In the FDA's analysis of medical adverse event reports to the FDA, recalled mesh products were the main cause of bowel perforation and obstruction complications.

If you are unsure about the specific mesh manufacturer and brand used in your surgery and have questions about your hernia repair, contact your surgeon or the facility where your surgery was performed to obtain the information from your medical record.

Section 30.8

Inguinal Hernia

This section includes text excerpted from "Inguinal Hernia," National Institute of Diabetes and Digestive and Kidney Diseases (NIDDK), June 2014.

An inguinal hernia happens when contents of the abdomen—usually fat or part of the small intestine—bulge through a weak area in the lower abdominal wall. The abdomen is the area between the chest and the hips. The area of the lower abdominal wall is also called the inguinal or groin region.

Two types of inguinal hernias are:

- indirect inguinal hernias, which are caused by a defect in the abdominal wall that is congenital, or present at birth

- direct inguinal hernias, which usually occur only in male adults and are caused by a weakness in the muscles of the abdominal wall that develops over time

Inguinal hernias occur at the inguinal canal in the groin region.

Inguinal Canal

The inguinal canal is a passage through the lower abdominal wall. People have two inguinal canals—one on each side of the lower abdomen. In males, the spermatic cords pass through the inguinal canals and connect to the testicles in the scrotum—the sac around the testicles. The spermatic cords contain blood vessels, nerves, and a duct, called the spermatic duct, that carries sperm from the testicles to the penis. In females, the round ligaments, which support the uterus, pass through the inguinal canals.

Causes of Inguinal Hernias

The cause of inguinal hernias depends on the type of inguinal hernia.

- **Indirect inguinal hernias.** A defect in the abdominal wall that is present at birth causes an indirect inguinal hernia.

  During the development of the fetus in the womb, the lining of the abdominal cavity forms and extends into the inguinal canal. In males, the spermatic cord and testicles descend out from inside the abdomen and through the abdominal lining to the scrotum through the inguinal canal. Next, the abdominal lining usually closes off the entrance to the inguinal canal a few weeks before or after birth. In females, the ovaries do not descend out from inside the abdomen, and the abdominal lining usually closes a couple of months before birth.

  Sometimes the lining of the abdomen does not close as it should, leaving an opening in the abdominal wall at the upper part of the inguinal canal. Fat or part of the small intestine may slide into the inguinal canal through this opening, causing a hernia. In females, the ovaries may also slide into the inguinal canal and cause a hernia.

Indirect hernias are the most common type of inguinal hernia. Indirect inguinal hernias may appear in 2 to 3 percent of male children; however, they are much less common in female children, occurring in less than 1 percent.

- **Direct inguinal hernias.** Direct inguinal hernias usually occur only in male adults as aging and stress or strain weaken the abdominal muscles around the inguinal canal. Previous surgery in the lower abdomen can also weaken the abdominal muscles.

  Females rarely form this type of inguinal hernia. In females, the broad ligament of the uterus acts as an additional barrier behind the muscle layer of the lower abdominal wall. The broad ligament of the uterus is a sheet of tissue that supports the uterus and other reproductive organs.

Risk Factors of Inguinal Hernias

Males are much more likely to develop inguinal hernias than females. About 25 percent of males and about 2 percent of females will develop an inguinal hernia in their lifetimes. Some people who have an inguinal hernia on one side will have or will develop a hernia on the other side.

People of any age can develop inguinal hernias. Indirect hernias can appear before age 1 and often appear before age 30; however, they may appear later in life. Premature infants have a higher chance of developing an indirect inguinal hernia. Direct hernias, which usually only occur in male adults, are much more common in men older than age 40 because the muscles of the abdominal wall weaken with age.

People with a family history of inguinal hernias are more likely to develop inguinal hernias. Studies also suggest that people who smoke have an increased risk of inguinal hernias.

Signs and Symptoms of Inguinal Hernias

The first sign of an inguinal hernia is a small bulge on one or, rarely, on both sides of the groin—the area just above the groin crease between the lower abdomen and the thigh. The bulge may increase in size over time and usually disappears when lying down.

Other signs and symptoms can include:

- discomfort or pain in the groin—especially when straining, lifting, coughing, or exercising—that improves when resting

463

- feelings such as weakness, heaviness, burning, or aching in the groin

- a swollen or an enlarged scrotum in men or boys

Indirect and direct inguinal hernias may slide in and out of the abdomen into the inguinal canal. A healthcare provider can often move them back into the abdomen with gentle massage.

Complications of Inguinal Hernias

Inguinal hernias can cause the following complications:

- **Incarceration.** An incarcerated hernia happens when part of the fat or small intestine from inside the abdomen becomes stuck in the groin or scrotum and cannot go back into the abdomen. A healthcare provider is unable to massage the hernia back into the abdomen.

- **Strangulation.** When an incarcerated hernia is not treated, the blood supply to the small intestine may become obstructed, causing "strangulation" of the small intestine. This lack of blood supply is an emergency situation and can cause the section of the intestine to die.

Diagnosis of Inguinal Hernias

A healthcare provider diagnoses an inguinal hernia with:

- a medical and family history

- a physical exam

- imaging tests, including X-rays

Medical and family history. Taking a medical and family history may help a healthcare provider diagnose an inguinal hernia. Often the symptoms that the patient describes will be signs of an inguinal hernia.

Physical exam. A physical exam may help diagnose an inguinal hernia. During a physical exam, a healthcare provider usually examines the patient's body. The healthcare provider may ask the patient to stand and cough or strain so the healthcare provider can feel for a bulge caused by the hernia as it moves into the groin or scrotum. The healthcare provider may gently try to massage the hernia back into its proper position in the abdomen.

Imaging tests. A healthcare provider does not usually use imaging tests, including X-rays, to diagnose an inguinal hernia unless he or she:

- is trying to diagnose a strangulation or an incarceration

- cannot feel the inguinal hernia during a physical exam, especially in patients who are overweight

- is uncertain if the hernia or another condition is causing the swelling in the groin or other symptoms

Specially trained technicians perform imaging tests at a healthcare provider's office, an outpatient center, or a hospital.

A radiologist—a doctor who specializes in medical imaging—interprets the images. A patient does not usually need anesthesia.

Tests may include the following:

- Abdominal X-ray

- Computerized tomography (CT) scan

- Abdominal ultrasound

Treatment of Inguinal Hernias

Repair of an inguinal hernia via surgery is the only treatment for inguinal hernias and can prevent incarceration and strangulation. healthcare providers recommend surgery for most people with inguinal hernias and especially for people with hernias that cause symptoms. Research suggests that men with hernias that cause few or no symptoms may be able to safely delay surgery until their symptoms increase. Men who delay surgery should watch for symptoms and see a healthcare provider regularly. healthcare providers usually recommend surgery for infants and children to prevent incarceration. Emergent, or immediate, surgery is necessary for incarcerated or strangulated hernias.

A general surgeon—a doctor who specializes in abdominal surgery—performs hernia surgery at a hospital or surgery center, usually on an outpatient basis. Recovery time varies depending on the size of the hernia, the technique used, and the age and health of the person.

Hernia surgery is also called herniorrhaphy. The two main types of surgery for hernias are:

- **Open hernia repair.** During an open hernia repair, a healthcare provider usually gives a patient local anesthesia in the abdomen with sedation; however, some patients may have:

- sedation with a spinal block, in which a healthcare provider injects anesthetics around the nerves in the spine, making the body numb from the waist down

- general anesthesia

The surgeon makes an incision in the groin, moves the hernia back into the abdomen, and reinforces the abdominal wall with stitches. Usually the surgeon also reinforces the weak area with a synthetic mesh or "screen" to provide additional support.

- **Laparoscopic hernia repair.** A surgeon performs laparoscopic hernia repair with the patient under general anesthesia. The surgeon makes several small, half-inch incisions in the lower abdomen and inserts a laparoscope—a thin tube with a tiny video camera attached. The camera sends a magnified image from inside the body to a video monitor, giving the surgeon a close-up view of the hernia and surrounding tissue. While watching the monitor, the surgeon repairs the hernia using synthetic mesh or "screen."

People who undergo laparoscopic hernia repair generally experience a shorter recovery time than those who have an open hernia repair. However, the surgeon may determine that laparoscopy is not the best option if the hernia is large or if the person has had previous pelvic surgery.

Most adults experience discomfort and require pain medication after either an open hernia repair or a laparoscopic hernia repair. Intense activity and heavy lifting are restricted for several weeks. The surgeon will discuss when a person may safely return to work. Infants and children also experience some discomfort; however, they usually resume normal activities after several days.

Surgery to repair an inguinal hernia is quite safe, and complications are uncommon. People should contact their healthcare provider if any of the following symptoms appear:

- redness around or drainage from the incision

- fever

- bleeding from the incision

- pain that is not relieved by medication or pain that suddenly worsens

Possible long-term complications include:

- long-lasting pain in the groin

- recurrence of the hernia, requiring a second surgery

- damage to nerves near the hernia

Prevention Strategies for Inguinal Hernias

People cannot prevent the weakness in the abdominal wall that causes indirect inguinal hernias. However, people may be able to prevent direct inguinal hernias by maintaining a healthy weight and not smoking.

People can keep inguinal hernias from getting worse or keep inguinal hernias from recurring after surgery by:

- avoiding heavy lifting

- using the legs, not the back, when lifting objects

- preventing constipation and straining during bowel movements

- maintaining a healthy weight

- not smoking

Eating, Diet, and Nutrition

Researchers have not found that eating, diet, and nutrition play a role in causing inguinal hernias. A person with an inguinal hernia may be able to prevent symptoms by eating high-fiber foods. Fresh fruits, vegetables, and whole grains are high in fiber and may help prevent the constipation and straining that cause some of the painful symptoms of a hernia.

The surgeon will provide instructions on eating, diet, and nutrition after inguinal hernia surgery. Most people drink liquids and eat a light diet the day of the operation and then resume their usual diet the next day.

Chapter 31

Weight-Loss (Bariatric) Surgery

Chapter Contents

Section 31.1

Overview of Bariatric Surgery for Severe Obesity

This section includes text excerpted from "Weight Management—
Bariatric Surgery," National Institute of Diabetes and Digestive and
Kidney Diseases (NIDDK), August 11, 2016.

What Is Obesity?

Obesity is defined as having a body mass index (BMI) of 30 or more.
BMI is a measure of your weight in relation to your height. Class 1
obesity means a BMI of 30 to 35, Class 2 obesity is a BMI of 35 to 40,
and Class 3 obesity is a BMI of 40 or more. Classes 2 and 3, also known
as severe obesity, are often hard to treat with diet and exercise alone.

What Is Bariatric Surgery?

Bariatric surgery is an operation that helps you lose weight by
making changes to your digestive system. Some types of bariatric surgeries make your stomach smaller, allowing you to eat and drink less
at one time and making you feel full sooner. Other bariatric surgeries
also change your small intestine—the part of your body that absorbs
calories and nutrients from foods and beverages.

Bariatric surgery may be an option if you have severe obesity and
have not been able to lose weight or keep from gaining back any weight
you lost using other methods such as lifestyle treatment or medications. Bariatric surgery also may be an option if you have serious
health problems, such as type 2 diabetes or sleep apnea, related to
obesity. Bariatric surgery can improve many of the medical conditions
linked to obesity, especially type 2 diabetes.

Does Bariatric Surgery Always Work?

Studies show that many people who have bariatric surgery lose
about 15 to 30 percent of their starting weight on average, depending on the type of surgery they have. However, no method, including

surgery, is sure to produce and maintain weight loss. Some people who have bariatric surgery may not lose as much as they hoped. Over time, some people regain a portion of the weight they lost. The amount of weight people regain may vary. Factors that affect weight regain may include a person's level of obesity and the type of surgery he or she had.

Bariatric surgery does not replace healthy habits, but may make it easier for you to consume fewer calories and be more physically active. Choosing healthy foods and beverages before and after the surgery may help you lose more weight and keep it off long term. Regular physical activity after surgery also helps keep the weight off. To improve your health, you must commit to a lifetime of healthy lifestyle habits and following the advice of your healthcare providers.

How Much Does Bariatric Surgery Cost?

On average, bariatric surgery costs between $15,000 and $25,000, depending on what type of surgery you have and whether you have surgery-related problems. Costs may be higher or lower based on where you live. The amount your medical insurance will pay varies by state and insurance provider.

Medicare and some Medicaid programs cover three common types of bariatric surgery—gastric bypass, gastric band, and gastric sleeve surgery—if you meet certain criteria and have a doctor's recommendation. Some insurance plans may require you to use approved surgeons and facilities. Some insurers also require you to show that you were unable to lose weight by completing a nonsurgical weight-loss program or that you meet other requirements.

Your health insurance company or your regional Medicare or Medicaid office will have more information about bariatric surgery coverage, options, and requirements.

Types of Bariatric Surgery

The type of surgery that may be best to help a person lose weight depends on a number of factors. You should discuss with your doctor what kind of surgery might be best for you or your teen.

What Is the Difference between Open and Laparoscopic Surgery?

In open bariatric surgery, surgeons make a single, large cut in the abdomen. More often, surgeons now use laparoscopic surgery, in which they make several small cuts and insert thin surgical tools through the cuts. Surgeons also insert a small scope attached to a camera that projects images onto a video monitor. Laparoscopic surgery has fewer risks than open surgery and may cause less pain and scarring than open surgery. Laparoscopic surgery also may lead to a faster recovery.

Open surgery may be a better option for certain people. If you have a high level of obesity, have had stomach surgery before, or have other complex medical problems, you may need open surgery.

What Are The Surgical Options?

In the United States, surgeons use three types of operations most often:

- laparoscopic adjustable gastric band

- gastric sleeve surgery, also called sleeve gastrectomy

- gastric bypass

Surgeons use a fourth operation, biliopancreatic diversion with duodenal switch, less often.

Laparoscopic Adjustable Gastric Band

In this type of surgery, the surgeon places a ring with an inner inflatable band around the top of your stomach to create a small pouch. This makes you feel full after eating a small amount of food. The band has a circular balloon inside that is filled with salt solution. The surgeon can adjust the size of the opening from the pouch to the rest of your stomach by injecting or removing the solution through a small device called a port placed under your skin.

After surgery, you will need several follow-up visits to adjust the size of the band opening. If the band causes problems or is not helping you lose enough weight, the surgeon may remove it.

The U.S. Food and Drug Administration (FDA) has approved use of the gastric band for people with a BMI of 30 or more who also have at least one health problem linked to obesity, such as heart disease or diabetes.

Gastric Sleeve

In gastric sleeve surgery, also called vertical sleeve gastrectomy, a surgeon removes most of your stomach, leaving only a banana-shaped section that is closed with staples. Like gastric band surgery, this surgery reduces the amount of food that can fit in your stomach, making you feel full sooner. Taking out part of your stomach may also affect gut hormones or other factors such as gut bacteria that may affect appetite and metabolism. This type of surgery cannot be reversed because some of the stomach is permanently removed.

Gastric Bypass

Gastric bypass surgery, also called Roux-en-Y gastric bypass, has two parts. First, the surgeon staples your stomach, creating a small pouch in the upper section. The staples make your stomach much smaller, so you eat less and feel full sooner.

Next, the surgeon cuts your small intestine and attaches the lower part of it directly to the small stomach pouch. Food then bypasses most of the stomach and the upper part of your small intestine so your body absorbs fewer calories. The surgeon connects the bypassed section farther down to the lower part of the small intestine. This bypassed section is still attached to the main part of your stomach, so digestive juices can move from your stomach and the first part of your small intestine into the lower part of your small intestine. The bypass also changes gut hormones, gut bacteria, and other factors that may affect appetite and metabolism. Gastric bypass is difficult to reverse, although a surgeon may do it if medically necessary.

Duodenal Switch

This surgery, also called biliopancreatic diversion with duodenal switch, is more complex than the others. The duodenal switch involves two separate surgeries. The first is similar to gastric sleeve surgery. The second surgery redirects food to bypass most of your small intestine. The surgeon also reattaches the bypassed section to the last part of the small intestine, allowing digestive juices to mix with food.

This type of surgery allows you to lose more weight than the other three. However, this surgery is also the most likely to cause surgery-related problems and a shortage of vitamins, minerals, and protein in your body. For these reasons, surgeons do not perform this surgery as often.

What Should I Expect before Surgery?

Before surgery, you will meet with several healthcare providers, such as a dietitian, a psychiatrist or psychologist, an internist, and a bariatric surgeon.

Table 31.1. Most Common Weight-Loss Surgeries

	Gastric Band	Gastric Sleeve	Gastric Bypass
What It Is	Surgeon places an inflatable band around top part of stomach, creating a small pouch with an adjustable opening.	Surgeon removes about 80 percent of stomach, creating a long, banana-shaped pouch.	Surgeon staples top part of stomach, creating a small pouch and attaching it to middle part of small intestine.
Pros	• Can be adjusted and reversed. • Short hospital stay and low risk of surgery-related problems. • No changes to intestines. • Lowest chance of vitamin shortage.	• Greater weight loss than gastric band. • No changes to intestines. • No objects placed in body. • Short hospital stay.	• Greater weight loss than gastric band. • No objects placed in body.
Cons	• Less weight loss than other types of bariatric surgery. • Frequent follow-up visits to adjust band; some people may not adapt to band. • Possible future surgery to remove or replace a part or all of the band system.	• Cannot be reversed. • Chance of vitamin shortage. • Higher chance of surgery-related problems than gastric band. • Chance of acid reflux.	• Difficult to reverse. • Higher chance of vitamin shortage than gastric band or gastric sleeve. • Higher chance of surgery-related problems than gastric band. • May increase risk of alcohol use disorder.

- The doctor will ask about your medical history, do a thorough physical exam, and order blood tests. If you are a smoker, he or she will likely ask you to stop smoking at least 6 weeks before your surgery.

- The surgeon will tell you more about the surgery, including how to prepare for it and what type of follow-up you will need.

- The dietitian will explain what and how much you will be able to eat and drink after surgery and help you to prepare for how your life will change after surgery.

- The psychiatrist or psychologist may do an assessment to see if bariatric surgery is an option for you.

These healthcare providers also will advise you to become more active and adopt a healthy eating plan before and after surgery. In some cases, losing weight and bringing your blood sugar levels closer to normal before surgery may lower your chances of having surgery-related problems.

Some bariatric surgery programs have groups you can attend before and after surgery that can help answer questions about the surgery and offer support.

What Should I Expect after Surgery?

After surgery, you will need to rest and recover. Although the type of follow-up varies by type of surgery, you will need to take supplements that your doctor prescribes to make sure you are getting enough vitamins and minerals.

Walking and moving around the house may help you recover more quickly. Start slowly and follow your doctor's advice about the type of physical activity you can do safely. As you feel more comfortable, add more physical activity.

After surgery, most people move from a liquid diet to a soft diet such as cottage cheese, yogurt, or soup, and then to solid foods over several weeks. Your doctor, nurse, or dietitian will tell you which foods and beverages you may have and which ones you should avoid. You will need to eat small meals and chew your food well.

How Much Weight Can I Expect to Lose?

The amount of weight people lose after bariatric surgery depends on the individual and on the type of surgery he or she had. A study following people for 3 years after surgery found that those who had gastric band surgery lost an average of about 45 pounds. People who had gastric bypass lost an average of 90 pounds. Most people regained some weight over time, but weight regain was usually small compared to their initial weight loss.

Researchers know less about the long-term results of gastric sleeve surgery, but the amount of weight loss seems to be similar to or slightly less than gastric bypass.

Your weight loss could be different. Remember, reaching your goal depends not just on the surgery but also on sticking with healthy lifestyle habits throughout your life.

Weight-Loss Devices

The FDA has approved several new weight-loss devices that do not permanently change your stomach or small intestine. These devices cause less weight loss than bariatric surgery, and some are only temporary. Researchers haven't studied any of them over a long period of time and don't know the long-term risks and benefits.

The electrical stimulation system uses a device implanted in your abdomen, by way of laparoscopic surgery, that blocks nerve activity between your stomach and brain. The device works on the vagus nerve, which helps signal the brain that the stomach feels full or empty.

The gastric balloon system consists of one or two balloons placed in your stomach through a tube inserted through your mouth. Your doctor or nurse will give you a sedative before the procedure. Once the balloons are in your stomach, doctors inflate them with salt water so they take up space in your stomach and help you feel fuller. You will need to have the balloons removed after 6 months or a year.

A new device uses a pump to drain part of the food in your stomach after a meal. The device includes a tube that goes from the inside of your stomach to a port on the outside of your abdomen. The port is a small valve that fits over the opening in your abdomen. About 20 to 30 minutes after eating, you attach tubing from the port to the pump and open the valve. The pump drains your stomach contents through a tube into the toilet, so that your body doesn't absorb about 30 percent of calories you ate. You can have the device removed at any time.

Section 31.2

Bariatric Surgery: Potential Candidates, Benefits, and Side Effects

This section includes text excerpted from "Bariatric Surgery— Potential Candidates for Bariatric Surgery," National Institute of Diabetes and Digestive and Kidney Diseases (NIDDK), July 2016.

Potential Candidates for Bariatric Surgery

Who Is a Good Adult Candidate for Bariatric Surgery?

Bariatric surgery may be an option for adults who have:

- a body mass index (BMI) of 40 or more, OR

- a BMI of 35 or more with a serious health problem linked to obesity, such as type 2 diabetes, heart disease, or sleep apnea

- a BMI of 30 or more with a serious health problem linked to obesity, for the gastric band only

Having surgery to lose weight is a serious decision. If you are thinking about having bariatric surgery, you should know what's involved. Your answers to the following questions may help you decide if surgery is an option for you:

- Have you been unable to lose weight or keep it off using nonsurgical methods such as lifestyle changes or drug treatment?

- Do you understand what the operation involves and its risks and benefits?

- Do you understand how your eating and physical activity patterns will need to change after you have surgery?

- Can you commit to following lifelong healthy eating and physical activity habits, medical follow-up, and the need to take extra vitamins and minerals?

Who Is A Good Teen Candidate For Bariatric Surgery?

Doctors sometimes use bariatric surgery to treat teens with severe obesity who also have obesity-related health problems. Bariatric surgery often improves health problems that could grow worse in adulthood if the teen remains obese.

Surgery may be an option for teens who have gone through puberty and reached their adult height, and have:

- a BMI of 35 or more with serious obesity-related health problems, such as type 2 diabetes or severe sleep apnea, OR

- a BMI of 40 or more with less severe health problems, such as high blood pressure or high cholesterol

Studies suggest that bariatric surgery is fairly safe for teens and can improve health problems such as type 2 diabetes for at least 3 years after surgery. Teens who took part in a study that followed them for 3 years after surgery lost an average of 90 pounds and kept most of the weight off. They also reported improved quality of life related to their weight. Researchers continue to study the long-term effects, which currently are unknown.

Like adults, teens who are thinking about weight-loss surgery should be prepared for the lifestyle changes they will need to make after the surgery. A surgical center that focuses on the unique needs of youth may help the teen patient prepare for and adjust to these changes. Parents and caregivers also should be prepared and ready to support their child.

Bariatric Surgery Benefits

What Are the Benefits of Bariatric Surgery?

Bariatric surgery can help you lose weight and improve many health problems related to obesity. These health problems include:

- type 2 diabetes
- high blood pressure
- unhealthy cholesterol levels
- sleep apnea
- urinary incontinence
- body pain
- knee and hip pain

478

You may be better able to move around and be physically active after surgery. You might also notice your mood improve and feel like your quality of life is better.

Bariatric Surgery Side Effects

What Are The Side Effects of Bariatric Surgery?

Side effects may include:

- bleeding

- infection

- leaking from the site where the sections of the stomach or small intestine, or both, are stapled or sewn together

- diarrhea

- blood clots in the legs that can move to the lungs and heart

Rarely, surgery-related problems can lead to death.

Other side effects may occur later. Your body may not absorb nutrients well, especially if you don't take your prescribed vitamins and minerals. Not getting enough nutrients can cause health problems, such as anemia and osteoporosis. Gallstones can occur after rapid weight loss. Some doctors prescribe medicine for about 6 months after surgery to help prevent gallstones. Gastric bands can erode into the stomach wall and need to be removed.

Other problems that could occur later include strictures and hernias. Strictures—narrowing of the new stomach or connection between the stomach and small intestine—make it hard to eat solid food and can cause nausea, vomiting, and trouble swallowing. Doctors treat strictures with special instruments to expand the narrowing. Two kinds of hernias may occur after bariatric surgery—at the incision site or in the abdomen. Doctors repair hernias with surgery.

Some research suggests that bariatric surgery, especially gastric bypass, may change the way your body absorbs and breaks down alcohol, and may lead to more alcohol-related problems after surgery.

Chapter 32

Gynecologic and Obstetric Surgery

Chapter Contents

Section 32.1

Hysterectomy

This section includes text excerpted from "Hysterectomy,"
Office on Women's Health (OWH), U.S. Department of
Health and Human Services (HHS), September 9, 2014.

A hysterectomy is a surgery to remove a woman's uterus (also
known as the womb). The uterus is where a baby grows when a woman
is pregnant. During the surgery the whole uterus is usually removed.
Your doctor may also remove your fallopian tubes and ovaries. After
a hysterectomy, you no longer have menstrual periods and cannot
become pregnant.

Why Would I Need a Hysterectomy?

Sometimes a hysterectomy may be medically necessary. But sometimes you can try medicines or other treatments first. Talk with your
doctor about all of your treatment options.

You may need a hysterectomy if you have one of the following:

- **Uterine fibroids.** Uterine fibroids are noncancerous growths in
  the uterine wall. In some women, they can cause pain and long-
  term heavy bleeding. Uterine fibroids tend to shrink after menopause, so you may choose to wait. Your doctor may also try other
  procedures, like myomectomy or endometrial ablation, before a
  hysterectomy.

- **Heavy or unusual vaginal bleeding.** Changes in hormone
  levels, infection, cancer or fibroids can cause heavy, prolonged
  bleeding. Hormonal birth control may help to lighten heavy
  bleeding, correct irregular bleeding and relieve pain.

- **Uterine prolapse.** This is when the uterus slips from its usual
  place down into the vagina. This is more common in women who
  have had several vaginal births, but it can also happen after
  menopause or because of obesity. You can try Kegel exercises
  (squeezing the pelvic floor muscles) to help restore tone to the
  muscle holding the uterus in place. Your doctor may also insert

a pessary (rubber or plastic object) into your vagina to hold your uterus in place.

- **Endometriosis.** Endometriosis happens when the tissue that lines the uterus grows outside of the uterus on the ovaries. This can cause severe pain and bleeding between periods. Your doctor can prescribe medicine or do surgery to remove the scar tissue or growths without harming surrounding tissue.

- **Adenomyosis.** In this condition, the tissue that lines the uterus grows inside the walls of the uterus where it doesn't belong. The uterine walls thicken and cause severe pain and heavy bleeding. Hormonal birth control may help.

- **Cancer (or precancer) of the uterus, ovary, cervix, or endometrium.** Hysterectomy may be the best option if you cancer in these organs.

Will the Hysterectomy Cause Me to Enter Menopause?

All women who have a hysterectomy will stop getting their period. Whether you will have other symptoms of menopause after a hysterectomy depends on whether your doctor removes your ovaries during the surgery. If you keep your ovaries during the hysterectomy, you should not have other menopausal symptoms right away.

If both ovaries are removed during the hysterectomy, you will no longer have periods and you may have other menopausal symptoms right away. Because your hormone levels drop quickly without ovaries, your symptoms may be stronger than with natural menopause.

What Changes Can I Expect after a Hysterectomy?

Hysterectomy is a major surgery, so recovery can take a few weeks. But for most women, the biggest change is a better quality of life. You should have relief from the symptoms that made the surgery necessary.

Other changes that you may experience after a hysterectomy include:

- **Menopause.** You will no longer have periods. If your ovaries are removed during the hysterectomy, you may have other menopause symptoms.

- **Change in sexual feelings.** Some women have vaginal dryness or less interest in sex after a hysterectomy, especially if the ovaries are removed.

- **Increased risk for other health problems.** If both ovaries are removed, this may put you at higher risk for certain conditions such as: bone loss, heart disease, and urinary incontinence (leaking of urine). Talk to your doctor about how to prevent these problems.

- **Sense of loss.** Some women may feel grief or depression over the loss of fertility or the change in their bodies. Talk to your doctor if you have symptoms of depression, including feelings of sadness, a loss of interest in food or things you once enjoyed, or less energy, that last longer than a few weeks after your surgery.

Section 32.2

Dilation and Curettage (D&C)

"Dilation and Curettage (D&C),"
© 2017 Omnigraphics. Reviewed June 2017.

What Is Dilation and Curettage (D&C)?

Dilation and curettage, also known as a D&C is a surgical procedure in which abnormal tissues are scraped from the lining (endometrium) of the uterus. It is an outpatient surgery and most women can return home the same day. In dilation and curettage, the cervix is dilated and a spoon-shaped instrument, called a curette, is used to scrape and remove the abnormal tissue. A variation of this procedure is Dilation and Evacuation (D&E) in which the contents of the uterus are removed using suction force.

Why Is D&C Advised?

Dilation and curettage serves diagnostic and therapeutic purposes. It is usually done for:

- Investigating abnormal or excessive uterine bleeding.

- Removal of fibroids (mostly noncancerous connective and muscle tissue growths in the uterus).

- Removal of polyps (growths attached to the inner wall of the uterus).

- Removal of hyperplasia (abnormal growth in the lining of the uterus).

- Examination of potentially cancerous tissue.

- Medical termination of pregnancy, (up to 14 weeks of gestation) also called an abortion.

- Abortion of abnormal fetus (having birth defects).

- Removal of placental and other tissues after miscarriage.

- Removal of remnant placental tissue, postpartum.

- Therapeutic abortion (termination of pregnancy that is dangerous to the mother).

- To determine the cause of infertility.

- Other reasons as seen fit by a doctor.

How Does One Prepare for D&C?

Make arrangements at home to take care of daily activities before you leave for the procedure. Ask someone to drive you home after surgery and arrange for a help when you're recovering. You will be informed as to when you need to stop eating before surgery in order to prevent vomiting during surgery. Inform the hospital about any allergies and medications that you are taking. You will not have to take regular medication on the day of surgery. You will be asked to avoid aspirin because it increases risk of bleeding. If you are allergic to local and general anesthetic agents, iodine, latex or tape, volunteer this information in advance. If you are a smoker, you should quit at least 8 weeks before surgery. Surgery leads to complications and healing time is increased in smokers. Follow instructions given to you by doctors and medical staff. Carry a sanitary napkin to wear when leaving for home.

How Is D&C Performed?

The patient is given sedation for relaxation. D&C is usually done under partial anesthesia, but in certain circumstances, at the request of the patient, she may be fully anesthetized. The patient also will be positioned with both legs harnessed onto stirrups. Prior to surgery, the cervix is dilated with a laminaria stick, which is a thick rod that is inserted in the cervix that absorbs fluid and dilates the cervix so that the uterus can be accessed. Medications are used to numb and soften the cervix to aid dilation. A speculum is then placed into the vagina and clamped into place. Once the cervix has dilated to one and a half inch, the surgeon uses a curette to scrape and clean the abnormal tissue from the uterus. Sometimes tissue samples are sent to the laboratory for analysis. The procedure results in cramps similar to menstrual cramps, which are usually controlled by pain medication.

What Are the Risks and Side Effects of D&C?

- You may experience problems with anesthesia such as nausea or vomiting.
- Abdominal pain or cramping.
- Infection or bleeding.
- Perforation of the uterus or bowel and damage to the cervix.
- Scar tissue may develop in the uterus.
- Foul-smelling discharge.
- Fever or chills.
- Inability to get pregnant after surgery.

Enquire with your medical practitioner about the risks applicable to you and other concerns prior to surgery.

What Happens after the Procedure?

The type of recovery varies along with the kind of procedure applied in your case. You will need to recover from anesthesia and be kept under observation initially. Once your blood pressure, pulse, and breathing have returned to normal you will be taken to recovery and then discharged. Have another person drive you home in case you are discharged on the same day. Sufficient rest will be required if you were anesthetized. After surgery, you will experience spotting or slight vaginal bleeding for a few days. Wear a sanitary napkin. You will also experience cramping. You will be advised not to douche or use tampons and engage in sexual intercourse for a short period of time. Restrictions will be placed on intense physical activity such as lifting heavy objects.

What Is the Follow-Up Required after D&C?

The endometrial lining will rebuild in a few days after surgery and regular menstrual periods will commence in due course of time. If you need pain medication, speak to your doctor. Aspirin could increase chances of bleeding and is not advised. Your cervix is under risk of bacterial infection until it is fully healed. Contact the clinic if you suffer from severe abdominal pain, fever, chills, or foul-smelling discharge.

References

1. "Dilation and Curettage (D and C)," The Johns Hopkins University, n.d.

2. "Dilation and Curettage (D&C)," University of Rochester Medical Center, n.d.

3. "Dilation and Curettage (D and C)," The Cleveland Clinic Foundation, n.d.

4. "Dilation and Curettage (D and C)," Memorial Sloan Kettering Cancer Center, April 3, 2017.

Section 32.3

Cesarean Section (C-Section)

This section includes text excerpted from "Labor and Delivery," *Eunice Kennedy Shriver* National Institute of Child Health and Human Development (NICHD), December 17, 2014.

A C-section, short for cesarean section, is also called cesarean birth. Cesarean birth is the delivery of a baby through surgical cuts in a woman's abdomen and uterus. The uterus is then closed with stitches that later dissolve. Stitches or staples also close the skin on the belly.

When Is Cesarean Delivery Needed?

Cesarean delivery may be necessary in the following circumstances:

- **A pregnancy with two or more fetuses (multiple pregnancy).** A cesarean delivery may be needed if labor has started too early (preterm labor), if the fetuses are not in good positions in the uterus for natural delivery, or if there are other problems.

- **Labor is not progressing.** Contractions may not open the cervix enough for the baby to move into the vagina.

- **The infant's health is in danger.** The umbilical cord, which connects the fetus to the uterus, may become pinched, or the fetus may have an abnormal heart rate. In these cases, a C-section allows the baby to be delivered quickly to address and resolve the baby's health problems.

- **Problems with the placenta.** Sometimes the placenta is not formed or working correctly, is in the wrong place in the uterus, or is implanted too deeply or firmly in the uterine wall. This can cause problems, such as depriving the fetus of needed oxygen and nutrients or vaginal bleeding.

- **The baby is too large.** Women with gestational diabetes, especially if their blood sugar levels are not well controlled, are at increased risk for having large infants. And larger infants are at risk for complications during delivery. These include shoulder dystocia, when the infant's head is delivered through the vagina but the shoulders are stuck.

- **The baby is breech, or in a breech presentation,** meaning the baby is coming out feet first instead of head first.

- **The mother has an infection,** such as human immunodeficiency virus (HIV) or herpes, that could be passed to the baby during vaginal birth. Cesarean delivery could help prevent transmission of the virus to the infant.

- **The mother has a medical condition.** A C-section enables the healthcare provider to better manage the mother's health issues.

Women who have a cesarean delivery may be given pain medication with an epidural block, a spinal block, or general anesthesia. An epidural block numbs the lower part of the body through an injection in the spine. A spinal block also numbs the lower part of the body but through an injection directly into the spinal fluid. Women who receive general anesthesia, often used for emergency cesarean deliveries, will not be awake during the surgery.

What Are the Risks of a Cesarean Section (C-Section)?

Cesarean birth is a type of surgery, meaning it has risks and possible complications for both mother and infant.

Possible risks from a C-section (which are also associated with vaginal birth) include:

- infection

- blood loss

- blood clots in the legs, pelvic organs, or lungs

- injury to surrounding structures, such as the bowel or bladder

- reaction to medication or anesthesia used

A woman who has a C-section also may have to stay in the hospital longer. The more C-sections a woman has, the greater her risk for certain medical problems and problems with future pregnancies, such as uterine rupture and problems with the placenta.

Can a C-Section Be Requested?

Some women may want to have a cesarean birth even if vaginal delivery is an option. Women should discuss this option in detail with their healthcare provider before making a final decision about a C-section.

As is true for vaginal births, unless there is a medical necessity, delivery should not occur before 39 weeks of pregnancy (called full term).

Section 32.4

Episiotomy

Text in this section is from "Episiotomy," © 2017 American Pregnancy Association. Reprinted with permission.

An **episiotomy** is a surgical incision used to enlarge the vaginal opening to help deliver a baby.

What Are Some Circumstances That Would Require an Episiotomy?

An episiotomy may be needed for any of the following reasons:

- Birth is imminent and the perineum hasn't had time to stretch slowly
- The baby's head is too large for the vaginal opening
- The baby is in distress
- The mother needs a forcep or vacuum assisted delivery
- The baby is in a breech presentation and there is a complication during delivery
- The mother isn't able to control her pushing

How Is an Episiotomy Performed?

If you have already had an epidural, you will probably not need any further anesthetic. If otherwise, it will be necessary to utilize a local anesthetic called a pudendal block in your perineum. The *mediolateral* cut is angled down, away from the vagina and the perineum, into the muscle.

The *midline* cut is performed by cutting straight down into the perineum, between the vagina and anus.

How Can I Prevent the Need to Have an Episiotomy?

The following measures can reduce the need for an episiotomy:

- Good nutrition—healthy skin stretches more easily!

- Kegels (exercise for your pelvic floor muscles)
- A slowed second stage of labor where pushing is controlled
- Warm compresses and support during delivery
- Use of perineum massage techniques
- Avoiding lying on your back while pushing

Can Episiotomies Be Harmful?

Episiotomies have the following potential side effects:

- Infection
- Bruising
- Swelling
- Bleeding
- Extended healing time
- Painful scarring that might require a period of abstinence from sexual intercourse
- Future problems with incontinence

What Are Some Pain Relief Options for Episiotomies and Tears?

If you end up having an episiotomy, or any tearing of the vaginal opening, you can try some of the following solutions to help ease the pain.

- Cold packs on the perineum. Ask your healthcare provider about special maxi pads that have built in cold packs.
- Take a sitz bath—a portable bath that you place over a toilet that allows warm water to cover the wound.
- Use medication such as Tucks Medicated Pads.
- Use a personal lubricant such as KY Jelly when you resume sexual intercourse.
- After using the bathroom, wash yourself with a squirt bottle instead of wiping. Patting dry instead of wiping can also help.

What If I Want to Avoid Having an Episiotomy?

Clearly state in your birth plan that you do not want an episiotomy unless absolutely necessary. Also, discuss the issue with your health-care provider during routine prenatal care.

Section 32.5

Female Sterilization

This section includes text excerpted from "Female Sterilization," U.S. Department of Health and Human Services (HHS), August 16, 2016.

What Is Female Sterilization?

Female sterilization permanently prevents women from becoming pregnant. There are two different procedures to achieve this goal, tubal ligation and tubal implants. They both work by blocking the fallopian tubes (tubes that lead from a woman's ovaries into the uterus or womb) so that sperm cannot meet with and fertilize an egg.

Because these methods cannot be undone, they are only recommended for women who are sure they never want to have a baby or who do not want to have more children

Tubal ligation. The fallopian tubes are cut, sealed, or tied. With this method, very tiny cuts (called incisions) are made in the abdomen or belly. This is also known as having "tubes tied" or tubal ligation. Surgical sterilization works to prevent pregnancy right away.

Tubal implant. A very small spring-like coil is placed into each fallopian tube. The coils cause scar tissue to form in the tubes, thereby blocking the tubes. This method does not involve cuts or incisions. Instead, a healthcare provider uses a thin tube to thread the small coils through the vagina and uterus into the fallopian tubes, where the coils will stay.

With the tubal implant, it will take up to three months for the scar tissue to fully block the tubes. So, it is important to use a back-up type of birth control (like a condom or the birth control shot) until your healthcare provider says it is not needed. You will go back to the health center or office for an exam and be checked to make sure the coils are in the right place and the tubes are blocked. This may require a special type X-ray where dye is placed into the uterus to make sure the tubes are blocked.

How Do I Get It?

Female sterilization is a relatively simple outpatient surgery done in a health center, doctor's office, or hospital. It can be performed under local or general anesthesia, depending on the method used to perform sterilization. You will go home the same day.

Advantages of Female Sterilization

- Safe and highly effective approach to preventing pregnancy.
- Lasts a lifetime, so no need to worry about birth control again.
- Quick recovery.
- No significant long-term side effects.
- Your male partner doesn't have to know about it or do anything different.

Drawbacks of Female Sterilization

- Does not protect against sexually transmitted infections (STIs), including human immunodeficiency virus (HIV)
- Some risk of infection, pain, or bleeding
- Very rarely, the tubes can grow back together. When this happens there is a risk for pregnancy. In some cases, this leads to tubal or ectopic pregnancy—when the pregnancy happens in the fallopian tubes, which is a life-threatening condition.
- Some women later change their mind and wish they could have a child or additional children.

Quick Facts on Female Sterilization

Effectiveness in preventing pregnancy

- Out of 100 women who have a sterilization procedure each year, less than one may become pregnant.

Sexually transmitted infection (STI) protection

- No

Office visit required

- Yes, done by a healthcare provider as an outpatient procedure (you go home the same day)

Section 32.6

Uterine Fibroid Surgery

This section includes text excerpted from "Uterine Fibroids," Office on Women's Health (OWH), U.S. Department of Health and Human Services (HHS), January 15, 2015.

What Are Fibroids?

Fibroids are muscular tumors that grow in the wall of the uterus (womb). Fibroids are almost always benign (not cancerous). Not all women with fibroids have symptoms. Women who do have symptoms

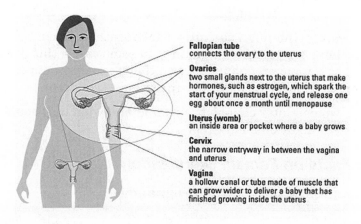

Fallopian tube
connects the ovary to the uterus

Ovaries
two small glands next to the uterus that make hormones, such as estrogen, which spark the start of your menstrual cycle, and release one egg about once a month until menopause

Uterus (womb)
an inside area or pocket where a baby grows

Cervix
the narrow entryway in between the vagina and uterus

Vagina
a hollow canal or tube made of muscle that can grow wider to deliver a baby that has finished growing inside the uterus

Figure 32.1. *Uterine Fibroids*

often find fibroids hard to live with. Some have pain and heavy menstrual bleeding. Treatment for uterine fibroids depends on your symptoms.

Another medical term for fibroids is leiomyoma or just "myoma." Fibroids are almost always benign (not cancerous). Fibroids can grow as a single tumor, or there can be many of them in the uterus. They can be as small as an apple seed or as big as a grapefruit. In unusual cases they can become very large.

Why Should Women Know about Fibroids?

About 20 percent to 80 percent of women develop fibroids by the time they reach age 50. Fibroids are most common in women in their 40s and early 50s. Not all women with fibroids have symptoms. Women who do have symptoms often find fibroids hard to live with. Some have pain and heavy menstrual bleeding. Fibroids also can put pressure on the bladder, causing frequent urination, or the rectum, causing rectal pressure. Should the fibroids get very large, they can cause the abdomen (stomach area) to enlarge, making a woman look pregnant.

Who Gets Fibroids?

There are factors that can increase a woman's risk of developing fibroids.

- **Age.** Fibroids become more common as women age, especially during the 30s and 40s through menopause. After menopause, fibroids usually shrink.

- **Family history.** Having a family member with fibroids increases your risk. If a woman's mother had fibroids, her risk of having them is about three times higher than average.

- **Ethnic origin.** African-American women are more likely to develop fibroids than white women.

- **Obesity.** Women who are overweight are at higher risk for fibroids. For very heavy women, the risk is two to three times greater than average.

- **Eating habits.** Eating a lot of red meat (e.g., beef) and ham is linked with a higher risk of fibroids. Eating plenty of green vegetables seems to protect women from developing fibroids.

Where Can Fibroids Grow?

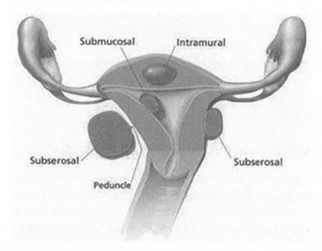

Figure 32.2. *Fibroids, Based on Where They Grow*

Most fibroids grow in the wall of the uterus. Doctors put them into three groups based on where they grow:

- **Submucosal** fibroids grow into the uterine cavity.

- **Intramural** fibroids grow within the wall of the uterus.

- **Subserosal** fibroids grow on the outside of the uterus.

Some fibroids grow on stalks that grow out from the surface of the uterus or into the cavity of the uterus. They might look like mushrooms. These are called pedunculated fibroids.

What Are Symptoms of Fibroids?

Most fibroids do not cause any symptoms, but some women with fibroids can have:

- heavy bleeding (which can be heavy enough to cause anemia) or painful periods

- feeling of fullness in the pelvic area (lower stomach area)

- enlargement of the lower abdomen

- frequent urination

- pain during sex

- lower back pain
- complications during pregnancy and labor, including a six-time greater risk of cesarean section
- reproductive problems, such as infertility, which is very rare

What Causes Fibroids?

No one knows for sure what causes fibroids. Researchers think that more than one factor could play a role. These factors could be:

- hormonal (affected by estrogen and progesterone levels)
- genetic (runs in families)

They grow rapidly during pregnancy, when hormone levels are high. They shrink when anti-hormone medication is used. They also stop growing or shrink once a woman reaches menopause.

Can Fibroids Turn into Cancer?

Fibroids are almost always benign (not cancerous). Rarely (less than one in 1,000) a cancerous fibroid will occur. This is called leiomyosarcoma. Doctors think that these cancers do not arise from an already-existing fibroid. Having fibroids does not increase the risk of developing a cancerous fibroid. Having fibroids also does not increase a woman's chances of getting other forms of cancer in the uterus.

What If I Become Pregnant and Have Fibroids?

Women who have fibroids are more likely to have problems during pregnancy and delivery. This doesn't mean there will be problems. Most women with fibroids have normal pregnancies. The most common problems seen in women with fibroids are:

- **Cesarean section.** The risk of needing a c-section is six times greater for women with fibroids.
- **Baby is breech.** The baby is not positioned well for vaginal delivery.
- **Labor fails to progress.**
- **Placental abruption**. The placenta breaks away from the wall of the uterus before delivery. When this happens, the fetus does not get enough oxygen.

- **Preterm delivery.**

Talk to your obstetrician if you have fibroids and become pregnant. All obstetricians have experience dealing with fibroids and pregnancy. Most women who have fibroids and become pregnant do not need to see an OB who deals with high-risk pregnancies.

How Do I Know for Sure That I Have Fibroids?

Your doctor may find that you have fibroids when you see her or him for a regular pelvic exam to check your uterus, ovaries, and vagina. The doctor can feel the fibroid with her or his fingers during an ordinary pelvic exam, as a (usually painless) lump or mass on the uterus. Often, a doctor will describe how small or how large the fibroids are by comparing their size to the size your uterus would be if you were pregnant. For example, you may be told that your fibroids have made your uterus the size it would be if you were 16 weeks pregnant. Or the fibroid might be compared to fruits, nuts, or a ball, such as a grape or an orange, an acorn or a walnut, or a golf ball or a volleyball.

Your doctor can do imaging tests to confirm that you have fibroids. These are tests that create a "picture" of the inside of your body without surgery. These tests might include:

- **Ultrasound**: Uses sound waves to produce the picture. The ultrasound probe can be placed on the abdomen or it can be placed inside the vagina to make the picture.

- **Magnetic resonance imaging (MRI)**: Uses magnets and radio waves to produce the picture

- **X-rays**: Uses a form of radiation to see into the body and produce the picture

- **CAT scan (CT)**: Takes many X-ray pictures of the body from different angles for a more complete image

- **Hysterosalpingogram (HSG) or sonohysterogram**: An HSG involves injecting X-ray dye into the uterus and taking X-ray pictures. A sonohysterogram involves injecting water into the uterus and making ultrasound pictures.

You might also need surgery to know for sure if you have fibroids. There are two types of surgery to do this:

- **Laparoscopy.** The doctor inserts a long, thin scope into a tiny incision made in or near the navel. The scope has a bright light and a camera. This allows the doctor to view the uterus and other organs on a monitor during the procedure. Pictures also can be made.

- **Hysteroscopy.** The doctor passes a long, thin scope with a light through the vagina and cervix into the uterus. No incision is needed. The doctor can look inside the uterus for fibroids and other problems, such as polyps. A camera also can be used with the scope.

What Questions Should I Ask My Doctor If I Have Fibroids?

- How many fibroids do I have?
- What size is my fibroid(s)?
- Where is my fibroid(s) located (outer surface, inner surface, or in the wall of the uterus)?
- Can I expect the fibroid(s) to grow larger?
- How rapidly have they grown (if they were known about already)?
- How will I know if the fibroid(s) is growing larger?
- What problems can the fibroid(s) cause?
- What tests or imaging studies are best for keeping track of the growth of my fibroids?
- What are my treatment options if my fibroid(s) becomes a problem?
- What are your views on treating fibroids with a hysterectomy versus other types of treatments?

A second opinion is always a good idea if your doctor has not answered your questions completely or does not seem to be meeting your needs.

How Are Fibroids Treated?

Most women with fibroids do not have any symptoms. For women who do have symptoms, there are treatments that can help. Talk with your doctor about the best way to treat your fibroids. She or he will consider many things before helping you choose a treatment. Some of these things include:

- whether or not you are having symptoms from the fibroids

- if you might want to become pregnant in the future

- the size of the fibroids

- the location of the fibroids

- your age and how close to menopause you might be

If you have fibroids but do not have any symptoms, you may not need treatment. Your doctor will check during your regular exams to see if they have grown.

Medications

If you have fibroids and have mild symptoms, your doctor may suggest taking medication. Over-the-counter drugs such as ibuprofen or acetaminophen can be used for mild pain. If you have heavy bleeding during your period, taking an iron supplement can keep you from getting anemia or correct it if you already are anemic.

Several drugs commonly used for birth control can be prescribed to help control symptoms of fibroids. Low-dose birth control pills do not make fibroids grow and can help control heavy bleeding. The same is true of progesterone-like injections (e.g., Depo-Provera®). An IUD (intrauterine device) called Mirena® contains a small amount of progesterone-like medication, which can be used to control heavy bleeding as well as for birth control.

Other drugs used to treat fibroids are "gonadotropin releasing hormone agonists" (GnRHa). The one most commonly used is Lupron®. These drugs, given by injection, nasal spray, or implanted, can shrink your fibroids. Sometimes they are used before surgery to make fibroids easier to remove. Side effects of GnRHas can include hot flashes, depression, not being able to sleep, decreased sex drive, and joint pain. Most women tolerate GnRHas quite well. Most women do not get a period when taking GnRHas. This can be a big relief to women who have heavy bleeding. It also allows women with anemia to recover to a normal blood count. GnRHas can cause bone thinning, so their use is generally limited to six months or less. These drugs also are very expensive, and some insurance companies will cover only some or none of the cost. GnRHas offer temporary relief from the symptoms of fibroids; once you stop taking the drugs, the fibroids often grow back quickly.

Surgery

If you have fibroids with moderate or severe symptoms, surgery may be the best way to treat them. Here are the options:

- **Myomectomy**: Surgery to remove fibroids without taking out the healthy tissue of the uterus. It is best for women who wish to have children after treatment for their fibroids or who wish to keep their uterus for other reasons. You can become pregnant after myomectomy. But if your fibroids were imbedded deeply in the uterus, you might need a cesarean section to deliver. Myomectomy can be performed in many ways. It can be major surgery (involving cutting into the abdomen) or performed with laparoscopy or hysteroscopy. The type of surgery that can be done depends on the type, size, and location of the fibroids. After myomectomy new fibroids can grow and cause trouble later. All of the possible risks of surgery are true for myomectomy. The risks depend on how extensive the surgery is.

- **Hysterectomy**: Surgery to remove the uterus. This surgery is the only sure way to cure uterine fibroids. Fibroids are the most common reason that hysterectomy is performed. This surgery is used when a woman's fibroids are large, if she has heavy bleeding, is either near or past menopause, or does not want children. If the fibroids are large, a woman may need a hysterectomy that involves cutting into the abdomen to remove the uterus. If the fibroids are smaller, the doctor may be able to reach the uterus through the vagina, instead of making a cut in the abdomen. In some cases hysterectomy can be performed through the laparoscope. Removal of the ovaries and the cervix at the time of hysterectomy is usually optional. Women whose ovaries are not removed do not go into menopause at the time of hysterectomy. Hysterectomy is a major surgery. Although hysterectomy is usually quite safe, it does carry a significant risk of complications. Recovery from hysterectomy usually takes several weeks.

- **Endometrial ablation**: The lining of the uterus is removed or destroyed to control very heavy bleeding. This can be done with laser, wire loops, boiling water, electric current, microwaves, freezing, and other methods. This procedure usually is considered minor surgery. It can be done on an outpatient basis or even in a doctor's office. Complications can occur, but are uncommon with most of the methods. Most people recover quickly.

About half of women who have this procedure have no more menstrual bleeding. About three in 10 women have much lighter bleeding. But, a woman cannot have children after this surgery.

- **Myolysis**: A needle is inserted into the fibroids, usually guided by laparoscopy, and electric current or freezing is used to destroy the fibroids.

- **Uterine Fibroid Embolization (UFE), or Uterine Artery Embolization (UAE)**: A thin tube is thread into the blood vessels that supply blood to the fibroid. Then, tiny plastic or gel particles are injected into the blood vessels. This blocks the blood supply to the fibroid, causing it to shrink. UFE can be an outpatient or inpatient procedure. Complications, including early menopause, are uncommon but can occur. Studies suggest fibroids are not likely to grow back after UFE, but more long-term research is needed. Not all fibroids can be treated with UFE. The best candidates for UFE are women who:

  - have fibroids that are causing heavy bleeding

  - have fibroids that are causing pain or pressing on the bladder or rectum

  - don't want to have a hysterectomy

  - don't want to have children in the future

What New Treatments Are Available for Uterine Fibroids?

The following methods are not yet standard treatments, so your doctor may not offer them or health insurance may not cover them.

- **Radiofrequency ablation** uses heat to destroy fibroid tissue without harming surrounding normal uterine tissue. The fibroids remain inside the uterus but shrink in size. Most women go home the same day and can return to normal activities within a few days.

- **Anti-hormonal drugs** may provide symptom relief without bone-thinning side effects.

Chapter 33

Kidney Transplant

What Is a Kidney Transplant and How Does It Work?

A kidney transplant is surgery to place a healthy kidney from a donor into your body. A donor is a person who has just died or a living person, most often a family member. A kidney from someone who has just died is a deceased donor kidney. A kidney from a living person is a living donor kidney. If you do not have a living donor who can give you a kidney, your transplant team will place you on a national waiting list for a kidney from a deceased donor. The United Network for Organ Sharing (UNOS) maintains the waiting list. The transplanted kidney takes over the job of filtering your blood. Your body normally attacks anything it sees as foreign, so you need to take medicines called immunosuppressants to keep your body from attacking the new kidney.

Surgeons place most transplanted kidneys in the lower abdomen, near the groin. The surgeon connects the artery and vein from the donor kidney to an artery and a vein in your body so your blood flows through your new kidney. The surgeon attaches the ureter from the donor kidney to your bladder, letting urine flow from the new kidney to your bladder. The new kidney may start working right away or may take up to a few weeks to make urine. If the new kidney does not start working right away, you will need dialysis treatments to filter wastes and extra salt and fluid from your body until it does start working.

This chapter includes text excerpted from "Kidney Transplant," National Institute of Diabetes and Digestive and Kidney Diseases (NIDDK), May 2016.

Unless your damaged kidneys cause infections or high blood pressure or are cancerous, they can remain in your body.

Chronic Kidney Disease and Kidney Failure

Every day, your kidneys filter about 120 to 150 quarts of blood to produce about 1 to 2 quarts of urine, composed of wastes and extra fluid. Chronic kidney disease (CKD) means your kidneys are not filtering as well as they should. CKD usually does not get better and may lead to kidney failure over time. When your kidneys fail, harmful wastes and extra salt and fluid buildup in your body. You then need treatment to replace the work your damaged kidneys have stopped doing. Treatment options include:

- hemodialysis

- peritoneal dialysis

- a kidney transplant

These treatments can help you stay well. Some people live with kidney disease for years without needing to go on dialysis or get a transplant. Others progress quickly to kidney failure. Left untreated, kidney failure will lead to coma, seizures, and death.

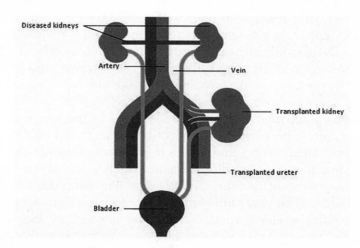

Figure 33.1. *Kidney Transplantation*

Surgeons place most transplanted kidneys in the lower abdomen, near the groin. Unless your damaged kidneys cause infections or high blood pressure or are cancerous, they can remain in the body.

What Are the Steps in the Transplant Process?

The transplant process has many steps.

Talking with Your Healthcare Provider

The first step is to talk with your healthcare provider about whether you are a candidate for a transplant. Transplantation is not for everyone. Your healthcare provider may tell you that you are not healthy enough for surgery or that you have a condition that would make transplantation unlikely to succeed. If you are a good candidate for a transplant, your healthcare provider will refer you to a transplant center.

Medical, Psychological, and Social Evaluation at a Transplant Center

The next step is a thorough physical, psychological, and social evaluation at the transplant center, where you will meet members of your transplant team. Your pretransplant evaluation may require several visits to the transplant center over the course of weeks or even months.

You will need to have blood tests as well as other tests to check your heart and other organs. Your blood type and other matching factors help determine whether your body will accept an available donor kidney.

Your transplant team will make sure you are healthy enough for surgery. Some medical conditions or illnesses could make transplantation less likely to succeed.

In addition, your team will make sure you can understand and follow the schedule for taking the medicines needed after surgery. Team members need to be sure that you are mentally prepared for the responsibilities of caring for a transplanted kidney.

If a family member or friend wants to donate a kidney, that person will need a health exam to test whether the kidney is a good match.

Who Is on My Transplant Team?

Your transplant team has many members, including your:

- **Surgeon**: The doctor who places the kidney in your body.

- **Nephrologist**: A doctor who specializes in kidney health. The nephrologist may work in partnership with a nurse practitioner or a physician's assistant.

- **Transplant coordinator**: A specially trained nurse who will be your point of contact, arrange your appointments, and educate you before and after the transplant.

- **Social worker**: A person who is trained to help people solve problems in their daily lives, such as finding employment, affordable housing, or daycare.

- **Dietitian**: A person who is an expert in food and nutrition. Dietitians teach people about the foods they should eat and how to plan healthy meals.

Placement on the Waiting List

If your medical evaluation shows you are a good candidate for a transplant, your transplant center will submit your name to be placed on the national waiting list for a kidney from a deceased donor. The Organ Procurement and Transplantation Network (OPTN) has a computer network that links all regional organ-gathering organizations — known as organ procurement organizations — and transplant centers. The United Network for Organ Sharing (UNOS), a private, nonprofit organization, runs the OPTN under a contract with the Federal Government. When UNOS officially adds you to the waiting list, UNOS will notify you and your transplant team.

UNOS allows you to register with multiple transplant centers to increase your chances of receiving a kidney. Each transplant center usually requires a separate medical evaluation.

Waiting Period

UNOS gives preference to people who have been on the waiting list the longest. However, other factors — such as your age, where you live, and your blood type — may make your wait longer or shorter. Wait times can range from a few months to several years.

If you have a living donor, you do not need to be placed on the waiting list and can schedule the surgery when it is convenient for you and your donor.

While you are on the waiting list, notify the transplant center of changes in your health. Also, let the transplant center know if you move or change phone numbers. The center will need to find you immediately when a kidney becomes available.

While you wait for a kidney, you will have blood drawn once a month. The sample will be sent to the transplant center. The center must have a recent sample of your blood for comparison with any kidney that becomes available.

Organ procurement organizations identify potential organs for transplant and coordinate with the national network. When a deceased donor kidney becomes available, the organ procurement organization notifies UNOS and creates a computer-generated list of suitable recipients.

Whether you are receiving your kidney from a deceased donor or a living donor, the transplant team considers three factors in matching kidneys with potential recipients. These matching factors help predict whether your body's immune system—which protects your body from infection by identifying and destroying bacteria, viruses, and other potentially harmful foreign substances—will accept or reject the new kidney.

- **Blood type.** Your blood type A, B, AB, or O must be compatible with the donor's. Blood type is the most important matching factor. Some transplant centers have developed techniques for transplanting kidneys that are not matched by blood type.

- **Human leukocyte antigens.** These six antigens are proteins that help your immune system tell the difference between your own body's tissues and foreign substances. You may still receive a kidney if the antigens do not completely match, as long as your blood type is compatible with the organ donor's blood type and other tests show no problems with matching.

- **Cross-matching antigens.** The cross-match is the last test performed before a kidney transplant can take place. A lab technician mixes a small sample of your blood with a sample of the organ donor's blood in a tube to see if the mixture causes a reaction. If no reaction occurs—called a negative cross-match—the transplant can proceed.

Transplant Surgery

If you are on a waiting list for a deceased donor kidney, you must go to the hospital as soon as you receive notification that a kidney is available. If a family member or friend is donating the kidney you will receive, you will schedule the operation in advance. Your transplant team will operate on you and your donor at the same time, usually in side-by-side rooms. One surgeon will perform the nephrectomy— the removal of the kidney from the donor—while another prepares you for placement of the donated kidney. In some centers, the same surgeon performs both operations. You will receive general anesthesia to make you sleep during the operation. The surgery usually takes 3 or 4 hours.

Recovery from Surgery

After surgery, you will probably feel sore and groggy when you wake up. However, many people who have a transplant report feeling much better immediately after surgery. Even if you wake up feeling great, you will typically need to stay in the hospital for several days to recover from surgery, and longer if you have any complications. You will have regular follow-up visits after leaving the hospital.

If you have a living donor, the donor will probably also stay in the hospital for several days. However, a new technique for removing a kidney for donation uses a smaller incision and may make it possible for the donor to leave the hospital in 2 to 3 days.

What Do I Need to Know about Care after My Transplant?

Often, rejection begins before any signs appear. The signs of rejection include indications that your kidney is not working as well as it should—for example, high blood pressure or swelling because your kidney is not getting rid of extra salt and fluid in your body. Advances in immunosuppressants have made other signs of rejection—such as fever, soreness in the lower abdomen where the new kidney is, and a decrease in the amount of urine you make—rare. If you have any of these symptoms, tell your transplant team. You will receive stronger doses of your immunosuppressants and additional medicines to help keep your body from rejecting your new kidney.

Even if you do everything you should, your body may still reject the new kidney, and you may need to go on dialysis. Unless your transplant team determines that you are no longer a good candidate for transplantation, you can go back on the waiting list for another kidney.

What Are Signs That My Body Is Rejecting My New Kidney?

Blood tests help you know your new kidney is working. Before you leave the hospital, you will schedule an appointment with your transplant team at the transplant center. At that appointment, a healthcare provider will draw blood to be tested. The tests show how well your kidneys are removing wastes from your blood. At first, you may return to the transplant center every 2 weeks, then every month. Eventually, you will need to return to the transplant center only once every 6 months or once every year, after your transplant team has determined that your kidney is doing its job.

Your blood tests may show that your kidney is not removing wastes from your blood as well as it should. You may have other signs that your body is rejecting your new kidney. If these problems occur, your transplant surgeon or nephrologist may order a kidney biopsy. Biopsy is a procedure that involves taking a small piece of tissue for examination under a microscope. Your transplant surgeon or nephrologist performs the biopsy in the transplant center or a hospital. The healthcare provider will give you light sedation and local anesthetic; however, in some cases, a patient may require general anesthesia. A pathologist—a doctor who specializes in diagnosing diseases—examines the tissue in a lab. The test can show whether your body is rejecting your new kidney.

How Do I Know My New Kidney Is Working Properly?

Blood tests help you know your new kidney is working. Before you leave the hospital, you will schedule an appointment with your transplant team at the transplant center. At that appointment, a healthcare provider will draw blood to be tested. The tests show how well your kidneys are removing wastes from your blood. At first, you may return to the transplant center every 2 weeks, then every month. Eventually, you will need to return to the transplant center only once every 6 months or once every year, after your transplant team has determined that your kidney is doing its job.

Your blood tests may show that your kidney is not removing wastes from your blood as well as it should. You may have other signs that your body is rejecting your new kidney. If these problems occur, your transplant surgeon or nephrologist may order a kidney biopsy. Biopsy is a procedure that involves taking a small piece of tissue for examination under a microscope. Your transplant surgeon or nephrologist performs the biopsy in the transplant center or a hospital. The healthcare provider will give you light sedation and local anesthetic; however, in some cases, a patient may require general anesthesia. A pathologist—a doctor who specializes in diagnosing diseases—examines the tissue in a lab. The test can show whether your body is rejecting your new kidney.

What Are the Side Effects of Immunosuppressants?

Some immunosuppressants may change your appearance. Your face may get fuller; you may gain weight or develop acne or facial hair. Not all people have these problems, and those who do can use diet, makeup, and hair removal to minimize changes in appearance.

Immunosuppressants weaken your immune system, which can lead to infections. In some people over long periods of time, a weakened immune system can increase their risk of developing cancer. Some immunosuppressants cause cataracts, diabetes, extra stomach acid, high blood pressure, and bone disease. When used over time, these medicines may also cause liver or kidney damage in some people. Your transplant team will order regular tests to monitor the levels of immunosuppressants in your blood and to measure your liver and kidney function.

What Financial Help Is Available to Pay for a Kidney Transplant?

United States citizens who have kidney failure are eligible to receive Medicare, the Federal Government insurance program. Treatment for kidney failure costs a lot; however, Medicare pays much of the cost, usually up to 80 percent. Often, private insurance pays the rest. For people who are not eligible for Medicare or who still need help with the portion Medicare does not cover, states have Medicaid programs that provide funds for healthcare based on financial need. Your social worker can help you locate resources for financial help.

What Help Is Available to Pay for Kidney Transplant Medicines?

Through patient-assistance programs, prescription drug companies give discounts to people who can show they cannot afford the cost of their prescribed medicines. Social workers can help patients complete applications to these programs.

The Partnership for Prescription Assistance has a website that directs patients, caregivers, and doctors to more than 275 public and private patient-assistance programs, including more than 150 programs offered by pharmaceutical companies.

Medicare has also compiled information to help beneficiaries pay pharmaceutical expenses.

NeedyMeds is a nonprofit organization that helps people find appropriate patient-assistance programs. The NeedyMeds website (www.needymeds.org) provides a directory of patient-assistance programs that can be searched by a medicine's brand or generic name or by a program or company name. Applications for these programs are usually available online.

Eating, Diet, and Nutrition

The diet for transplant patients has more choices than the diet for dialysis patients, although you may still have to cut back on some foods. Your diet will probably change as your medicines, test results, weight, and blood pressure change.

- **You may need to count calories.** Your medicines may give you a bigger appetite and cause you to gain weight.

- **You may have to eat less sodium.** Your medicines may cause your body to retain sodium, leading to high blood pressure.

Chapter 34

Urological Surgery

Chapter Contents

Section 34.1

Circumcision

This section contains text excerpted from the following sources: Text
beginning with the heading "What Is Circumcision?" is excerpted
from "Circumcision," Office on Women's Health (OWH), U.S.
Department of Health and Human Services (HHS), February 1, 2017;
Text under the heading "Trends in Male Newborn Circumcisions
in U.S. Hospitals" is excerpted from "Circumcisions Performed
in U.S. Community Hospitals," Agency for Healthcare Research
and Quality (AHRQ), U.S. Department of Health and Human
Services (HHS), February 2012. Reviewed June 2017.

What Is Circumcision?

If you have a baby boy, you likely will be asked whether you want
him to be circumcised. Circumcision is the removal of the foreskin,
which is the skin that covers the tip of the penis. It's a good idea to
think about this before going into labor because it is often offered
before a new baby leaves the hospital.

The American Academy of Pediatrics (AAP) does not recommend
routine circumcision because the medical benefits do not outweigh the
risks. But parents also need to consider their religious, cultural, and
personal preferences when making the choice to circumcise their son.

What Are the Benefits of Circumcision?

There are medical benefits and risks to circumcision. Possible benefits include:

- A lower risk of urinary tract infections (UTIs). Keep in mind
  that UTIs affect only 1 percent or less of men who are not
  circumcised.

- A lower risk of penile cancer. Keep in mind that penile cancer is
  very rare in both men who are or are not circumcised.

- A possible lower risk of sexually transmitted infections (STIs).
  Keep in mind that practicing safe sex, including using a condom,
  is the best protection against STIs.

What Are the Risks of Circumcision?

The risks of circumcision include:

- Pain. If you decide to have your baby circumcised, you can ask that a numbing medicine be put on your baby's penis to lessen the pain.

- A low risk of bleeding or infection.

These risks are higher when circumcision is performed on older babies, boys, and men. Talk to your doctor if you have concerns about the risks or possible benefits.

Trends in Male Newborn Circumcisions in U.S. Hospitals

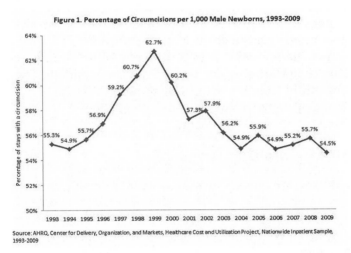

Figure 1. Percentage of Circumcisions per 1,000 Male Newborns, 1993-2009

Source: AHRQ, Center for Delivery, Organization, and Markets, Healthcare Cost and Utilization Project, Nationwide Inpatient Sample, 1993-2009

Figure 34.1. *Percentage of Circumcisions per 1,000 Male Newborns, 1993-2009.*

Between 1993 and 1999, the rate of male newborn circumcisions performed in the hospital increased by 13 percent, from 55.3 to 62.7 percent of male newborn hospital stays. However, between 1999 and 2004, the rate of male newborn circumcisions decreased by 12 percent, from 62.7 to 54.9 percent of male newborn hospital stays. This coincides with the American Academy of Pediatrics (AAP) policy statement on circumcision published in 1999. From 2004 to 2009, the rate of male newborn circumcisions remained relatively stable in the range of 55 to 56 percent of male newborns in the hospital.

515

Section 34.2

Prostate Cancer Surgery

This section includes text excerpted from "Prostate
Cancer Treatment (PDQ®)—Patient Version," National
Cancer Institute (NCI), July 7, 2016.

Prostate Cancer

Prostate cancer is a disease in which malignant (cancer) cells form in the tissues of the prostate. The prostate is a gland in the male reproductive system. It lies just below the bladder (the organ that collects and empties urine) and in front of the rectum (the lower part of the intestine). It is about the size of a walnut and surrounds part of the urethra (the tube that empties urine from the bladder). The prostate gland makes fluid that is part of the semen. Prostate cancer is most common in older men. In the United States, about 1 out of 5 men will be diagnosed with prostate cancer.

Signs of Prostate Cancer

Signs of prostate cancer include a weak flow of urine or frequent urination.

These and other signs and symptoms may be caused by prostate cancer or by other conditions. Check with your doctor if you have any of the following:

- Weak or interrupted ("stop-and-go") flow of urine.

- Sudden urge to urinate.

- Frequent urination (especially at night).

- Trouble starting the flow of urine.

- Trouble emptying the bladder completely.

- Pain or burning while urinating.

- Blood in the urine or semen.

- A pain in the back, hips, or pelvis that doesn't go away.

- Shortness of breath, feeling very tired, fast heartbeat, dizziness, or pale skin caused by anemia.

Other conditions may cause the same symptoms. As men age, the prostate may get bigger and block the urethra or bladder. This may cause trouble urinating or sexual problems. The condition is called benign prostatic hyperplasia (BPH), and although it is not cancer, surgery may be needed. The symptoms of benign prostatic hyperplasia or of other problems in the prostate may be like symptoms of prostate cancer.

Diagnose Prostate Cancer

The following tests and procedures may be used:

- Physical exam and history
- Digital rectal exam (DRE)
- Prostate-specific antigen (PSA) test
- Transrectal ultrasound
- Transrectal magnetic resonance imaging (MRI)
- Biopsy

Stages of Prostate Cancer

After prostate cancer has been diagnosed, tests are done to find out if cancer cells have spread within the prostate or to other parts of the body.

The process used to find out if cancer has spread within the prostate or to other parts of the body is called staging. The information gathered from the staging process determines the stage of the disease. It is important to know the stage in order to plan treatment. The results of the tests used to diagnose prostate cancer are often also used to stage the disease. (See the General Information section.) In prostate cancer, staging tests may not be done unless the patient has symptoms or signs that the cancer has spread, such as bone pain, a high PSA level, or a high Gleason score.

The following tests and procedures also may be used in the staging process:

- Bone scan
- Magnetic resonance imaging (MRI)

517

- CAT scan
- Pelvic lymphadenectomy
- Seminal vesicle biopsy
- ProstaScint scan

The stage of the cancer is based on the results of the staging and diagnostic tests, including the prostate-specific antigen (PSA) test and the Gleason score. The tissue samples removed during the biopsy are used to find out the Gleason score. The Gleason score ranges from 2–10 and describes how different the cancer cells look from normal cells and how likely it is that the tumor will spread. The lower the number, the less likely the tumor is to spread.

The following are prostate cancer stages:

Stage I

In stage I, cancer is found in the prostate only. The cancer:

- is found by needle biopsy (done for a high PSA level) or in a small amount of tissue during surgery for other reasons (such as benign prostatic hyperplasia). The PSA level is lower than 10 and the Gleason score is 6 or lower; or

- is found in one-half or less of one lobe of the prostate. The PSA level is lower than 10 and the Gleason score is 6 or lower; or

- cannot be felt during a digital rectal exam and cannot be seen in imaging tests. Cancer is found in one-half or less of one lobe of the prostate. The PSA level and the Gleason score are not known.

Stage II

In stage II, cancer is more advanced than in stage I, but has not spread outside the prostate. Stage II is divided into stages IIA and IIB.

In stage IIA, cancer:

- is found by needle biopsy (done for a high PSA level) or in a small amount of tissue during surgery for other reasons (such as benign prostatic hyperplasia). The PSA level is lower than 20 and the Gleason score is 7; or

- is found by needle biopsy (done for a high PSA level) or in a small amount of tissue during surgery for other reasons (such as benign prostatic hyperplasia). The PSA level is at least 10 but lower than 20 and the Gleason score is 6 or lower; or

- is found in one-half or less of one lobe of the prostate. The PSA level is at least 10 but lower than 20 and the Gleason score is 6 or lower; or

- is found in one-half or less of one lobe of the prostate. The PSA level is lower than 20 and the Gleason score is 7; or

- is found in more than one-half of one lobe of the prostate.

In stage IIB, cancer:

- is found in opposite sides of the prostate. The PSA can be any level and the Gleason score can range from 2 to 10; or

- cannot be felt during a digital rectal exam and cannot be seen in imaging tests. The PSA level is 20 or higher and the Gleason score can range from 2 to 10; or

- cannot be felt during a digital rectal exam and cannot be seen in imaging tests. The PSA can be any level and the Gleason score is 8 or higher.

Stage III

In stage III, cancer has spread beyond the outer layer of the prostate and may have spread to the seminal vesicles. The PSA can be any level and the Gleason score can range from 2 to 10.

Stage IV

In stage IV, the PSA can be any level and the Gleason score can range from 2 to 10. Also, cancer:

- has spread beyond the seminal vesicles to nearby tissue or organs, such as the rectum, bladder, or pelvic wall; or

- may have spread to the seminal vesicles or to nearby tissue or organs, such as the rectum, bladder, or pelvic wall. Cancer has spread to nearby lymph nodes; or

- has spread to distant parts of the body, which may include lymph nodes or bones. Prostate cancer often spreads to the bones.

Treatment for Patients with Prostate Cancer

Different types of treatment are available for patients with prostate cancer. Some treatments are standard (the currently used treatment), and some are being tested in clinical trials. A treatment clinical trial is a research study meant to help improve current treatments or obtain information on new treatments for patients with cancer. When clinical trials show that a new treatment is better than the standard treatment, the new treatment may become the standard treatment. Patients may want to think about taking part in a clinical trial. Some clinical trials are open only to patients who have not started treatment.

Surgery

Patients in good health whose tumor is in the prostate gland only may be treated with surgery to remove the tumor. The following types of surgery are used:

- **Radical prostatectomy:** A surgical procedure to remove the prostate, surrounding tissue, and seminal vesicles. There are two types of radical prostatectomy:

  - **Retropubic prostatectomy:** A surgical procedure to remove the prostate through an incision (cut) in the abdominal wall. Removal of nearby lymph nodes may be done at the same time.

  - **Perineal prostatectomy:** A surgical procedure to remove the prostate through an incision (cut) made in the perineum (area between the scrotum and anus). Nearby lymph nodes may also be removed through a separate incision in the abdomen.

- **Pelvic lymphadenectomy:** A surgical procedure to remove the lymph nodes in the pelvis. A pathologist views the tissue under a microscope to look for cancer cells. If the lymph nodes contain cancer, the doctor will not remove the prostate and may recommend other treatment.

- **Transurethral resection of the prostate (TURP):** A surgical procedure to remove tissue from the prostate using a resectoscope (a thin, lighted tube with a cutting tool) inserted through the urethra. This procedure is done to treat benign prostatic hypertrophy and it is sometimes done to relieve symptoms caused by a tumor before other cancer treatment is given. TURP may also be done in men whose tumor is in the prostate only and who cannot have a radical prostatectomy.

In some cases, nerve-sparing surgery can be done. This type of surgery may save the nerves that control erection. However, men with large tumors or tumors that are very close to the nerves may not be able to have this surgery.

Possible problems after prostate cancer surgery include the following:

- Impotence.

- Leakage of urine from the bladder or stool from the rectum.

- Shortening of the penis (1 to 2 centimeters). The exact reason for this is not known.

- Inguinal hernia (bulging of fat or part of the small intestine through weak muscles into the groin). Inguinal hernia may occur more often in men treated with radical prostatectomy than in men who have some other types of prostate surgery, radiation therapy, or prostate biopsy alone. It is most likely to occur within the first 2 years after radical prostatectomy.

Radiation Therapy and Radiopharmaceutical Therapy

Radiation therapy is a cancer treatment that uses high-energy X-rays or other types of radiation to kill cancer cells or keep them from growing. There are different types of radiation therapy:

- External radiation therapy uses a machine outside the body to send radiation toward the cancer. Conformal radiation is a type of external radiation therapy that uses a computer to make a 3-dimensional (3-D) picture of the tumor and shapes the radiation beams to fit the tumor. This allows a high dose of radiation to reach the tumor and causes less damage to nearby healthy tissue.

Hypofractionated radiation therapy may be given because it has a more convenient treatment schedule. Hypofractionated radiation therapy is radiation treatment in which a larger than usual total dose of radiation is given once a day over a shorter period of time (fewer days) compared to standard radiation therapy. Hypofractionated radiation therapy may have worse side effects than standard radiation therapy, depending on the schedules used.

- Internal radiation therapy uses a radioactive substance sealed in needles, seeds, wires, or catheters that are placed directly into or near the cancer. In early-stage prostate cancer, the radioactive seeds are placed in the prostate using needles that are inserted through the skin between the scrotum and rectum. The placement of the radioactive seeds in the prostate is guided by images from transrectal ultrasound or computed tomography (CT). The needles are removed after the radioactive seeds are placed in the prostate.

- Radiopharmaceutical therapy uses a radioactive substance to treat cancer. Radiopharmaceutical therapy includes the following:

  - Alpha emitter radiation therapy uses a radioactive substance to treat prostate cancer that has spread to the bone. A radioactive substance called radium-223 is injected into a vein and travels through the bloodstream. The radium-223 collects in areas of bone with cancer and kills the cancer cells.

The way the radiation therapy is given depends on the type and stage of the cancer being treated. External radiation therapy, internal radiation therapy, and radiopharmaceutical therapy are used to treat prostate cancer.

Men treated with radiation therapy for prostate cancer have an increased risk of having bladder and/or gastrointestinal cancer.

Radiation therapy can cause impotence and urinary problems.

Hormone Therapy

Hormone therapy is a cancer treatment that removes hormones or blocks their action and stops cancer cells from growing. Hormones are substances made by glands in the body and circulated in the bloodstream. In prostate cancer, male sex hormones can cause prostate cancer to grow. Drugs, surgery, or other hormones are used to reduce the amount of male hormones or block them from working.

Hormone therapy for prostate cancer may include the following:

- Luteinizing hormone-releasing hormone agonists can stop the testicles from making testosterone. Examples are leuprolide, goserelin, and buserelin.

- Antiandrogens can block the action of androgens (hormones that promote male sex characteristics), such as testosterone. Examples are flutamide, bicalutamide, enzalutamide, and nilutamide.

- Drugs that can prevent the adrenal glands from making androgens include ketoconazole and aminoglutethimide.

- Orchiectomy is a surgical procedure to remove one or both testicles, the main source of male hormones, such as testosterone, to decrease the amount of hormone being made.

- Estrogens (hormones that promote female sex characteristics) can prevent the testicles from making testosterone. However, estrogens are seldom used today in the treatment of prostate cancer because of the risk of serious side effects.

Hot flashes, impaired sexual function, loss of desire for sex, and weakened bones may occur in men treated with hormone therapy. Other side effects include diarrhea, nausea, and itching.

Chemotherapy

Chemotherapy is a cancer treatment that uses drugs to stop the growth of cancer cells, either by killing the cells or by stopping them from dividing. When chemotherapy is taken by mouth or injected into a vein or muscle, the drugs enter the bloodstream and can reach cancer cells throughout the body (systemic chemotherapy). When chemotherapy is placed directly into the cerebrospinal fluid, an organ, or a body cavity such as the abdomen, the drugs mainly affect cancer cells in those areas (regional chemotherapy). The way the chemotherapy is given depends on the type and stage of the cancer being treated.

Biologic Therapy

Biologic therapy is a treatment that uses the patient's immune system to fight cancer. Substances made by the body or made in a laboratory are used to boost, direct, or restore the body's natural defenses against cancer. Sipuleucel-T is a type of biologic therapy used to treat prostate cancer that has metastasized (spread to other parts of the body).

Bisphosphonate Therapy

Bisphosphonate drugs, such as clodronate or zoledronate, reduce bone disease when cancer has spread to the bone. Men who are treated with antiandrogen therapy or orchiectomy are at an increased risk of bone loss. In these men, bisphosphonate drugs lessen the risk of bone fracture (breaks). The use of bisphosphonate drugs to prevent or slow the growth of bone metastases is being studied in clinical trials.

Section 34.3

Urinary Incontinence Surgery

This section contains text excerpted from the following sources: Text beginning with the heading "What Is Urinary Incontinence (UI) in Men?" is excerpted from "Bladder Control Problems in Men (Urinary Incontinence)," National Institute of Diabetes and Digestive and Kidney Diseases (NIDDK), November 2015; Text beginning with the heading "What Is Stress Urinary Incontinence?" is excerpted from "Stress Urinary Incontinence (SUI)," U.S. Food and Drug Administration (FDA), September 5, 2013. Reviewed June 2017.

What Is Urinary Incontinence (UI) in Men?

Urinary incontinence (UI) is the loss of bladder control, resulting in the accidental leakage of urine from the body. For example, a man may feel a strong, sudden need, or urgency, to urinate just before losing a large amount of urine, called urgency incontinence.

UI can be slightly bothersome or totally debilitating. For some men, the chance of embarrassment keeps them from enjoying many activities, including exercising, and causes emotional distress. When people are inactive, they increase their chances of developing other health problems, such as obesity and diabetes.

What Causes UI in Men?

Urinary incontinence in men results when the brain does not properly signal the bladder, the sphincters do not squeeze strongly enough, or both. The bladder muscle may contract too much or not enough because of a problem with the muscle itself or the nerves controlling the bladder muscle. Damage to the sphincter muscles themselves or the nerves controlling these muscles can result in poor sphincter function. These problems can range from simple to complex.

A man may have factors that increase his chances of developing UI, including:

- **Birth defects**: Problems with development of the urinary tract

- **A history of prostate cancer**: Surgery or radiation treatment for prostate cancer can lead to temporary or permanent UI in men

UI is not a disease. Instead, it can be a symptom of certain conditions or the result of particular events during a man's life. Conditions or events that may increase a man's chance of developing UI include:

- **Benign prostatic hyperplasia (BPH)**: A condition in which the prostate is enlarged yet not cancerous. In men with BPH, the enlarged prostate presses against and pinches the urethra. The bladder wall becomes thicker. Eventually, the bladder may weaken and lose the ability to empty, leaving some urine in the bladder. The narrowing of the urethra and incomplete emptying of the bladder can lead to UI.

- **Chronic coughing**: Long-lasting coughing increases pressure on the bladder and pelvic floor muscles.

- **Neurological problems**: Men with diseases or conditions that affect the brain and spine may have trouble controlling urination.

- **Physical inactivity**: Decreased activity can increase a man's weight and contribute to muscle weakness.

- **Obesity**: Extra weight can put pressure on the bladder, causing a need to urinate before the bladder is full.

- **Older age**: Bladder muscles can weaken over time, leading to a decrease in the bladder's capacity to store urine.

How Is UI in Men Treated?

Surgery

As a last resort, surgery to treat urgency incontinence in men includes the artificial urinary sphincter (AUS) and the male sling. A healthcare professional performs the surgery in a hospital with regional or general anesthesia. Most men can leave the hospital the same day, although some may need to stay overnight.

- **Artificial urinary sphincter (AUS).** An AUS is an implanted device that keeps the urethra closed until the man is ready to urinate. The device has three parts: a cuff that fits around the urethra, a small balloon reservoir placed in the abdomen, and a pump placed in the scrotum—the sac that holds the testicles. The cuff contains a liquid that makes it fit tightly around the urethra to prevent urine from leaking. When it is time to urinate, the man squeezes the pump with his fingers to deflate the cuff. The liquid moves to the balloon reservoir and lets urine flow through the urethra. When the bladder is empty, the cuff automatically refills in the next 2 to 5 minutes to keep the urethra tightly closed.

- **Male sling.** A healthcare professional performs a sling procedure, also called urethral compression procedure, to add support to the urethra, which can sometimes better control urination. Through an incision in the tissue between the scrotum and the rectum, also called the perineum, the healthcare professional uses a piece of human tissue or mesh to compress the urethra against the pubic bone. The surgeon secures the ends of the tissue or mesh around the pelvic bones. The lifting and compression of the urethra sometimes provides better control over urination.

What Is Stress Urinary Incontinence (SUI)?

Stress urinary incontinence (SUI) is a leakage of urine during moments of physical activity that increases abdominal pressure, such as coughing, sneezing, laughing, or exercise. SUI is the most common type of urinary incontinence in women.

SUI can happen when pelvic tissues and muscles, which support the bladder and urethra, become weak and allow the bladder "neck" (where the bladder and urethra intersect) to descend during bursts of physical activity. This descent can prevent the urethra from working properly to control the flow of urine. SUI can also occur when the sphincter muscle that controls the urethra weakens. The weakened sphincter muscle is not able to stop the flow of urine under normal circumstances and when there is an increase in abdominal pressure. Weakness may occur from pregnancy, childbirth, aging, or prior pelvic surgery. Other risk factors for SUI include chronic coughing or straining, obesity and smoking.

It is important for you to consult with your healthcare provider for proper diagnosis of SUI.

What Are the Treatment Options for Women with SUI?

Women have both nonsurgical and surgical options to treat SUI.

Not every woman with SUI will need surgery. Some factors you should consider before deciding whether to undergo surgery include:

- the severity of your SUI symptoms and their effect on your daily activities;

- your desire for future pregnancy as vaginal delivery can cause recurrence of SUI symptoms, which could require future surgery

Nonsurgical Treatment Options

Examples of nonsurgical treatment options for SUI include:

- **Pelvic Floor Exercises:** A type of exercise to strengthen the pelvic floor by contracting and relaxing the muscles that surround the opening of the urethra, vagina, and rectum. These exercises, commonly referred to as Kegel exercises, improve the muscles' strength and function and may help to hold urine in the bladder longer.

- **Pessary:** A removable device that is inserted into the vagina against the vaginal wall and urethra to support the bladder neck. This helps reposition the urethra to reduce SUI.

- **Transurethral Bulking Agents:** Collagen injections around the urethra that make the space around the urethra thicker, thus helping to control urine leakage. The effects may not be permanent.

- **Behavioral Modification:** This includes avoiding activities that trigger episodes of leaking.

Surgical Treatment Options

Surgery to decrease or prevent urine leakage can be done through the vagina or abdomen. The urethra or bladder neck is supported with either stitches alone or with tissue surgically removed from other parts of the body such as the abdominal wall or leg (fascial sling), with tissue from another person (donor tissue) or with material such as surgical mesh (mesh sling).

Surgical mesh in the form of a "sling" (sometimes called "tape") is permanently implanted to support the urethra or bladder neck in order to correct SUI. This is commonly referred to as a "sling procedure."

The use of surgical mesh slings to treat SUI provides a less invasive approach than nonmesh repairs, which require a larger incision in the abdominal wall. The multi-incision sling procedure can be performed using three incisions, in two ways: with one vaginal incision and two lower abdominal incisions, called retropubic; or with one vaginal incision and two groin/thigh incisions, called transobturator. There is also a "mini-sling" procedure that utilizes a shorter piece of surgical mesh, which may be done with only one incision.

Section 34.4

Urinary Diversion

This section includes text excerpted from "Urinary Diversion," National Institute of Diabetes and Digestive and Kidney Diseases (NIDDK), September 2013. Reviewed June 2017.

What Is Urinary Diversion?

Urinary diversion is a surgical procedure that reroutes the normal flow of urine out of the body when urine flow is blocked. Urine flow may be blocked because of:

- an enlarged prostate

- injury to the urethra

- birth defects of the urinary tract

- kidney, ureter, or bladder stones

- tumors of the genitourinary tract—which includes the urinary tract and reproductive organs—or adjacent tissues and organs

- conditions causing external pressure to the urethra or one or both ureters

Bladder removal or a malfunctioning bladder may also cause blocked urine flow. When urine cannot flow out of the body, it can accumulate in the bladder, ureters, and kidneys. As a result, body wastes and extra water do not empty from the body, potentially resulting in pain, urinary tract infections, kidney failure, or, if left untreated, death. Urinary diversion can be temporary or permanent, depending on the reason for the procedure.

What Is a Nephrostomy?

A nephrostomy involves a small tube inserted through the skin directly into a kidney. The nephrostomy tube drains urine from the kidney into an external drainage pouch. Nephrostomy tubes are often used for less than a week after a percutaneous nephrolithotomy—a surgical procedure to break up and remove a kidney stone.

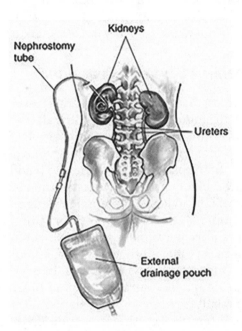

Figure 34.2. *Nephrostomy Tube and External Drainage Pouch*

This treatment is often used when a kidney stone is quite large or in a location that does not permit effective use of other treatments. For this procedure, a surgeon makes a tiny incision in the back and creates a tunnel into one of the kidneys. As the kidney heals after surgery, the nephrostomy provides an alternative route for urine drainage until normal urinary flow resumes. A person may also need a nephrostomy if narrowing, blockage, or inflammation of the ureters keeps urine from draining properly. Under these circumstances, the nephrostomy may stay in place for several weeks until the problem is resolved.

What Is Urinary Catheterization?

Urinary catheterization involves placing a thin, flexible tube—called a catheter—into the bladder to drain urine. Two methods of urinary catheterization include insertion of a catheter through the urethra or through an incision in the skin. For the first method, a special type of catheter, called a Foley catheter, is inserted through the urethra. A Foley catheter has a water-filled balloon on the end that a healthcare provider inserts into the bladder to keep the catheter in place. For the second method, called a suprapubic catheterization, a catheter is inserted through an incision in the skin beneath the belly button directly into the bladder. Urinary catheters may remain in place for several days or weeks while tissues heal after urinary tract surgery or treatment of urinary blockage.

What Is Permanent Urinary Diversion?

Permanent urinary diversion requires surgery to reroute urine flow to an external pouch through an opening in the wall of the abdomen, called a stoma, or to a surgically created internal reservoir. Stomas range from three-fourths of an inch to 3 inches wide. Surgeons perform permanent urinary diversion when a patient has a damaged bladder or no longer has a bladder. Advanced bladder cancer ranks as the most common reason for bladder removals. Bladder damage may result from nerve damage, birth defects, or chronic—or long-lasting—inflammation. Nerve damage severe enough to require permanent urinary diversion generally occurs from multiple sclerosis, among other diseases; spinal cord injuries; and damage caused by pelvic trauma or radiation injury. The most common birth defect requiring bladder surgery is spina bifida. Chronic bladder inflammation can result from severe cases of interstitial cystitis or chronic urinary retention. Interstitial cystitis is a condition that causes the bladder to become swollen and irritated, leading to decreased bladder capacity. Urinary retention is the inability to empty the bladder completely.

What Is a Urostomy?

A urostomy is a stoma that connects to the urinary tract and makes it possible for urine to drain out of the body when regular urination cannot occur. The stoma has no muscle, so it cannot control urine flow, causing a continuous flow. An external pouch collects urine flowing through the stoma. Ileal conduit and cutaneous ureterostomy are the two main types of urostomy.

Ileal Conduit

An ileal conduit uses a section of the bowel—usually the small intestine—surgically removed from the digestive tract and repositioned to serve as a passage, or conduit, for urine from the ureters to a stoma. One end of the conduit attaches to the ureters; the other end attaches to the stoma. The surgeon reconnects the bowel where the section was removed so that it functions normally. The urine flows through the newly formed ileal conduit and the stoma into an external pouch.

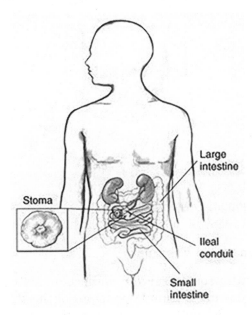

Figure 34.3. *Ileal Conduit and Stoma*

Cutaneous Ureterostomy

In cutaneous ureterostomy, the surgeon detaches one or both ureters and attaches them directly to a stoma. This type of urostomy is not as common as an ileal conduit because of a higher complication rate and the need for follow-up surgery. A surgeon performs cutaneous ureterostomy when the bowel cannot be used to create a stoma because of certain diseases and conditions or exposure to high doses of radiation.

What Is Continent Urinary Diversion?

Continent urinary diversion is an internal reservoir that a surgeon creates from a section of the bowel. Urine flows through the ureters into the reservoir and is drained by the patient. Continent urinary diversion does not require an external pouch. Continent urinary diversion consists of two main types, continent cutaneous reservoir and bladder substitute.

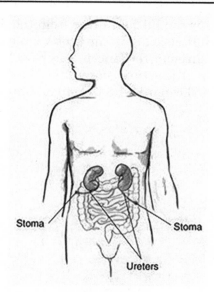

Figure 34.4. *Cutaneous Ureterostomy*

Continent Cutaneous Reservoir

A continent cutaneous reservoir connects to a stoma. A surgically created valve keeps urine from flowing out of the stoma. The patient inserts a catheter through the continent stoma to drain urine from the reservoir several times throughout the day. The stoma is very small—less than 1 inch wide—and sometimes can be hidden in the belly button.

Bladder Substitute

For a bladder substitute, also called a neobladder, a surgeon creates an internal reservoir that connects to the ureters at one end and to the urethra at the other. Since this type of reservoir connects to the urethra, urine empties from the reservoir in a more natural process, just as a person with a normal urinary tract would do when going to the bathroom with a natural bladder. However, the bladder substitute does not function as well as a natural bladder. In some cases, a catheter must be inserted through the urethra to completely empty the reservoir. A patient with this type of permanent diversion may have a higher chance of urinary incontinence—the accidental loss of urine. Only certain people qualify for this type of diversion, and surgeons carefully select eligible patients.

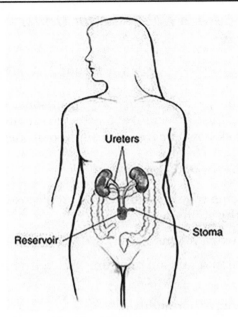

Figure 34.5. *Continent Cutaneous Reservoir*

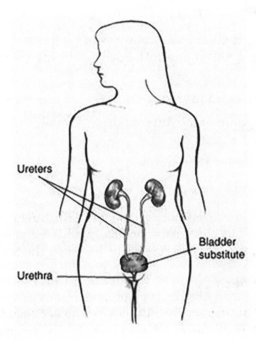

Figure 34.6. *Bladder Substitute*

What Special Care Is Needed after Urinary Diversion Surgery?

After urinary diversion surgery, a wound, ostomy, and continence (WOC) nurse or an enterostomal therapist helps patients learn how to take care of their permanent urinary diversions. WOC nurses and enterostomal therapists specialize in ostomy care and rehabilitation. Patients should ask how to care for their stomas and pouches.

Caring for a Continent Stoma

A continent stoma requires daily care. Care focuses on maintaining a clean and healthy stoma by:

- wiping away extra mucus
- washing the stoma and surrounding skin with mild soap and water
- rinsing the stoma thoroughly
- drying the stoma completely

Caring for a Noncontinent Stoma

A noncontinent stoma also requires basic daily care. Care focuses on maintaining a suitable and healthy skin area for attachment of the pouch by:

- wiping away extra mucus
- washing the stoma and surrounding skin with mild soap and water
- rinsing the stoma thoroughly
- drying the stoma completely

Patients should inspect their stoma and skin and notify their healthcare providers of any changes, specifically evidence of skin breakdown, typically in an area where urine leaks between the pouch and stoma.

Caring for a Pouch

A person with an ileal conduit or with cutaneous ureterostomy also works with WOC nurses or enterostomal therapists to learn how to care for an external pouch. The pouch system usually consists of two pieces—a barrier that sticks to the skin, known as a wafer, and a disposable plastic bag or pouch that attaches to the barrier. Sometimes the barrier and pouch are one unit. The barrier protects the skin from urine and is designed to be as gentle as possible on the skin. The length of time the barrier stays sealed to the skin depends on many things, such as whether the barrier fits properly, the condition of the skin around the stoma, the patient's physical activity level, and the shape of the body around the stoma.

The pouch has a drain valve at the bottom so the patient can empty it into a toilet without removing the pouch from the stoma. During the day, most patients need to empty the pouch about as often as they used the bathroom before having urinary diversion surgery. Patients should empty the pouch when it is about one-third to one-half full. At night, patients can attach a piece of flexible tubing to the drain valve on the pouch to let urine flow into a bigger pouch during sleep.

Patients should rinse and clean the pouch daily and change it every 5 to 7 days. When changing a pouch, patients need to clean the skin around the stoma with a wet towelette or washcloth. The skin should be completely dry before applying a new pouch. If the constant flow of urine from the stoma irritates the skin, patients can use protective skin wipes or an ostomy powder designed to protect the skin around the stoma.

Wearing a urostomy pouch does not require special clothing. Modern pouches are designed to lie flat against the body so they aren't

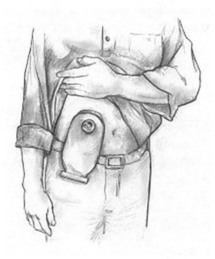

Figure 34.7. *Urostomy Pouch*

noticeable under most clothing. A patient can tuck the pouch inside elastic undergarments or between undergarments and outer clothing. A simple pouch cover adds comfort by absorbing sweat and keeping the plastic pouch from resting against the skin. Cotton knit or stretch undergarments may give extra support and security. Some people with urostomies wear a belt that attaches to the pouch system and wraps around the waist. The belt supports the pouch system and, for some people, provides a sense of security.

Caring for a Continent Cutaneous Reservoir

For a continent cutaneous reservoir, patients learn how to insert a catheter through the stoma or urethra to drain the internal reservoir. Patients can drain the reservoir by inserting the catheter while standing in front of the toilet or sitting on the toilet. During the first few weeks after urinary diversion surgery, patients need to drain the internal reservoir every couple of hours. Over time, the reservoir capacity will increase and patients will be able to go 4 to 6 hours between reservoir drainings. Patients should wash their hands with soap and water each time they use a catheter. Before and after catheterization, patients should clean the stoma and skin around it with a wet towelette or washcloth and completely dry the stoma and skin.

The reservoir is made from part of the bowel, so it may produce mucus that normally lines the digestive tract. To clear this mucus, patients may need to irrigate, or flush out, the reservoir using a syringe with sterile water or normal saline. Patients should talk with a WOC nurse, an enterostomal therapist, or a urologist—a doctor who specializes in the urinary tract—about how often they should irrigate the reservoir.

Infection

Bacteria often enter urostomies and continent urinary diversions and begin growing in number. At times, bacterial overgrowth causes a symptomatic urinary tract infection. Symptoms of infection may include:

- fever
- milky urine or urine containing extra mucus
- strong-smelling urine
- back pain

- poor appetite

- nausea

- vomiting

Patients with symptoms of infection should call their healthcare providers at once. Drinking eight full glasses of water every day can help prevent infection by flushing out bacteria and keeping bacterial counts low. Patients should talk with their healthcare providers about appropriate times to have their urine tested and when to have treatment with antibiotics. Urine testing and infection treatment play a critical role in successful long-term care with minimal complications.

Activities

To help the stoma heal, patients need to restrict their activities, including driving and heavy lifting, during the first 2 to 3 weeks after urinary diversion surgery. Once the stoma has healed, patients should be able to do most of the activities they enjoyed before urinary diversion surgery, even swimming and other water sports. The only exceptions may be contact sports such as football or karate. Patients whose jobs include strenuous physical activities should talk with their healthcare providers and employers about making adjustments to their job responsibilities.

Relationships

Patients may worry that people will have negative reactions to their urinary diversion. Most people will never know patients are wearing a pouch or have a continent urinary diversion. Friends and relatives are likely to be aware of the patient's health problems. However, only a spouse, intimate partner, or primary caretaker needs to know the details of the urinary diversion. Patients can choose how much they share about their condition.

Urinary diversion surgery may reduce sexual function, especially when the bladder has been removed because of cancer. Patients who have good sexual function may resume sexual activities after urinary diversion surgery as soon as their healthcare providers say it is safe. Patients should talk with their healthcare providers about any concerns they have about maintaining a satisfying sexual relationship. Healthcare providers can give information about ways to protect the stoma during sexual activity. Patients may want to ask about specially designed apparel to enhance intimacy for people with urostomies. Communicating with a sexual partner is essential. Patients should share their concerns and wishes and listen carefully to their partner's concerns.

Eating, Diet, and Nutrition

After urinary diversion surgery, patients will likely be able to resume their normal diet. Some foods, such as asparagus and seafood, may cause urine to have a stronger odor, which may be noticeable when emptying a pouch. If odor is a concern, patients should talk with their healthcare providers about changes in diet. Patients should also talk with their healthcare providers about their dietary needs. Some patients with continent urinary reservoirs have a chance of vitamin B deficiency and may require lifelong vitamin B injections. This requirement is only for a specific type of diversion and should be discussed with the healthcare provider in detail.

Section 34.5

Vasectomy (Male Sterilization)

This section includes text excerpted from "Male Sterilization," U.S. Department of Health and Human Services (HHS), August 16, 2016.

What Is Vasectomy?

Vasectomy or male sterilization is a procedure performed on a man that will permanently keep him from being able to get a woman pregnant.

Vasectomy is an outpatient procedure done under local anesthesia. After the local anesthesia is injected, the healthcare provider then makes tiny cuts (incisions) in the scrotum, the sac that holds the testes or "balls." The vas deferens—two tubes that carry sperm to the penis—are then cut, tied or blocked.

Some men receive a no-scalpel vasectomy where, instead of cutting the skin of the scrotum, very tiny holes are made. The tubes that carry sperm are pulled through the holes and tied off and cut. A no-scalpel vasectomy does not require stitches.

After a vasectomy, a man will still produce semen, the fluid that comes out of his penis when he has sex. A man will need to return to his health provider after about three months to be tested to make sure there are no more sperm in his semen. It takes about three months to clear the sperm out of the system. A man should use another type of birth control (like a condom) until his healthcare provider tells him there are no longer any sperm in his semen.

There may be surgery available to reverse a vasectomy, but men should consider the procedure permanent. Before a vasectomy, men can also freeze their sperm for future use if they choose.

Where Can I Get a Vasectomy?

A vasectomy can be done in a medical office or clinic. It is an out-patient procedure, so a man can go home the same day.

While not all family planning clinics perform vasectomies, your local family planning clinic may be able to tell you where vasectomy is available in your area.

How Effective Is Vasectomy?

Out of 100 women each year whose partner has had a vasectomy, less than one may get pregnant.

Advantages of Vasectomy

- The man's partner doesn't have to know about it or do anything different.

- Lifts the contraceptive burden from the woman.

- Safe and highly effective approach to preventing pregnancy.

- Lasts a lifetime, so no need to worry about birth control again.

- The procedure is simple to do and usually involves only a little bit of discomfort.

- Quick recovery time after the procedure.

- Most cost-effective of all birth control methods.

Drawbacks of Vasectomy

- Provides no protection against sexually transmitted infections (STIs), including HIV.

- Requires a visit to a clinic or medical office.

- Risk of swelling, bruising, and tenderness for a short time after the procedure.

- Very rarely, the tubes that carry sperm can grow back together. When this happens there is a risk of pregnancy.

Some men, or their partners, later change their minds and wish they could have a child or additional children.

Chapter 35

Cosmetic and Reconstructive Surgery

Chapter Contents

Section 35.1

Cosmetic Surgery: Things to Consider

This section includes text excerpted from "Cosmetic Surgery," girlshealth.gov, Office on Women's Health (OWH), April 15, 2014.

People might have cosmetic surgery for a number of reasons, including to remove acne scars, change their noses, and make their breasts smaller or bigger. But if there's something you don't like about your body, your best bet is to try to work on how you feel about it. Your attitude can make a big difference. Try to focus on what you like about yourself. And remember that you've got lots more to offer the world than just how you look.

Risks of Cosmetic Surgery

People who have cosmetic surgery face many of the same risks as anyone having surgery. These include:

- Infection

- Not healing well

- Damage to nerves

- Bleeding

- Not being happy with the results

- Risks from anesthesia, such as lung problems

You face additional concerns if you're considering surgery to make your breasts bigger through breast implants. (Keep in mind that you usually can't have this surgery until you're 18). For one, these surgeries usually need to be done over at some point. Also, breast implant risks include dimples and wrinkles that won't go away, pain, and an implant breaking. There are other possible problems, too, including that you might not be able to breastfeed when you have a baby and it could be harder to see signs of breast cancer in a mammogram (breast X-ray).

What I Need to Know about Cosmetic Surgery

Here are a few key points to keep in mind if you are thinking about plastic surgery:

- Talk to your parents or guardians about any surgery and any concerns you have about how your body looks.

- Don't rely on surgery to change your life in a huge way.

- Make sure any doctor you consider is qualified for the surgery you're considering and is certified by the American Board of Plastic Surgery (ABPS).

- Some doctors won't perform certain procedures if they don't think you're old enough. For example, it is usually not a good idea to have cosmetic surgery while your body is still growing.

- Health insurance usually does not cover the cost of plastic surgery.

If I Feel Unhappy about My Body

Most people want to look good, and in your teen years you've got lots going on with your body. How you feel about how you look is called body image, and it can affect how you feel about yourself overall.

It's not always easy to have a positive body image, but you can work on it. One way is to ignore magazines and TV shows that say you need to look a certain way. Try to hang out with people who have healthy attitudes about how they look and who support and accept you. And remember to focus on what you like about yourself—inside and out.

If how parts of your body look bothers you a huge amount and you can't stop thinking about them, you could have body dysmorphic disorder (BDD). People with BDD spend a lot of time and energy looking at their flaws and trying to hide them. They also may ask friends to reassure them about their looks and sometimes want a lot of cosmetic surgery. BDD is an illness, and you can get help. If you or a friend may have BDD, talk to an adult you trust, such as your parent or guardian, school counselor, doctor, or nurse.

Section 35.2

Liposuction

This section includes text excerpted from
"The Skinny on Liposuction," U.S. Food and Drug
Administration (FDA), March 27, 2017.

Liposuction is the most popular form of cosmetic surgery in the United States, according to the American Society for Aesthetic Plastic Surgery (ASAPS).

If you are considering joining the millions of people worldwide who have had liposuction, U.S. Food and Drug Administration's (FDA) Center for Devices and Radiological Health (CDRH), which regulates the medical products used in liposuction, suggests you consider the following before having the surgery:

- Liposuction is intended only for body contouring. It is not intended as a means of weight loss.

- During liposuction, body fat is removed from under the skin with the use of vacuum suction—either with a hollow pen-like instrument called a "cannula," or an ultrasonic probe that breaks fat up into small pieces and then removes it.

- While physicians may perform liposuction on the abdomen, hips, thighs, calves, arms, buttocks, back, neck, or face, it has never been cleared for use on the neck or face.

- Liposuction is also used in medical procedures such as reduction of men's breast size and removing fat tumors (lipomas).

Who Can Perform Liposuction Surgery?

Plastic surgeons and dermatologists often perform liposuction, but any licensed physician may perform the procedure.

While some physicians' professional societies recommend it, no standardized training is required for conducting liposuction. You may want to base your decision to have liposuction on whether or not a doctor has had specialized training in the procedure, and has successfully performed it before.

Liposuction may be performed in a doctor's office, surgical center or hospital. Because it is a surgical procedure, it is important that:

- it be performed in a clean environment

- there is access to emergency medical equipment or a nearby hospital emergency room.

Remember, even the best-screened patients under the care of the best-trained and experienced physicians may experience complications as a result of liposuction.

What Are the Risks?

- **Infections** can become serious issues. Keep the wounds clean.

- **Embolisms** may occur when loosened fat enters the blood through blood vessels ruptured during liposuction. Pieces of fat can wind up in the lungs, or even the brain. Fat emboli may cause permanent disability or, in some cases, be fatal.

- **Puncture wounds in the organs** (visceral perforations) may require surgery for repair. They can also prove fatal.

- **Seroma** is a pooling of serum, the straw-colored liquid from your blood, in areas where tissue has been removed.

- **Paresthesias** (changes in sensation that may be caused by nerve compression) is an altered sensation at the site of the liposuction. This may either be in the form of an increased sensitivity (pain), or numbness in the area. In some cases, these changes in sensation may be permanent.

- **Swelling,** in some cases, may persist for weeks or months after liposuction.

- **Skin necrosis** occurs when the skin above the liposuction site changes color and falls off. Large areas of skin necrosis may become infected with bacteria or microorganisms.

- **Burns** can occur during ultrasound-assisted liposuction if the ultrasound probe becomes hot.

- **Fluid imbalance** may impact you after you go home. The condition can result in serious ailments such as heart problems, excess fluid collecting in the lungs, or kidney problems.

- **Toxicity from anesthesia** due to the use of lidocaine, a skin-numbing drug, can cause lightheadedness, restlessness, drowsiness, a ringing in the ears, slurred speech, a metallic taste in the mouth, numbness of the lips and tongue, shivering, muscle twitching and convulsions. Lidocaine toxicity may cause the heart to stop.

- **Scars** at the site of the incision are usually small and fade with time, although some may be larger or more prominent.

- **Bumpy or wavy appearances** can occur at the liposuction site after the procedure.

More Factors to Consider

Will You Like Your Looks after Liposuction?

The cosmetic effect after liposuction may be very good and many patients report being satisfied. However, your appearance afterward may not be what you expected or wanted. Some physicians counsel their patients that reasonable expectations are important.

The Results May Not Be Permanent

If you gain weight after liposuction surgery, the fat may return to sites where you had liposuction or to other sites.

Liposuction Is Not for Everyone

You are probably not a good candidate for liposuction surgery if cost is an issue. Most medical insurance will not pay for cosmetic liposuction, and the cost may be significant. You are also probably not a good candidate if you are overweight or obese and trying to lose weight, if you have a disease or are on medication that affects wound healing, or if your skin elasticity is inadequate. Lack of skin elasticity can cause the area the fat was removed from to be baggy after liposuction.

There Are Alternatives

These include changing your diet to lose excess body fat, exercising, accepting your body and appearance as it is, or using clothing or makeup to downplay or emphasize body or facial features.

Make sure you understand the procedure and what you can expect

It is important for you to read the patient information that your doctor provides so that you understand the risks involved. Ask about potential problems that could occur, and ask about the physician's experience in performing liposuction.

How Accurate Is the Advertising?

Be wary of advertisements that say or imply you will have a perfect appearance after liposuction. Remember that advertisements are meant to sell you a product or service. Also, don't base your decision simply on cost.

Don't Be Pressured

Take your time to decide whether liposuction is right for you and whether you are willing to take the risks of the surgery for its benefits.

Section 35.3

Surgery for Skin Cancer

This section includes text excerpted from "Skin Cancer Treatment (PDQ®)—Patient Version," National Cancer Institute (NCI), July 22, 2016.

Skin Cancer

Skin cancer is a disease in which malignant (cancer) cells form in the tissues of the skin.

The skin is the body's largest organ. It protects against heat, sunlight, injury, and infection. Skin also helps control body temperature and stores water, fat, and vitamin D. The skin has several layers, but the two main layers are the epidermis (upper or outer layer) and the dermis (lower or inner layer). Skin cancer begins in the epidermis, which is made up of three kinds of cells:

- **Squamous cells:** Thin, flat cells that form the top layer of the epidermis.

- **Basal cells:** Round cells under the squamous cells.

- **Melanocytes:** Cells that make melanin and are found in the lower part of the epidermis. Melanin is the pigment that gives skin its natural color. When skin is exposed to the sun, melanocytes make more pigment and cause the skin to darken.

Skin cancer can occur anywhere on the body, but it is most common in skin that is often exposed to sunlight, such as the face, neck, hands, and arms.

Types of Skin Cancer

There are different types of cancer that start in the skin.
The most common types are basal cell carcinoma and squamous cell carcinoma, which are nonmelanoma skin cancers. Nonmelanoma skin cancers rarely spread to other parts of the body. Melanoma is a much rarer type of skin cancer. It is more likely to invade nearby tissues and spread to other parts of the body. Actinic keratosis is a skin condition that sometimes becomes squamous cell carcinoma.

Skin Cancer Surgery

One or more of the following surgical procedures may be used to treat nonmelanoma skin cancer or actinic keratosis:

- **Mohs micrographic surgery.** The tumor is cut from the skin in thin layers. During surgery, the edges of the tumor and each layer of tumor removed are viewed through a microscope to check for cancer cells. Layers continue to be removed until no more cancer cells are seen. This type of surgery removes as little normal tissue as possible and is often used to remove skin cancer on the face.

- **Simple excision.** The tumor is cut from the skin along with some of the normal skin around it.

- **Shave excision.** The abnormal area is shaved off the surface of the skin with a small blade.

- **Electrodesiccation and curettage.** The tumor is cut from the skin with a curette (a sharp, spoon-shaped tool). A needle-shaped electrode is then used to treat the area with an electric current that stops the bleeding and destroys cancer cells that remain around the edge of the wound. The process may be repeated one to three times during the surgery to remove all of the cancer.

- **Cryosurgery.** A treatment that uses an instrument to freeze and destroy abnormal tissue, such as carcinoma in situ. This type of treatment is also called cryotherapy.

- **Laser surgery.** A surgical procedure that uses a laser beam (a narrow beam of intense light) as a knife to make bloodless cuts in tissue or to remove a surface lesion such as a tumor.

- **Dermabrasion.** Removal of the top layer of skin using a rotating wheel or small particles to rub away skin cells.

- **Laser surgery.** A surgical procedure that uses a laser beam (a narrow beam of intense light) as a knife to make bloodless cuts in tissue or to remove a surface lesion such as a tumor.

- **Dermabrasion.** Removal of the top layer of skin using a rotating wheel or small particles to rub away skin cells.

Chapter 36

Gender Reassignment Surgery

Gender dysphoria or gender identity disorder, sometimes used synonymously with Transsexualism, refers to "discomfort or distress that is caused by a discrepancy between a person's gender identity and that person's sex assigned at birth (and the associated gender role and/or primary and secondary sex characteristics)."

Distress can be severe, resulting in higher prevalence of depression and anxiety. Treatment for gender dysphoria varies based on individualized assessment for each patient, but generally includes some combination of psychotherapy, cross-sex hormonal therapy, and surgical intervention. The goals of treatment for gender dysphoria are to minimize dysphoria and help patients function in society in their desired gender role.

What Is Gender Reassignment Surgery?

Gender reassignment is the only treatment for gender dysphoria that has shown significant benefits in numerous research trials and meta-analyses over the past half century. Overall, gender reassignment surgeries have been found safe, effective, and necessary in treating gender dysphoria. Feelings of regret are extremely rare and, where present, mostly transient. Access to transition-related care not only

This section includes text excerpted from "Summary of Clinical Evidence for Gender," Centers for Medicare and Medicaid Services (CMS), January 2, 2016.

results in reduction of dysphoria and improved psychological outcomes, but is also linked to improved primary care outcomes.

Categories of Gender Reassignment Surgery

The category of gender reassignment surgery (GRS) includes:

1. Breast/chest surgeries;

2. Genital surgeries;

3. Other surgeries.

Female-To-Male (FTM) Surgery

For the Female-to-Male (FTM) patient, surgical procedures may include the following:

1. **Breast/chest surgery**. Subcutaneous mastectomy, nipple grafts, chest reconstruction;

2. **Genital surgery**. Hysterectomy/salpingo-oophorectomy, metoidioplasty, phalloplasty (employing a pedicled or free vascularized flap), reconstruction of the fixed part of the urethra, vaginectomy, vulvectomy, scrotoplasty, and implantation of erection and/or testicular prostheses;

3. **Other**. Voice surgery (rare), liposuction, and lipofilling.

Male-To-Female (MTF) Surgery

For the Male-to-Female (MTF) patient, surgical procedures may include the following:

1. **Breast/chest surgery**. Mammaplasty;

2. **Genital surgery**. Orchiectomy, penectomy, vaginoplasty, clitoroplasty, vulvoplasty, labiaplasty, urethroplasty, prostatectomy;

3. **Other surgeries**. Reconstructive facial feminization surgery, liposuction, lipofilling, voice surgery, thyroid cartilage reduction, electrolysis or laser hair removal, and hair reconstruction.

Surgeries for Female-to-Male (FTM) Individuals

Breast / Chest Surgery

Mastectomy for transgender men is necessary for many in order to resolve gender dysphoria. When bilateral (double-incision) mastectomy is performed, nipple grafts are a necessary component of the surgery; when "keyhole" (periareolar incision) is performed, nipple grafts are less likely necessary, but may be required in some cases. Both procedures are highly effective, and in either type, reconstruction of the chest to approximate a normal male chest is a necessary component.

In follow-up studies, transgender men who have undergone mastectomy report very low rates of complication and high rates of satisfaction; scarring is generally within expected limits and necrosis of nipple grafts is rare. Chest reconstruction surgery in combination with hormone therapy has been shown to be more effective in alleviating gender dysphoria than hormones alone. Quality of life is higher among transgender men who have undergone chest reconstruction than those who have not.

Genital Surgeries

Three procedures may be indicated for transgender men whose gender dysphoria affects the genitals. Hysterectomy may be performed with or without salpingectomy and oophorectomy; the procedures are safe, with complication rates comparable to the nontransgender population, and effective in reducing gender dysphoria. If dysphoria related to external genitals is present, patients should receive individualized assessment to determine if metoidioplasty or phalloplasty will be more effective in reducing gender dysphoria. Both procedures are highly effective in treating gender dysphoria and have acceptable complication rates when weighed against the benefits for some patients; when complications do occur, they are often relatively minor and can be easily treated. Phalloplasty may be safely performed using either a free or pedicled flap technique. Urethral lengthening is required as a component of phalloplasty and is often necessary for metoidioplasty. Scrotoplasty and testicular implants may be necessary components of phalloplasty and metoidioplasty if individualized assessment determines the results would better resolve dysphoria.

Surgeries for Male-to-Female (MTF) Individuals

Breast / Chest Surgery

In transgender women who undergo hormone therapy, maximal breast development is generally reached within 2 years; while in some hormone therapy alone is sufficient to achieve breast size appropriate to age and body habitus, in 40–70 percent, breast reconstruction may be necessary in order for the individual to pass as female and thereby reduce or resolve gender dysphoria.

Mammaplasty in transgender women serves a primarily therapeutic purpose and should be considered reconstructive rather than cosmetic. In a recent cohort study, psychosocial well-being improved after breast reconstruction, indicating that the procedure is effective in reducing gender dysphoria. Safety is a paramount issue underscoring the necessity of access to breast reconstruction as well, as transgender women who are unable to access safe methods of breast reconstruction sometimes resort to injection of nonmedical grade silicone to obtain breast shape and size.

Genital Surgeries

Genital surgeries for transgender women generally fall into two types: orchiectomy, performed alone or as part of vaginoplasty, and procedures associated with vaginoplasty (penectomy, vaginoplasty, clitoroplasty, vulvoplasty, labiaplasty, urethroplasty, and rarely prostatectomy).

Whether or not assessment indicates vaginoplasty is necessary to resolve an individual's gender dysphoria, orchiectomy may be indicated separately.

Vaginoplasty has been shown to be necessary, safe, and effective in treating gender dysphoria. The procedure may be performed using skin grafts or flaps; the most common technique involves inversion of an anteriorly pedicled penile skin flap in combination with a small dorsally based scrotal flap.

Follow-up studies indicate high satisfaction, improved sexual, physical, and psychosocial health, and reduction of gender dysphoria. Follow-up studies have found complications including dehissance, prolonged vaginal bleeding, vaginal pain, anorgasmia, rectal-vaginal fistula, vaginal stenosis, urethral stenosis, clitoral necrosis, vaginal prolapse, and vaginal hair; complication rates are acceptable when weighed against the benefits for some patients. Prevaginoplasty electrolysis is necessary to prevent vaginal hair.

Chapter 37

Organ Transplant Surgeries

Chapter Contents

Section 37.1

How Organ Allocation Works and Transplant Process

This section includes text excerpted from "About Transplantation," Health Resources and Services Administration (HRSA), January 15, 2016.

More than 120,000 people in the United States are waiting to receive a life-giving organ transplant. Health Resources and Services Administration (HRSA) simply doesn't have enough donated organs to transplant everyone in need, so it balances factors of:

- justice (fair consideration of candidates' circumstances and medical needs), and

- medical utility (trying to increase the number of transplants performed and the length of time patients and organs survive).

Many factors used to match organs with patients in need are the same for all organs, but the system must accommodate some unique differences for each organ.

The First Step

Before an organ is allocated, all transplant candidates on the waiting list that are incompatible with the donor because of blood type, height, weight and other medical factors are automatically screened from any potential matches. Then, the computer application determines the order that the other candidates will receive offers, according to national policies.

Geography Plays a Part

There are 58 local donor service areas and 11 regions that are used for U.S. organ allocation. Hearts and lungs have less time to be transplanted, so HRSA uses a radius from the donor hospital instead of regions when allocating those organs.

The Right-Sized Organ

Proper organ size is critical to a successful transplant, which means that children often respond better to child-sized organs. Although pediatric candidates have their own unique scoring system, children essentially are first in line for other children's organs.

Factors in Organ Allocation

Blood type and other medical factors weigh into the allocation of every donated organ, but, other factors are unique to each organ-type.

Kidney

- Waiting time
- Donor/recipient immune system incompatibility
- Pediatric status
- Prior living donor
- How far from donor hospital
- Survival benefit

Heart

- Medical need
- How far from donor hospital

Lung

- Survival benefit
- Medical urgency
- Waiting time
- Distance from donor hospital

Liver

- Medical need
- Distance from donor hospital

Preserving Organs

Donated organs require special methods of preservation to keep them viable between the time of procurement and transplantation.

Common Maximum Organ Preservation Times

- Heart, lung: 4–6 hours

- Liver: 8–12 hours

- Pancreas: 12–18 hours

- Kidney: 24–36 hours

The Transplant Team

There are many people at the transplant center who work to make a transplant successful. Each person on the "transplant team" is an expert in a different area. The transplant team includes all or some of the following professionals:

- **Clinical transplant coordinators** have responsibility for the patient's evaluation, treatment, and follow-up care.

- **Transplant physicians** are doctors who manage the patient's medical care, tests, and medications. He or she does not perform surgery. The transplant physician works closely with the transplant coordinator to coordinate the patient's care until transplanted, and in some centers, provides follow-up care to the recipient.

- **Transplant surgeons** perform the transplant surgery and may provide the follow-up care for the recipient. The transplant surgeon has special training to perform transplants.

- **Financial coordinators** have detailed knowledge of financial matters and hospital billing. The financial coordinator works with other members of the transplant team, insurers, and administrative personnel to coordinate and clarify the financial aspects of the patient's care before, during, and after the transplant.

- **Social workers** help the patient and their family understand and cope with a variety of issues associated with a patient's illness and/or the various side-effects of the transplant itself. In some cases, the social worker may perform some of the financial coordinator duties as well.

Transplant Process

Transplant data show that more and more people receive transplants every year and that many people with transplants are living longer after receiving their organ(s) than ever before.

Waiting Times

Waiting times vary widely for many reasons. The shortage of organs causes most patients to wait for a transplant. The amount of time a patient waits does not show how well a transplant center or optical parametric oscillator (OPO) is doing its job. Each patient's situation is different. Some patients are more ill than others when they are put on the transplant waiting list. Some patients get sick more quickly than other patients, or respond differently to treatments. Patients may have medical conditions that make it harder to find a good match for them.

How long a patient waits depends on many factors. These can include:

- blood type (some are rarer than others)
- tissue type
- height and weight of transplant candidate
- size of donated organ
- medical urgency
- time on the waiting list
- the distance between the donor's hospital and the potential donor organ
- how many donors there are in the local area over a period of time and
- the transplant center's criteria for accepting organ offers

Depending on the kind of organ needed, some factors are more important than others.

Patient Notification

Potential recipients often contact the Organ Procurement and Transplantation Network's (OPTN) to ask if they are on the National Patient Waiting list. Unfortunately, the OPTN cannot provide this information. A patient's presence and status on the waiting list should be discussed with the patient's transplant team.

- The transplant program must notify patients in writing within ten business days of registration that the patient has been placed on the national transplant waiting list (including the date the patient was listed), or

- The transplant program must notify the patient in writing ten days after completion of the evaluation that the patient will not be placed on the patient waiting list.

- Once listed, if the patient is removed from the waiting list for any reason other than transplantation or death, the transplant program must notify the patient in writing within ten business days that the patient has been removed from the list.

This policy is intended to improve communication between transplant centers and their patients and to help patients better understand the listing and transplant process.

Options to Consider

As an informed participant, it is important that transplant candidates know their treatment options. Some patients choose to list at hospitals in different parts of the country, change hospitals, and transfer their waiting time to a different center or receive a transplant from a living donor.

- **Multiple Listing.** Sometimes patients choose to register for a transplant at more than one hospital. When a patient lists at a transplant hospital, they are generally considered for organs from a donor in that local area first. If a patient is put on the list at more than one transplant hospital, they will be considered for donor organs that become available in more than one local area.

National transplant policy allows a patient to register for a transplant at more than one transplant hospital. However, each hospital may have its own rules for allowing its patients to be on the list at another hospital. Patients should ask each hospital whether it allows its patients to list at more than one transplant hospital. Being listed in more than one area does not guarantee an organ will become available faster than for patients registered at only one transplant hospital. Generally, each transplant center will require the patient to go through a separate evaluation, even if the patient is already listed at another hospital.

- **Transferring Waiting Time.** Patients may switch to a different transplant hospital and transfer their waiting time to that hospital. Waiting time from the original center is added to the time collected at the new hospital.

The transplant teams at the first hospital and the new hospital will be responsible for coordinating the exchange of information and notifying United Network for Organ Sharing (UNOS) of the transfer of waiting time. Patients should ask each hospital if transferred waiting time will be accepted.

- **Variability among Transplant Centers.** Hospitals can vary widely in the number of transplants they perform and the characteristics of the donor and recipient pool. Organ procurement organizations can vary widely in the number and types of donors they receive each year.

- **Living Donation.** In addition to deceased organ donation, patients may also receive organs from living donors. With more than 100,000 people currently waiting for a transplant in the United States, the need for donor organs is far greater than the supply. Living donation offers an alternative for individuals awaiting transplantation.

Section 37.2

Organ Transplant Patients and Fungal Infections

This section includes text excerpted from "Organ Transplant Patients and Fungal Infections," Centers for Disease Control and Prevention (CDC), January 25, 2017.

As an organ transplant patient, you have new opportunities for a healthy and full life. You may also have some new health challenges. One of those challenges is avoiding infections. While anti-rejection medication helps your accept the new organ by lowering your body's immune system response, it can also put you at greater risk for fungal infections.

What You Need to Know about Fungal Infections

Fungal infections can range from mild to life-threatening. Some fungal infections are mild skin rashes, but others can be deadly, like fungal pneumonia. Because of this, it's important to seek treatment as soon as possible to try to avoid serious infection.

Fungal infections can look like bacterial or viral infections. If you're taking medicine to fight a bacterial or viral infection and you aren't getting better, ask your doctor about testing you for a fungal infection.

Fungal infections may be more common in certain types of transplants. Some experts think that fungal infections may be most common in small bowel transplant patients, followed by lung, liver, and heart transplant patients.

Where you live (geography) matters. Some disease-causing fungi are more common in certain parts of the world. If you have had an organ transplant and live in or visit these areas, you're more likely to get these infections than the general population.

Your hospital stay matters. After your transplant, you may need to stay in the hospital for a long time. While there, you may need procedures that can increase your chance of getting a fungal infection.

Fungal infections can happen any time after your surgery. Fungal infections can happen days, weeks, months, or years after the transplant surgery.

Some types of fungal infections are more common than others in solid organ transplant patients. In the United States, invasive candidiasis is most common, followed by aspergillosis and cryptococcosis, but other types of fungal infections are also possible. For lung transplant patients, aspergillosis is most common.

Indoor mold. You may be at higher risk for getting sick from indoor mold.

Preventing Fungal Infections in Organ Transplant Patients

Fungi are difficult to avoid because they are a natural part of the environment. Fungi live outdoors in soil, on plants, trees, and other vegetation. They are also on many indoor surfaces and on your skin. However, there may be some ways you to lower your chance of getting a serious fungal infection.

Learn about fungal infections. There are different types of fungal infections. Learning about them can help you and your healthcare provider recognize the symptoms early, which may prevent serious illness.

Get additional medical care if necessary. Fungal infections often resemble other illnesses. Visiting your healthcare provider may help with faster diagnosis and may prevent serious illness.

Antifungal medication. Your healthcare provider may prescribe medication to prevent fungal infections. Scientists are still learning about which transplant patients are at highest risk and how to best prevent fungal infections.

Protect yourself from the environment. As you recover from your surgery and start doing your normal activities again, there may be some ways to lower your chances of getting a serious fungal infection by trying to avoid disease-causing fungi in the environment. It's important to note that although these actions are recommended, they have not been proven to prevent fungal infections.

- Try to avoid areas with a lot of dust like construction or excavation sites.

- Stay inside during dust storms.

- Stay away from areas with bird and bat droppings. This includes places like chicken coops and caves.

- Wear gloves when handling materials such as soil, moss, or manure.

- Wear shoes, long pants, and a long-sleeved shirt when doing outdoor activities such as gardening, yard work, or visiting wooded areas.

Chapter 38

Emergency, Critical Care, or Traumatic Surgery

Chapter Contents

Section 38.1

Amputation

This section contains text excerpted from the following
sources: Text under the heading "What Is Amputation?" is excerpted
from "Amputation," Office on Women's Health (OWH), U.S.
Department of Health and Human Services (HHS), September 22,
2009. Reviewed June 2017; Text under the heading "Secondary
Complications" is excerpted from "Long-Term Care Following
Traumatic Amputation," U.S. Department of Veterans Affairs
(VA), December 1, 2012. Reviewed June 2017; Text under the
heading "Take Care of Yourself after an Amputation or Other
Surgery" is excerpted from "Take Care of Yourself after an
Amputation or Other Surgery," Centers for Disease Control and
Prevention (CDC), February 18, 2010. Reviewed June 2017;
Text beginning with the heading "Pain Following Amputation"
is excerpted from "VA/DoD Clinical Practice Guideline for the
Management of Upper Extremity Amputation Rehabilitation,"
U.S. Department of Veterans Affairs (VA), 2014.

What Is Amputation?

Amputation is the loss of a body part—usually a finger, toe, arm,
or leg. A traumatic amputation is when a part of your body is completely or partially cut off due to an accident or violence. With surgical
amputation, a limb or part of a limb is removed in a planned operation.
Some people need surgical amputation because of an illness, such as
diabetes or cancer.

You will start physical therapy as soon as possible after your surgery. At first, this involves gentle stretching and exercises to keep
muscles strong and joints healthy and promote good blood flow. Your
therapy will continue as your body heals. Later, you will practice activities such as moving from a bed to a wheelchair or getting dressed.
Therapy can last a long time.

Some people choose to wear a manmade limb, called a prosthesis.
Some prostheses can restore the function of the lost body part. For
example, many people who have had an amputation below the knee can
walk independently with a prosthesis. Some people choose prostheses

for cosmetic reasons. Many people practice with a temporary prosthesis before receiving a permanent one. Prosthetic fitting and adjustment can take time, but is important. A prosthesis that does not fit well can lead to inactivity or limited use.

Recovery from amputation can be a hard journey. Feelings of sadness, anger, and frustration are common. People who have limb loss are at higher risk of depression. People who have limb loss and chronic illness, such as diabetes, are even more likely to be depressed. If recovering from amputation is a struggle for you, talk to your doctor. Treatment with medicine or counseling can help you get through this tough time. Family and caregiver support can also help. Meeting with someone who has had an amputation and now uses a prosthesis can be very motivating.

Secondary Complications

Amputation of one or more limbs has a longitudinal impact on many areas outside of the residual limb itself. The two areas most commonly affected are the musculoskeletal and the cardiovascular systems. Many of the considerations in these areas gradually progress or worsen over time, whereas other conditions may be more intermittent. These conditions highlight the importance of comprehensive prevention strategies including proper nutrition, exercise, tobacco cessation, and wellness counseling for individuals with amputations. Wellness promotion and preventive measures should be part of one's lifestyle. Medical monitoring and education should be routine in amputation clinics and rehabilitation services.

Take Care of Yourself after an Amputation or Other Surgery

Any wound or cut from amputation or surgery can get infected. This happens when germs or dirt enters your body through an opening in your skin. After your surgery, pay attention to your body and watch for these problems that infections can cause:

- warmth
- redness and swelling
- white or yellow pus coming out of the wound or cut
- red lines under your skin running up towards your chest from the wound or cut

- sudden increase in pain

- soreness or tenderness that hurts a lot

Take good care of the part of your limb that's left; take special care of the cut where the limb was removed. Infection can lead to problems, a need for more surgeries, or even death. If you think you're getting an infection, take care of it as soon as you can. Follow the instructions your nurse or doctor gave you. If you're taking antibiotics, take all the pills, even if the redness or soreness gets better or goes away. Try to rest whenever possible. Put your limb up higher than your chest, if you can. This will help it heal. Seek medical help right quickly if you have any of these things:

- cold or cool skin or limb

- wound or area that smells bad

- feeling very tired or achy

- sore or cut has thick brown or gray discharge

- or skin around the sore or cut turns black or ugly

Remember, the best way to handle an infection is to stop it before it starts. Here are some things you can do:

- Wash your limb with mild soap and clean water, then rinse and pat dry. Do this every day or more if you sweat a lot or if it's red or sore.

- Wash anything that touches your skin, like socks, with mild soap and clean water, then rinse and dry. Don't put a wet sock or other cloth on your arm or leg.

- Use lotion to avoid flaking, peeling, and dry skin. Apply lotion at night, before going to bed. If you don't have any lotion, use fresh vegetable cooking oil, for example coconut or olive oil. Never use lard or used cooking oil.

- Eat healthy foods and drink plenty of water to keep your skin healthy.

Pain Following Amputation

There are several different types of pain that may be experienced after amputation, including:

- Immediate post-surgical pain: Pain experienced after any surgery where skin, muscle, bone, and nerves are cut.

- Residual limb pain (RLP): Pain that occurs specifically in the remaining tissue of the amputated limb. It is an expected symptom following amputation. This pain can reappear later due to poor prosthetic socket fit, bruising of the limb, chafing or rubbing of the skin, and other factors.

- Phantom limb pain (PLP): Pain in the missing part of the limb. It is the most difficult postamputation pain to manage as it is not well understood.

- Phantom limb sensations (PLS): Non-painful sensory perceptions that the amputated limb is still there, thus the term phantom limb. These are common and may be present throughout your lifetime.

- Associated musculoskeletal pain: Pain that occurs in body regions other than the amputated limb, such as the back, shoulder, or opposite limb and may be related to overuse/compensatory motions or fit and use of the prosthesis. These may be aggravated by your job, environment, and advancing age.

Pain Management

Due to the variety of pain symptoms following upper limb loss, multiple treatment approaches may result in the best outcome. Medications, as well as other treatment approaches, should be considered. Ask your doctor what medications can be prescribed to help with your pain as well as if there are other appropriate treatment options available. Always follow up with your doctor to assure your treatment regimen is both safe and effective.

Section 38.2

Chest Tube Thoracostomy

This section contains text excerpted from the following sources: Text in this section begins with excerpts from "Problems and Prevention: Chest Tube Insertion," Agency for Healthcare Research and Quality (AHRQ), U.S. Department of Health and Human Services (HHS), October 2014; Text beginning with the heading "Drainage Tube Placement" is excerpted from "IR Drainage Tube Placement," National Institutes of Health (NIH), September 2013. Reviewed June 2017.

If chest tubes are inserted incorrectly, patients can suffer adverse outcomes and even fatal complications, and clinicians can be exposed to injury or infection.

Chest tube insertion is a life-saving procedure used to relieve tension pneumothorax or hemothorax, the accumulation of air or blood (fluid) under pressure in the pleural space, seen most often in trauma patients. If performed incorrectly, patients can suffer adverse outcomes and even fatal complications, and clinicians can be exposed to injury or infection. Major sources of adverse outcomes include breaks in sterile technique, inadequate anesthesia, incorrect insertion techniques, and inadequate self-protection by clinicians.

Drainage Tube Placement

A drainage tube placement procedure removes fluid, infection, or air from your body. This procedure is called "minimally invasive" because the doctor will use small, spaghetti-like tubes (catheters) and wires—it is not surgery. However, potential complications may include bleeding, infection or pain. If you are scheduled for a "chest tube" placement to remove air or fluid from around your lung, you may have a chest X-ray done before you return to your room.

Preparation

What your doctor or healthcare provider will need to do or place orders for:

- A History and Physical (H&P) to be written no more than 30 days before the procedure
- Blood work including a CBC, Acute Care Panel, and Coags within 7 days of the procedure

What you will need to do:

- If you take aspirin, ibuprofen (Motrin), naproxen (Aleve) or blood-thinning medicines, ask your doctor at least a week before the procedure if you should continue taking them.
- Please do not eat anything after midnight on the day of the procedure. Please ask your doctor if you may drink a sip of clear liquids such as water, clear tea, or black coffee up to 2 hours before your procedure,
- Please ask your doctor if you should take your regular medications, at their usual time, with a sip of water before your procedure.

During the procedure, the radiologist may give you contrast dye through an intravenous (I.V.) catheter. This dye helps the radiologist see your blood vessels on X-rays so that he or she can place the catheter.

If you are allergic to I.V. contrast, you may need to take some medications before the procedure. These medications will enable you to receive the I.V. contrast safely. Your doctor will probably ask you to take these medications several times during the day before the procedure, often starting 13 hours before the procedure.

You may be asked to take these medications on one of these schedules:

- Prednisone by mouth, 13 hours before the procedure
- Prednisone by mouth, 7 hours before the procedure plus prednisone and benadryl (diphenhydramine) by mouth 1 hour before the procedure
- Prednisone and Benadryl (diphenhydramine) by mouth 1 hour before the procedure.

Note for patients with diabetes: If you take a medication for diabetes made with metformin, you must stop this medication for 48 hours after the procedure, and have a BUN/creatinine (blood work) to assess your kidney function BEFORE restarting this medicine. Your doctor will talk to you about the need to take other diabetes medications.

Immediately before the Procedure

When you arrive in Interventional Radiology, the radiologist and nurse will discuss the procedure with you and answer your questions. You will be asked to sign a consent form giving them permission to perform the procedure. Then, you will change into a hospital gown, if you are not already in one.

During the Procedure

- Any procedure where the skin is broken has a risk of infection or bleeding. To reduce these problems, your blood work will be checked to ensure your clotting function is adequate and cleanse your skin with antiseptic soap to decrease the risk of infection.

- An I.V. may be started, unless you already have one.

- Your nurse and/or interventional radiology technologist applies monitors to assess your "vital signs" (heart rhythm, breathing and blood pressure). Your skin is cleansed and draped with sterile towels. Do not touch the cleansed site or towels.

- You receive local anesthesia (numbing medicine) at the catheter insertion site. You may receive moderate sedation, medications given IV to keep you comfortable and relaxed.

- Your nurse monitors you throughout the procedure.

- The radiologist uses ultrasound and fluoroscopy (real-time X-Ray) to assist in visualizing the catheter placement for the procedure. The procedure generally lasts 1-2 hours or slightly more, depending upon the complexity of the procedure.

- The radiologist places a small spaghetti-like tube (catheter) into the area that needs to be drained.

- After the drainage tube is placed and secured with a stitch and a dressing is applied over the site.

After the Procedure

- You will return to your room on a stretcher or in a wheelchair, depending on the drainage catheter insertion site and how you feel.

- You should remain on bed rest or chair-rest, generally for 2 to 4 hours.

- Your nurse will check the site for bleeding, swelling and pain frequently while you are resting.

- Slowly resume your diet.

- Rest today and limit your physical activity.

- If you received sedation or anesthesia, do not drive a car, operate machinery, make legal/important decisions, or drink alcoholic beverages for at least 24 hours.

- Discuss with your physician when you should resume taking aspirin, ibuprofen (Motrin), naproxen (Aleve) or blood thinners.

- If you had a chest tube placed, the tube will be placed to a special container which may be attached to a suction tube on the wall of your room.

- If you had a chest tube placed, do not fly for several days (generally 2 to 3 days) after the tube is removed. Please discuss this with your doctor or primary care team.

Special Instructions

Notify your nurse or physician if you have any of these symptoms.

- Increasing redness, bleeding or swelling at the site

- Increasing or severe pain

- Weakness or dizziness

- Shortness of breath

- Difficulty breathing

- Fever/chills

If you have symptoms that you feel are significant or severe, and you cannot contact your primary care team, call 911 or go to your nearest Emergency Room.

Part Four

Managing Pain and Surgical Complications

Chapter 39

Pain Control and Surgery

You've probably been in pain at one time or another. Maybe you've had a headache or bruise—pain that doesn't last too long. But, many older people have ongoing pain from health problems like arthritis, cancer, diabetes, or shingles. They may even have many different kinds of pain.

Pain can be your body's way of warning you that something is wrong. Always tell the doctor where you hurt and exactly how it feels.

Acute Pain and Chronic Pain

There are two kinds of pain. Acute pain begins suddenly, lasts for a short time, and goes away as your body heals. You might feel acute pain after surgery or if you have a broken bone, infected tooth, or kidney stone.

Pain that lasts for several months or years is called chronic (or persistent) pain. This pain often affects older people. Examples include rheumatoid arthritis (RA) and sciatica. In some cases, chronic pain

---

This chapter contains text excerpted from the following sources: Text in this chapter begins with excerpts from "Pain: You Can Get Help," National Institute on Aging (NIA), National Institutes of Health (NIH), May 2015; Text beginning with the heading "What Happens If I Stop Medicines Suddenly?" is excerpted from "Tips for Decreasing Pain Medications after Surgery," U.S. Department of Veterans Affairs (VA), July 3, 2016; Text under the heading "Opioid Addiction" is excerpted from "Prescription Pain Medications (Opioids)," National Institute on Drug Abuse (NIDA) for Teens, May 30, 2017.

follows after acute pain from an injury or other health issue has gone away, like postherpetic neuralgia after shingles.

Living with any type of pain can be very hard. It can cause many other problems. For instance, pain can:

- Get in the way of your daily activities.

- Disturb your sleep and eating habits.

- Make it difficult to continue working.

- Cause depression or anxiety.

Describing Pain

Many people have a hard time describing pain. Think about these questions when you explain how the pain feels:

- Where does it hurt?

- When did it start? Does the pain come and go?

- What does it feel like? Is the pain sharp, dull, or burning? Would you use some other word to describe it?

- Do you have other symptoms?

- When do you feel the pain? In the morning? In the evening? After eating?

- Is there anything you do that makes the pain feel better or worse? For example, does using a heating pad or ice pack help? Does changing your position from lying down to sitting up make it better? Have you tried any over-the-counter medications for it?

Your doctor or nurse may ask you to rate your pain on a scale of 0 to 10, with 0 being no pain and 10 being the worst pain you can imagine. Or, your doctor may ask if the pain is mild, moderate, or severe. Some doctors or nurses have pictures of faces that show different expressions of pain. You point to the face that shows how you feel.

Attitudes about Pain

Everyone reacts to pain differently. Many older people have been told not to talk about their aches and pains. Some people feel they should be brave and not complain when they hurt. Other people are quick to report pain and ask for help.

Worrying about pain is a common problem. This worry can make you afraid to stay active, and it can separate you from your friends and family. Working with your doctor, you can find ways to continue to take part in physical and social activities despite being in pain.

Some people put off going to the doctor because they think pain is just part of aging and nothing can help. This is not true! It is important to see a doctor if you have a new pain. Finding a way to manage your pain is often easier if it is addressed early.

Treating Pain

Treating, or managing, chronic pain is important. The good news is that there are ways to care for pain. Some treatments involve medications, and some do not. Your doctor may make a treatment plan that is specific for your needs.

Most treatment plans do not just focus on reducing pain. They also include ways to support daily function while living with pain.

Pain doesn't always go away overnight. Talk with your doctor about how long it may take before you feel better. Often, you have to stick with a treatment plan before you get relief. It's important to stay on a schedule. Sometimes this is called "staying ahead" or "keeping on top" of your pain. As your pain lessens, you can likely become more active and will see your mood lift and sleep improve.

Medicines to Treat Pain

Your doctor may prescribe one or more of the following pain medications:

- **Acetaminophen** may help all types of pain, especially mild to moderate pain. Acetaminophen is found in over-the-counter and prescription medicines. People who drink a lot of alcohol or who have liver disease should not take acetaminophen. Be sure to talk with your doctor about whether it is safe for you to take and what would be the right dose.

- **Nonsteroidal anti-inflammatory drugs (NSAIDs)** include medications like aspirin, naproxen, and ibuprofen. Some types of NSAIDs can cause side effects, like internal bleeding, which make them unsafe for many older adults. For instance, you may not be able to take ibuprofen if you have high blood pressure or had a stroke. Talk to your doctor before taking NSAIDs to see if they are safe for you.

- **Narcotics** (also called opioids) are used for severe pain and require a doctor's prescription. They may be habit-forming. Examples of narcotics are codeine, morphine, and oxycodone.

- **Other medications** are sometimes used to treat pain. These include antidepressants, anticonvulsive medicines, local pain-killers like nerve blocks or patches, and ointments and creams.

As people age, they are at risk for developing more serious side effects from medication. It's important to take exactly the amount of pain medicine your doctor prescribes.

Mixing any pain medication with alcohol or other drugs, such as tranquilizers, can be dangerous. Make sure your doctor knows all the medicines you take, including over-the-counter drugs and herbal supplements, as well as the amount of alcohol you drink.

If you think the medicine is not working, don't change it on your own. Talk to your doctor or nurse. You might say, "I've been taking the medication as you directed, but it still hurts too much to play with my grandchildren. Is there anything else I can try?"

Pain Specialist

Some doctors receive extra training in pain management. If you find that your regular doctor can't help you, ask him or her for the name of a pain medicine specialist. You also can ask for suggestions from friends and family, a nearby hospital, or your local medical society.

What Other Treatments Help with Pain?

In addition to drugs, there are a variety of complementary and alternative approaches that may provide relief. Talk to your doctor about these treatments. It may take both medicine and other treatments to feel better.

- Acupuncture uses hair-thin needles to stimulate specific points on the body to relieve pain.

- Biofeedback helps you learn to control your heart rate, blood pressure, and muscle tension. This may help reduce your pain and stress level.

- Cognitive behavioral therapy is a form of short-term counseling that may help reduce your reaction to pain.

- Distraction can help you cope with pain by learning new skills that may take your mind off your discomfort.

- Electrical nerve stimulation uses electrical impulses in order to relieve pain.

- Guided imagery uses directed thoughts to create mental pictures that may help you relax, manage anxiety, sleep better, and have less pain.

- Hypnosis uses focused attention to help manage pain.

- Massage therapy can release tension in tight muscles.

- Physical therapy uses a variety of techniques to help manage everyday activities with less pain and teaches you ways to improve flexibility and strength.

Helping Yourself

There are things you can do yourself that might help you feel better. Try to:

- Keep a healthy weight. Putting on extra pounds can slow healing and make some pain worse. Keeping a healthy weight might help with knee pain, or pain in the back, hips, or feet.

- Be active. Try to keep moving. Pain might make you inactive, which can lead to a cycle of more pain and loss of function. Mild activity can help.

- Get enough sleep. It will improve healing and your mood.

- Avoid tobacco, caffeine, and alcohol. They can get in the way of your treatment and increase your pain.

- Join a pain support group. Sometimes, it can help to talk to other people about how they deal with pain. You can share your ideas and thoughts while learning from others.

- Participate in activities you enjoy. Taking part in activities that you find relaxing, like listening to music or doing art, might help take your mind off of some of the pain.

What Happens If I Stop Medicines Suddenly?

If you stop taking opioid pain meds suddenly, you may have symptoms of withdrawal 6–24 hours later, which can include:

- Shaking

- Fever/sweating for no reason

- Nausea (wanting to throw up)

- Vomiting (throwing up)

- Diarrhea

- More pain

- Feeling worried

- Feeling irritable

- Trouble sleeping or very tired

To Wean Off Medication Given for Surgery

There are two parts:

1. Increase the amount of time between doses.

    For example, if you are taking a pain med every 4 hours, stretch the time between doses:

    - Take same dose every 5–6 hours for 5–7 days.

    - Then, take same dose every 7–8 hours for 5–7 days.

2. Decrease the dose.

    For example, if you are taking 2 pills at a time, start taking 1 pill each time for 5–7 days.

    - If taking 1 pill each time, cut pill in half and only take a half each dose for 5–7 days.

    - Then, try to stop taking the medication completely.

Opioid Addiction

Prescription opioids usually come in pill form and are given to treat severe pain—for example, pain from dental surgery, serious sports injuries, or cancer. Opioids are also commonly prescribed to treat other kinds of pain that lasts a long time (chronic pain), but it is unclear if they are effective for long-term pain.

For most people, when opioids are taken as prescribed by a medical professional for a short time, they are relatively safe and can reduce pain effectively. However, dependence and addiction are still potential risks when taking prescription opioids. Dependence means you feel withdrawal symptoms when not taking the drug. Continued use can

can lead to addiction, where you continue to use despite negative consequences. These risks increase when these medications are misused. Prescription medications are some of the most commonly misused drugs by teens, after tobacco, alcohol, and marijuana.

Chapter 40

Assisted Breathing and Surgery

The Ventilator

A ventilator is a machine that supports breathing. These machines mainly are used in hospitals.

Ventilators:

- Get oxygen into the lungs.

- Remove carbon dioxide from the body. (Carbon dioxide is a waste gas that can be toxic.)

- Help people breathe easier.

- Breathe for people who have lost all ability to breathe on their own.

A ventilator often is used for short periods, such as during surgery when you're under general anesthesia. The term "anesthesia" refers to a loss of feeling and awareness. General anesthesia temporarily puts you to sleep. The medicines used to induce anesthesia can disrupt normal breathing. A ventilator helps make sure that you continue

This chapter includes text excerpted from "Ventilator/Ventilator Support," National Heart, Lung, and Blood Institute (NHLBI), February 1, 2011. Reviewed June 2017.

breathing during surgery. A ventilator also may be used during treatment for a serious lung disease or other condition that affects normal breathing.

Some people may need to use ventilators long term or for the rest of their lives. In these cases, the machines can be used outside of the hospital—in long-term care facilities or at home. A ventilator doesn't treat a disease or condition. It's used only for life support.

Who Needs a Ventilator?

Ventilators most often are used:

- During surgery if you're under anesthesia (that is, if you're given medicine that makes you sleep and/or causes a loss of feeling)

- If a disease or condition impairs your lung function

During Surgery

If you have general anesthesia during surgery, you'll likely be connected to a ventilator. The medicines used to induce anesthesia can disrupt normal breathing. A ventilator helps make sure that you continue breathing during surgery.

After surgery, you may not even know you were connected to a ventilator. The only sign may be a slight sore throat for a short time. The sore throat is caused by the tube that connects the ventilator to your airway. Once the anesthesia wears off and you begin breathing on your own, the ventilator is disconnected. The tube in your throat also is taken out. This usually happens before you completely wake up from surgery.

However, depending on the type of surgery you have, you could stay on a ventilator for a few hours to several days after your surgery. Most people who have anesthesia during surgery only need a ventilator for a short time, though.

For Impaired Lung Function

You may need a ventilator if a disease, condition, or other factor has impaired your breathing. Although you might be able to breathe on your own, it's very hard work. You may feel short of breath and uncomfortable. A ventilator can help ease the work of breathing. People who can't breathe on their own also use ventilators.

Many diseases, conditions, and factors can affect lung function. Examples include:

- Pneumonia and other infections.

- Chronic obstructive pulmonary disease (COPD) or other lung diseases.

- Upper spinal cord injuries, polio, amyotrophic lateral sclerosis (ALS), myasthenia gravis, and other diseases or factors that affect the nerves and muscles involved in breathing.

- Brain injury or stroke.

- Drug overdose.

A ventilator helps you breathe until you recover. If you can't recover enough to breathe on your own, you may need a ventilator for the rest of your life.

How a Ventilator Works

Ventilators blow air—or air with extra oxygen—into the airways and then the lungs. The airways are pipes that carry oxygen-rich air to your lungs. They also carry carbon dioxide, a waste gas, out of your lungs.

The airways include your:

- nose and linked air passages, called nasal cavities

- mouth

- larynx, or voice box

- trachea, or windpipe

- tubes called bronchial tubes or bronchi, and their branches

A ventilator blows air into your airways through a breathing tube. One end of the tube is inserted into your windpipe and the other end is attached to the ventilator. The breathing tube serves as an airway by letting air and oxygen from the ventilator flow into the lungs.

The process of inserting the tube into your windpipe is called intubation. Usually, the breathing tube is put into your windpipe through your nose or mouth. The tube is then moved down into your throat. A tube placed like this is called an endotracheal tube. In an emergency, you're given medicine to make you sleepy and ease the pain of the breathing tube being put into your windpipe. If it's not an emergency, the procedure is done in an operating room using anesthesia. (That is, you're given medicine that makes you sleep and/or causes a loss of feeling.)

An endotracheal tube is held in place by tape or with an endotracheal tube holder. This holder often is a strap that fits around the head. Sometimes the breathing tube is placed through a surgically made hole called a tracheostomy. The hole goes through the front of your neck and into your windpipe. The tube put into the hole sometimes is called a "trach" tube. The procedure to make a tracheostomy usually is done in an operating room. Anesthesia is used, so you won't be awake or feel any pain. Specially made ties or bands that go around the neck hold the trach tube in place.

Both types of breathing tubes pass through your vocal cords and affect your ability to talk. For the most part, endotracheal tubes are used for people who are on ventilators for shorter periods. The advantage of this tube is that it can be placed in an airway without surgery. Trach tubes are used for people who need ventilators for longer periods. For people who are awake, this tube is more comfortable than the endotracheal tube. Under certain conditions, a person who has a trach tube may be able to talk.

A ventilator uses pressure to blow air or a mixture of gases (like oxygen and air) into the lungs. This pressure is known as positive pressure. You usually exhale (breathe out) the air on your own, but sometimes the ventilator does this for you too. A ventilator can be set to "breathe" a set number of times a minute. Sometimes it's set so that you can trigger the machine to blow air into your lungs. But, if you fail to trigger it within a certain amount of time, the machine automatically blows air to keep you breathing.

Rarely, doctors recommend a ventilator called a chest shell. This type of ventilator works like an iron lung—an early ventilator used by many polio patients in the last century. However, the chest shell isn't as bulky and confining as the iron lung.

The chest shell fits snugly to the outside of your chest. A machine creates a vacuum between the shell and the chest wall. This causes your chest to expand, and air is sucked into your lungs. No breathing tube is used with a chest shell. When the vacuum is released, your chest falls back into place and the air in your lungs comes out. This cycle of vacuum and release is set at a normal breathing rate.

What to Expect While on a Ventilator

Ventilators normally don't cause pain. The breathing tube in your airway may cause some discomfort. It also affects your ability to talk and eat. If your breathing tube is a trach tube, you may be able to talk. (A trach tube is put directly into your windpipe through a hole in the front of your neck). Instead of food, your healthcare team may give you nutrients through a tube inserted into a vein. If you're on a ventilator for a long time, you'll likely get food through a nasogastric, or feeding, tube. The tube goes through your nose or mouth or directly into your stomach or small intestine through a surgically made hole.

A ventilator greatly restricts your activity and also limits your movement. You may be able to sit up in bed or in a chair, but you usually can't move around much.

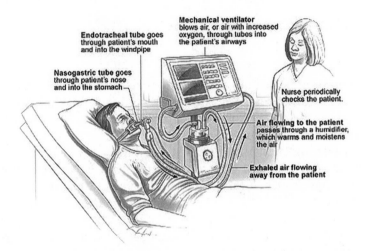

Figure 40.1. *Patient on a Ventilator*

The illustration shows a standard setup for a ventilator in a hospital room. The ventilator pushes warm, moist air (or air with increased oxygen) to the patient. Exhaled air flows away from the patient.

If you need to use a ventilator long term, you may be given a portable machine. This machine allows you to move around and even go outside, although you need to bring your ventilator with you. Sometimes the ventilator is set so that you can trigger the machine to blow air into your lungs. But, if you fail to trigger it within a certain amount of time, the machine automatically blows air to keep you breathing.

Ongoing Care

While you're on a ventilator, your healthcare team will closely watch you. The team may include doctors, nurses, and respiratory therapists.

You may need periodic chest X-rays and blood tests to check the levels of oxygen and carbon dioxide (blood gases) in your body. These tests help your healthcare team find out how well the ventilator is working for you. Based on the test results, they may adjust the ventilator's airflow and other settings as needed.

Also, a nurse or respiratory therapist will suction your breathing tube from time to time. This helps remove mucus from your lungs. Suctioning will cause you to cough, and you may feel short of breath for several seconds. You may get extra oxygen during suctioning to relieve shortness of breath.

Risks of Being on a Ventilator

Infections

One of the most serious and common risks of being on a ventilator is pneumonia. The breathing tube that's put in your airway can allow bacteria to enter your lungs. As a result, you may develop ventilator-associated pneumonia (VAP).

The breathing tube also makes it hard for you to cough. Coughing helps clear your airways of lung irritants that can cause infections. VAP is a major concern for people using ventilators because they're often already very sick. Pneumonia may make it harder to treat their other disease or condition. VAP is treated with antibiotics. You may need special antibiotics if the VAP is caused by bacteria that are resistant to standard treatment.

Another risk of being on a ventilator is a sinus infection. This type of infection is more common in people who have endotracheal tubes. (An endotracheal tube is put into your windpipe through your mouth or nose.) Sinus infections are treated with antibiotics.

Other Risks

Using a ventilator also can put you at risk for other problems, such as:

- **Pneumothorax.** This is a condition in which air leaks out of the lungs and into the space between the lungs and the chest wall. This can cause pain and shortness of breath, and it may cause one or both lungs to collapse.

- **Lung damage.** Pushing air into the lungs with too much pressure can harm the lungs.

- **Oxygen toxicity.** High levels of oxygen can damage the lungs.

These problems may occur because of the forced airflow or high levels of oxygen from the ventilator. Using a ventilator also can put you at risk for blood clots and serious skin infections. These problems tend to occur in people who have certain diseases and/or who are confined to bed or a wheelchair and must remain in one position for long periods. Another possible problem is damage to the vocal cords from the breathing tube. If you find it hard to speak or breathe after your breathing tube is removed, let your doctor know.

What to Expect When You're Taken Off of a Ventilator

"Weaning" is the process of taking you off of a ventilator so that you can start to breathe on your own. People usually are weaned after they've recovered enough from the problem that caused them to need the ventilator. Weaning usually begins with a short trial. You stay connected to the ventilator, but you're given a chance to breathe on your own. Most people are able to breathe on their own the first time weaning is tried. Once you can successfully breathe on your own, the ventilator is stopped. If you can't breathe on your own during the short trial, weaning will be tried at a later time. If repeated weaning attempts over a long time don't work, you may need to use the ventilator long term. After you're weaned, the breathing tube is removed. You may cough while this is happening. Your voice may be hoarse for a short time after the tube is removed.

Chapter 41

Managing Blood Loss with Blood Transfusions

Blood Transfusion

A blood transfusion is a safe, common procedure in which blood is given to you through an intravenous (IV) line in one of your blood vessels.

Blood transfusions are done to replace blood lost during surgery or due to a serious injury. A transfusion also may be done if your body can't make blood properly because of an illness. During a blood transfusion, a small needle is used to insert an IV line into one of your blood vessels. Through this line, you receive healthy blood. The procedure usually takes 1 to 4 hours, depending on how much blood you need.

Blood transfusions are very common. Each year, almost 5 million Americans need a blood transfusion. Most blood transfusions go well. Mild complications can occur. Very rarely, serious problems develop.

Important Information about Blood

The heart pumps blood through a network of arteries and veins throughout the body. Blood has many vital jobs. It carries oxygen and

This chapter includes text excerpted from "Blood Transfusion," National Heart, Lung, and Blood Institute (NHLBI), January 30, 2012. Reviewed June 2017.

other nutrients to your body's organs and tissues. Having a healthy supply of blood is important to your overall health. Blood is made up of various parts, including red blood cells, white blood cells, platelets, and plasma. Blood is transfused either as whole blood (with all its parts) or, more often, as individual parts.

Blood Types

Every person has one of the following blood types: A, B, AB, or O. Also, every person's blood is either Rh-positive or Rh-negative. So, if you have type A blood, it's either A positive or A negative. The blood used in a transfusion must work with your blood type. If it doesn't, antibodies (proteins) in your blood attack the new blood and make you sick.

Type O blood is safe for almost everyone. About 40 percent of the population has type O blood. People who have this blood type are called universal donors. Type O blood is used for emergencies when there's no time to test a person's blood type. People who have type AB blood are called universal recipients. This means they can get any type of blood. If you have Rh-positive blood, you can get Rh-positive or Rh-negative blood. But if you have Rh-negative blood, you should only get Rh-negative blood. Rh-negative blood is used for emergencies when there's no time to test a person's Rh type.

Blood Banks

Blood banks collect, test, and store blood. They carefully screen all donated blood for possible infectious agents, such as viruses, that could make you sick. Blood bank staff also screen each blood donation to find out whether it's type A, B, AB, or O and whether it's Rh-positive or Rh-negative. Getting a blood type that doesn't work with your own blood type will make you very sick. That's why blood banks are very careful when they test the blood. To prepare blood for a transfusion, some blood banks remove white blood cells. This process is called white cell or leukocyte reduction. Although rare, some people are allergic to white blood cells in donated blood. Removing these cells makes allergic reactions less likely.

Not all transfusions use blood donated from a stranger. If you're going to have surgery, you may need a blood transfusion because of blood loss during the operation. If it's surgery that you're able to schedule months in advance, your doctor may ask whether you would like to use your own blood, rather than donated blood. If you choose to use your own blood, you will need to have blood drawn one or more times prior to the surgery. A blood bank will store your blood for your use.

Alternatives to Blood Transfusions

Researchers are trying to find ways to make blood. There's currently no man-made alternative to human blood. However, researchers have developed medicines that may help do the job of some blood parts. For example, some people who have kidney problems can now take a medicine called erythropoietin that helps their bodies make more red blood cells. This means they may need fewer blood transfusions.

Surgeons try to reduce the amount of blood lost during surgery so that fewer patients need blood transfusions. Sometimes they can collect and reuse the blood for the patient.

Types of Blood Transfusions

Blood is transfused either as whole blood (with all its parts) or, more often, as individual parts. The type of blood transfusion you need depends on your situation. For example, if you have an illness that stops your body from properly making a part of your blood, you may need only that part to treat the illness.

Red Blood Cell Transfusions

Red blood cells are the most commonly transfused part of the blood. These cells carry oxygen from the lungs to your body's organs and tissues. They also help your body get rid of carbon dioxide and other waste products. You may need a transfusion of red blood cells if you've lost blood due to an injury or surgery. You also may need this type of transfusion if you have severe anemia due to disease or blood loss.

Anemia is a condition in which your blood has a lower than normal number of red blood cells. Anemia also can occur if your red blood cells don't have enough hemoglobin. Hemoglobin is an iron-rich protein that gives blood its red color. This protein carries oxygen from the lungs to the rest of the body.

Platelets and Clotting Factor Transfusions

Platelets and clotting factors help stop bleeding, including internal bleeding that you can't see. Some illnesses may cause your body to not make enough platelets or clotting factors. You may need regular transfusions of these parts of your blood to stay healthy. For example, if you have hemophilia, you may need a special clotting factor to replace the clotting factor you're lacking. Hemophilia is a rare, inherited bleeding disorder in which your blood doesn't clot normally.

If you have hemophilia, you may bleed for a longer time than others after an injury or accident. You also may bleed internally, especially in the joints (knees, ankles, and elbows).

Plasma Transfusions

Plasma is the liquid part of your blood. It's mainly water, but also contains proteins, clotting factors, hormones, vitamins, cholesterol, sugar, sodium, potassium, calcium, and more. If you have been badly burned or have liver failure or a severe infection, you may need a plasma transfusion.

Who Needs a Blood Transfusion?

Blood transfusions are very common. Each year, almost five million Americans need blood transfusions. This procedure is used for people of all ages.

Many people who have surgery need blood transfusions because they lose blood during their operations. For example, about one-third of all heart surgery patients have a transfusion. Some people who have serious injuries—such as from car crashes, war, or natural disasters—need blood transfusions to replace blood lost during the injury. Some people need blood or parts of blood because of illnesses.

You may need a blood transfusion if you have:

- A severe infection or liver disease that stops your body from properly making blood or some parts of blood.

- An illness that causes anemia, such as kidney disease or cancer. Medicines or radiation used to treat a medical condition also can cause anemia. There are many types of anemia, including aplastic, Fanconi, hemolytic, iron-deficiency, and sickle cell anemias and thalassemia.

- A bleeding disorder, such as hemophilia or thrombocytopenia.

Before Blood Transfusion

Before a blood transfusion, a technician tests your blood to find out what blood type you have (that is, A, B, AB, or O and Rh-positive or

Rh-negative). He or she pricks your finger with a needle to get a few drops of blood or draws blood from one of your veins. The blood type used in your transfusion must work with your blood type. If it doesn't, antibodies (proteins) in your blood attack the new blood and make you sick. Some people have allergic reactions even when the blood given does work with their own blood type. To prevent this, your doctor may prescribe a medicine to stop allergic reactions. If you have allergies or have had an allergic reaction during a past transfusion, your doctor will make every effort to make sure you're safe. Most people don't need to change their diets or activities before or after a blood transfusion. Your doctor will let you know whether you need to make any lifestyle changes prior to the procedure.

During Blood Transfusion

Blood transfusions take place in either a doctor's office or a hospital. Sometimes they're done at a person's home, but this is less common. Blood transfusions also are done during surgery and in emergency rooms.

A needle is used to insert an intravenous (IV) line into one of your blood vessels. Through this line, you receive healthy blood. The procedure usually takes 1 to 4 hours. The time depends on how much blood you need and what part of the blood you receive.

During the blood transfusion, a nurse carefully watches you, especially for the first 15 minutes. This is when allergic reactions are most likely to occur. The nurse continues to watch you during the rest of the procedure as well.

After Blood Transfusion

After a blood transfusion, your vital signs are checked (such as your temperature, blood pressure, and heart rate). The intravenous (IV) line is taken out. You may have some bruising or soreness for a few days at the site where the IV was inserted.

You may need blood tests that show how your body is reacting to the transfusion. Your doctor will let you know about signs and symptoms to watch for and report.

What Are the Risks of a Blood Transfusion?

Most blood transfusions go very smoothly. However, mild problems and, very rarely, serious problems can occur.

Allergic Reactions

Some people have allergic reactions to the blood given during transfusions. This can happen even when the blood given is the right blood type.

Allergic reactions can be mild or severe. Symptoms can include:

- anxiety

- chest and/or back pain

- trouble breathing

- fever, chills, flushing, and clammy skin

- a quick pulse or low blood pressure

- nausea (feeling sick to the stomach)

A nurse or doctor will stop the transfusion at the first signs of an allergic reaction. The healthcare team determines how mild or severe the reaction is, what treatments are needed, and whether the transfusion can safely be restarted.

Viruses and Infectious Diseases

Some infectious agents, such as human immunodeficiency virus (HIV), can survive in blood and infect the person receiving the blood transfusion. To keep blood safe, blood banks carefully screen donated blood.

The risk of catching a virus from a blood transfusion is very low.

- **HIV.** Your risk of getting HIV from a blood transfusion is lower than your risk of getting killed by lightning. Only about 1 in 2 million donations might carry HIV and transmit HIV if given to a patient.

- **Hepatitis B and C.** The risk of having a donation that carries hepatitis B is about 1 in 205,000. The risk for hepatitis C is 1 in 2 million. If you receive blood during a transfusion that contains hepatitis, you'll likely develop the virus.

- **Variant Creutzfeldt-Jakob disease (vCJD).** This disease is the human version of Mad Cow Disease. It's a very rare, yet fatal brain disorder. There is a possible risk of getting vCJD from a blood transfusion, although the risk is very low. Because of this, people who may have been exposed to vCJD aren't eligible blood donors.

Fever

You may get a sudden fever during or within a day of your blood transfusion. This is usually your body's normal response to white blood cells in the donated blood. Over-the-counter fever medicine usually will treat the fever. Some blood banks remove white blood cells from whole blood or different parts of the blood. This makes it less likely that you will have a reaction after the transfusion.

Iron Overload

Getting many blood transfusions can cause too much iron to buildup in your blood (iron overload). People who have a blood disorder like thalassemia, which requires multiple transfusions, are at risk for iron overload. Iron overload can damage your liver, heart, and other parts of your body. If you have iron overload, you may need iron chelation therapy. For this therapy, medicine is given through an injection or as a pill to remove the extra iron from your body.

Lung Injury

Although it's unlikely, blood transfusions can damage your lungs, making it hard to breathe. This usually occurs within about 6 hours of the procedure. Most patients recover. However, 5 to 25 percent of patients who develop lung injuries die from the injuries. These people usually were very ill before the transfusion. Doctors aren't completely sure why blood transfusions damage the lungs. Antibodies (proteins) that are more likely to be found in the plasma of women who have been pregnant may disrupt the normal way that lung cells work. Because of this risk, hospitals are starting to use men's and women's plasma differently.

Acute Immune Hemolytic Reaction

Acute immune hemolytic reaction is very serious, but also very rare. It occurs if the blood type you get during a transfusion doesn't match or work with your blood type. Your body attacks the new red blood cells, which then produce substances that harm your kidneys. The symptoms include chills, fever, nausea, pain in the chest or back, and dark urine. The doctor will stop the transfusion at the first sign of this reaction.

Delayed Hemolytic Reaction

This is a much slower version of acute immune hemolytic reaction. Your body destroys red blood cells so slowly that the problem can go unnoticed until your red blood cell level is very low. Both acute and delayed hemolytic reactions are most common in patients who have had a previous transfusion.

Graft-versus-Host Disease

Graft-versus-host disease (GVHD) is a condition in which white blood cells in the new blood attack your tissues. GVHD usually is fatal. People who have weakened immune systems are the most likely to get GVHD. Symptoms start within a month of the blood transfusion. They include fever, rash, and diarrhea. To protect against GVHD, people who have weakened immune systems should receive blood that has been treated so the white blood cells can't cause GVHD.

Chapter 42

Infection and Surgery

Chapter Contents

Section 42.1

Surgical Site Infections (SSI)

This section includes text excerpted from "What You
Should Know before Your Surgery," Centers for Disease
Control and Prevention (CDC), March 14, 2016.

Having any type of surgery can be stressful. You might be asking
yourself: What is the recovery process? How long will I be out of work?
What do I do after leaving the hospital or surgery center?

An important question you might not have thought of is: How do I
avoid getting a surgical site infection (SSI)?

What Is Surgical Site Infection (SSI)?

A SSI is an infection patient can get during or after surgery. SSIs
can happen on any part of the body where surgery takes place and can
sometimes involve only the skin. Other SSIs are more serious and can
involve tissues under the skin, organs, or implanted material.

These infections can make recovery from surgery more difficult
because they can cause additional complications, stress, and medical
cost. It is important that healthcare providers, patients, and loved
ones work together to prevent these infections.

Ensure Cleanliness of the Surgical Site

Patients should expect safe healthcare everywhere care is given,
including doctor's offices, surgery centers, physical/occupational clinics,
and other outpatient care practices. The healthcare providers need to
ensure that the surgical site is clean. They can:

- Clean their hands and arms up to the elbows with an antiseptic
  agent just before the surgery.

- Wear hair covers, masks, gowns, and gloves during surgery to
  keep the surgery area clean.

- Give you antibiotics before surgery starts when indicated.

- Clean the skin at the surgery site with a special soap that kills
  germs.

Preventing Surgical Site Infections

- Before your surgery, discuss other health problems, such as diabetes, with your doctor. These issues can affect your surgery and your treatment.

- Quit smoking. Patients who smoke get more infections.

- Follow your doctor's instructions for cleaning your skin before your surgery. For example, if your doctor recommends using a special soap before surgery, make sure you do so.

- Avoid shaving near where you will have surgery. Shaving with a razor can irritate your skin and make it easier to develop an infection. If someone tries to shave you before surgery, ask why this is necessary.

Postsurgery Recommendations to Protect against Surgical Site Infection

- Ask your provider to clean their hands before they examine you or check your wound.

- Do not allow visitors to touch the surgical wound or dressings.

- Ask family and friends to clean their hands before and after visiting you.

- Make sure you understand how to care for your wound before you leave the medical facility.

- Always clean your hands before and after caring for your wound.

- Make sure you know who to contact if you have questions or problems after you get home.

- If you have any symptoms of an infection, such as redness and pain at the surgery site, drainage, or fever, call your doctor immediately.

Section 42.2

Steps to Reduce Healthcare-Associated Infections (HAIs)

This section includes text excerpted from "Healthcare-Associated Infections," Office of Disease Prevention and Health Promotion (ODPHP), U.S. Department of Health and Human Services (HHS), February 6, 2016.

Healthcare-Associated Infections (HAIs)

Healthcare-associated infections (HAIs) are infections that patients get while receiving treatment for medical or surgical conditions, and many HAIs are preventable. Modern healthcare employs many types of invasive devices and procedures to treat patients and to help them recover. Infections can be associated with procedures (like surgery) and the devices used in medical procedures, such as catheters or ventilators. HAIs are important causes of morbidity and mortality in the United States and are associated with a substantial increase in healthcare costs each year. At any one time in the United States, 1 out of every 25 hospitalized patients are affected by an HAI.

HAIs occur in all types of care settings, including:

- Acute care hospitals

- Ambulatory surgical centers

- Dialysis facilities

- Outpatient care (e.g., physicians' offices and healthcare clinics)

- Long-term care facilities (e.g., nursing homes and rehabilitation facilities)

There are two major healthcare-associated infections; central line-associated bloodstream infections (CLABSI) and methicillin-resistant *Staphylococcus aureus* (MRSA) infections.

Common types of HAIs include:

- Catheter-associated urinary tract infections

- Surgical site infections
- Bloodstream infections
- Pneumonia
- *Clostridium difficile*

HAIs: A Significant Source of Complications

HAIs are a significant source of complications across the continuum of care and can be transmitted between different healthcare facilities. However, studies suggest that implementing existing prevention practices can lead to up to a 70 percent reduction in certain HAIs. Likewise, modeling data suggests that substantial reductions in resistant bacteria, like MRSA, can be achieved through coordinated activities between healthcare facilities in a given region. The financial benefit of using these prevention practices is estimated to be $25 billion to $31.5 billion in medical cost savings.

HAIs Risk Factors

Risk factors for HAIs can be grouped into three general categories: medical procedures and antibiotic use, organizational factors, and patient characteristics. The behaviors of healthcare providers and their interactions with the healthcare system also influence the rate of HAIs.

HAIs Prevention

Studies have shown that proper education and training of healthcare workers increases compliance with and adoption of best practices (e.g., infection control, hand hygiene, attention to safety culture, and antibiotic stewardship) to prevent HAIs. Examples of best practices by a healthcare provider include careful insertion, maintenance, and prompt removal of catheters, as well as the careful use of antibiotics. Another example of a best practice is decolonization of patients with an evidence-based method to reduce transmission of MRSA in hospitals.

Research suggests that many of these infections are preventable. Efforts are underway to expand implementation of strategies known to prevent HAIs, advance development of effective prevention tools, and explore new prevention approaches. Many efforts to prevent HAIs have focused on acute care settings. Increasingly, healthcare delivery, including complex procedures, is being shifted to outpatient settings, such as ambulatory surgical centers, end-stage renal disease facilities, and long-term care facilities. These settings often have limited capacity for oversight and infection control compared to hospital-based settings. Because patients with HAIs, including HAIs caused by antibiotic resistance organisms, often move between various types of healthcare facilities, prevention efforts must also expand across the continuum of care. Moreover, the challenges posed by antibiotic-resistant organisms and *C. difficile* are best addressed through coordinated action among healthcare facilities in a given region.

Section 42.3

Catheter-Associated Urinary Tract Infections (CAUTI)

This section contains text excerpted from the following sources: Text in this section begins with excerpts from "Healthcare-Associated Infections (HAI)—Frequently Asked Questions about Catheter-Associated Urinary Tract Infections," Centers for Disease Control and Prevention (CDC), October 2, 2015; Text under the heading "How Common Is UTI?" is excerpted from "Healthcare-Associated Infections (HAI)—Catheter-Associated Urinary Tract Infections (CAUTI)," Centers for Disease Control and Prevention (CDC), October 16, 2015.

A urinary tract infection (UTI) is an infection involving any part of the urinary system, including urethra, bladder, ureters, and kidney. UTIs are the most common type of healthcare-associated infection reported to the National Healthcare Safety Network (NHSN). Among UTIs acquired in the hospital, approximately 75 percent are associated with a urinary catheter, which is a tube inserted into the bladder through the urethra to drain urine. Between 15–25 percent of hospitalized patients receive urinary catheters during their hospital stay. The most important risk factor for developing a catheter-associated UTI (CAUTI) is prolonged use of the urinary catheter. Therefore, catheters should only be used for appropriate indications and should be removed as soon as they are no longer needed.

What Is a Urinary Catheter?

An indwelling urinary catheter is a drainage tube that is inserted into the urinary bladder through the urethra, is left in place, and is connected to a closed collection system. Alternative methods of urinary drainage may be employed in some patients. Intermittent ("in-and-out") catheterization involves brief insertion of a catheter into the bladder through the urethra to drain urine at intervals. An external catheter is a urine containment device that fits over or adheres to the genitalia and is attached to a urinary drainage bag. The most commonly used external catheter is a soft flexible sheath that fits over the penis ("condom" catheter). A suprapubic catheter is surgically inserted into the bladder through an incision above the pubis.

What Is a Urinary Tract Infection (UTI)?

A urinary tract infection (UTI) is an infection that involves any of the organs or structures of the urinary tract, including the kidneys, ureters, bladder, and urethra. Some of the common symptoms of a urinary tract infection are burning or pain in the lower abdomen (that is, below the stomach), fever, burning during urination, or an increase in the frequency of urination. UTIs are the most common type of healthcare-associated infection (HAI) and are most often caused by the placement or presence of a catheter in the urinary tract.

What Is a Catheter-Associated Urinary Tract Infection (CAUTI)?

A catheter-associated urinary tract infection (CAUTI) occurs when germs (usually bacteria) enter the urinary tract through the urinary catheter and cause infection. CAUTIs have been associated with increased morbidity, mortality, healthcare costs, and length of stay. The risk of CAUTI can be reduced by ensuring that catheters are used only when needed and removed as soon as possible; that catheters are placed using proper aseptic technique; and that the closed sterile drainage system is maintained.

Can CAUTIs Be Treated?

Yes, most CAUTIs can be treated with antibiotics and/or removal or change of the catheter. The healthcare provider will determine the best treatment for each patient.

What Are Some of the Things That Hospitals Are Doing to Prevent CAUTIs?

Hospitals should follow the recommendations in the 2009 Centers for Disease Control and Prevention (CDC) *Guideline for Prevention of Catheter-associated Urinary Tract Infections*. The guideline emphasizes the proper use, insertion, and maintenance of urinary catheters in different healthcare settings. It also presents effective quality improvement programs that healthcare facilities can use to prevent CAUTIs.

What Can Patients Do to Help Prevent CAUTI?

Patients with a urinary catheter can take the following precautions to prevent CAUTI:

- Understand why the catheter is needed and ask the healthcare provider frequently if the catheter is still needed.

- If the patient has a long-term catheter, they must clean their hands before and after touching the catheter.

- Check the position of the urine bag; it should always be below the level of the bladder.

- Do not tug or pull on the tubing.

- Do not twist or kink the catheter tubing.

How Common Is UTI?

UTIs are the most common type of healthcare-associated infection reported to the National Healthcare Safety Network (NHSN). Among UTIs acquired in the hospital, approximately 75 percent are associated with a urinary catheter, which is a tube inserted into the bladder through the urethra to drain urine. Between 15–25 percent of hospitalized patients receive urinary catheters during their hospital stay. The most important risk factor for developing a catheter-associated UTI (CAUTI) is prolonged use of the urinary catheter. Therefore, catheters should only be used for appropriate indications and should be removed as soon as they are no longer needed.

Section 42.4

Central Line-Associated Bloodstream Infection (CLABSI)

This section includes text excerpted from "Central Line-Associated Bloodstream Infections: Resources for Patients and Healthcare Providers," Centers for Disease Control and Prevention (CDC), February 7, 2011. Reviewed June 2017.

Central line-associated bloodstream infections (CLABSIs) result in thousands of deaths each year and billions of dollars in added costs to the U.S. healthcare system, yet these infections are preventable. Centers for disease control and prevention (CDC) is providing guidelines and tools to the healthcare community to help end CLABSIs.

Central Line

A central line (also known as a central venous catheter) is a catheter (tube) that doctors often place in a large vein in the neck, chest, or groin to give medication or fluids or to collect blood for medical tests. You may be familiar with intravenous catheters (also known as IVs) that are used frequently to give medicine or fluids into a vein near the skin's surface (usually on the arm or hand), for short periods of time. Central lines are different from IVs because central lines access a major vein that is close to the heart and can remain in place for weeks or months and be much more likely to cause serious infection. Central lines are commonly used in intensive care units.

Central Line-Associated Bloodstream Infection (CLABSI)

A central line-associated bloodstream infection (CLABSI) is a serious infection that occurs when germs (usually bacteria or viruses) enter the bloodstream through the central line. Healthcare providers must follow a strict protocol when inserting the line to make sure the line remains sterile and a CLABSI does not occur. In addition to inserting the central line properly, healthcare providers must use stringent infection control practices each time they check the line or change the dressing. Patients who get a CLABSI have a fever, and might also have red skin and soreness around the central line. If this happens, healthcare providers can do tests to learn if there is an infection present.

Role of Healthcare Provider in Preventing CLABSI

Healthcare providers can take the following steps to help prevent CLABSIs:

- Follow recommended central line insertion practices to prevent infection when the central line is placed, including:
  - Perform hand hygiene
  - Apply appropriate skin antiseptic
  - Ensure that the skin prep agent has completely dried before inserting the central line
  - Use all five maximal sterile barrier precautions:
    - Sterile gloves
    - Sterile gown
    - Cap
    - Mask
    - Large sterile drape
- Once the central line is in place:
  - Follow recommended central line maintenance practices
  - Wash their hands with soap and water or an alcohol-based hand rub before and after touching the line
- Remove a central line as soon as it is no longer needed. The sooner a catheter is removed, the less likely the chance of infection.

Role of Patients in Preventing CLABSI

Here are some ways patients can protect themselves from CLABSI:

- Research the hospital, if possible, to learn about its CLABSI rate.
- Speak up about any concerns so that healthcare personnel are reminded to follow the best infection prevention practices.

- Ask a healthcare provider if the central line is absolutely necessary. If so, ask them to help you understand the need for it and how long it will be in place.

- Pay attention to the bandage and the area around it. If the bandage comes off or if the bandage or area around it is wet or dirty, tell a healthcare worker right away.

- Don't get the central line or the central line insertion site wet.

- Tell a healthcare worker if the area around the catheter is sore or red or if the patient has a fever or chills.

- Do not let any visitors touch the catheter or tubing.

- The patient should avoid touching the tubing as much as possible.

- In addition, everyone visiting the patient must wash their hands—before and after they visit.

Section 42.5

Clostridium difficile (C. difficile) *Infections*

This section includes text excerpted from "Healthcare-Associated Infections—*Clostridium difficile* Infection Information for Patients," Centers for Disease Control and Prevention (CDC), February 24, 2015.

Clostridium difficile (*C. difficile*) is a bacterium that causes inflammation of the colon, known as colitis. People who have other illnesses or conditions requiring prolonged use of antibiotics, and the elderly, are at greater risk of acquiring this disease. The bacteria are found in the feces. People can become infected if they touch items or surfaces that are contaminated with feces and then touch their mouth or mucous membranes. Healthcare workers can spread the bacteria to patients or contaminate surfaces through hand contact.

General Information about Clostridium difficile (C. difficile)

Clostridium difficile (*C. difficile*) is a bacterium that causes inflammation of the colon, known as colitis.

People who have other illnesses or conditions requiring prolonged use of antibiotics, and the elderly, are at greater risk of acquiring this disease. The bacteria are found in the feces. People can become infected if they touch items or surfaces that are contaminated with feces and then touch their mouth or mucous membranes. Healthcare workers can spread the bacteria to patients or contaminate surfaces through hand contact.

Symptoms of C. difficile

Symptoms include:

- Watery diarrhea (at least three bowel movements per day for two or more days)
- Fever
- Loss of appetite
- Nausea
- Abdominal pain/tenderness

Transmission of C. difficile

Clostridium difficile is shed in feces. Any surface, device, or material (e.g., toilets, bathing tubs, and electronic rectal thermometers) that becomes contaminated with feces may serve as a reservoir for the *Clostridium difficile* spores. *Clostridium difficile* spores are transferred to patients mainly via the hands of healthcare personnel who have touched a contaminated surface or item. *Clostridium difficile* can live for long periods on surfaces.

Treatment of C. difficile Infection

Whenever possible, other antibiotics should be discontinued; in a small number of patients, diarrhea may go away when other antibiotics are stopped. Treatment of primary infection caused by *C. difficile* is an antibiotic such as metronidazole, vancomycin, or fidaxomicin. While metronidazole is not approved for treating *C. difficile* infections by the U.S. Food and Drug Administration (FDA), it has been commonly recommended and used for mild *C. difficile* infections; however, it should not be used for severe *C. difficile* infections. Whenever possible, treatment should be given by mouth and continued for a minimum of 10 days.

One problem with antibiotics used to treat primary *C. difficile* infection is that the infection returns in about 20 percent of patients. In a small number of these patients, the infection returns over and over and can be quite debilitating. While a first return of a *C. difficile* infection is usually treated with the same antibiotic used for primary infection, all future infections should be managed with oral vancomycin or fidaxomicin.

Transplanting stool from a healthy person to the colon of a patient with repeat *C. difficile* infections has been shown to successfully treat *C. difficile*. These "fecal transplants" appear to be the most effective method for helping patients with repeat *C. difficile* infections. This procedure may not be widely available and its longterm safety has not been established.

Section 42.6

Methicillin-Resistant Staphylococcus aureus *(MRSA)* Infections

This section includes text excerpted from "Methicillin-Resistant *Staphylococcus aureus* (MRSA)—General Information about MRSA in the Community," Centers for Disease Control and Prevention (CDC), February 9, 2016.

MRSA is methicillin-resistant *Staphylococcus aureus*, a type of staph bacteria that is resistant to several antibiotics. In the general community, MRSA most often causes skin infections. In some cases, it causes pneumonia (lung infection) and other issues. If left untreated, MRSA infections can become severe and cause sepsis—a life-threatening reaction to severe infection in the body.

In a healthcare setting, such as a hospital or nursing home, MRSA can cause severe problems such as bloodstream infections, pneumonia and surgical site infections.

Symptoms of *Methicillin-Resistant* Staphylococcus aureus *(MRSA)*

Sometimes, people with MRSA skin infections first think they have a spider bite. However, unless a spider is actually seen, the irritation is likely not a spider bite. Most staph skin infections, including MRSA, appear as a bump or infected area on the skin that might be:

- red

- swollen

- painful

- warm to the touch

- full of pus or other drainage

- accompanied by a fever

If you or someone in your family experiences these signs and symptoms, cover the area with a bandage, wash your hands, and contact your doctor. It is especially important to contact your doctor if signs and symptoms of an MRSA skin infection are accompanied by a fever.

Risk of Transmission of MRSA

Anyone can get MRSA on their body from contact with an infected wound or by sharing personal items, such as towels or razors, that have touched infected skin. MRSA infection risk can be increased when a person is in activities or places that involve crowding, skin-to-skin contact, and shared equipment or supplies. People including athletes, daycare and school students, military personnel in barracks, and those who recently received inpatient medical care are at higher risk.

Reducing Risk of MRSA

There are the steps you can take to reduce your risk of MRSA infection:

- Maintain good hand and body hygiene. Wash hands often, and clean your body regularly, especially after exercise.

- Keep cuts, scrapes, and wounds clean and covered until healed.

- Avoid sharing personal items such as towels and razors.

- Get care early if you think you might have an infection.

What Should I Do If I See These Symptoms?

If you or someone in your family experiences these signs and symptoms, cover the area with a bandage, wash your hands, and contact your doctor. It is especially important to contact your doctor if signs and symptoms of an MRSA skin infection are accompanied by a fever.

What Should I Do If I Think I Have a Skin Infection?

- You can't tell by looking at the skin if it is a staph infection (including MRSA).

- Contact your doctor if you think you have an infection. Finding infections early and getting care make it less likely that the infection will become severe.

- Do not try to treat the infection yourself by picking or popping the sore.

- Cover possible infections with clean, dry bandages until you can be seen by a doctor, nurse, or other healthcare provider.

Prevent Spreading of MRSA

- **Cover your wounds.** Keep wounds covered with clean, dry bandages until healed. Follow your doctor's instructions about proper care of the wound. Pus from infected wounds can contain MRSA so keeping the infection covered will help prevent the spread to others. Bandages and tape can be thrown away with the regular trash. Do not try to treat the infection yourself by picking or popping the sore.

- **Clean your hands often.** You, your family, and others in close contact should wash their hands often with soap and water or use an alcohol-based hand rub, especially after changing the bandage or touching the infected wound.

- **Do not share personal items.** Personal items include towels, washcloths, razors, and clothing, including uniforms.

- **Wash used sheets, towels, and clothes with water and laundry detergent.** Use a dryer to dry them completely.

- **Wash clothes according to manufacturer's instructions on the label.** Clean your hands after touching dirty clothes.

Prevalence of MRSA

Studies show that about one in three people carry staph in their nose, usually without any illness. Two in 100 people carry MRSA.

615

There are no data showing the total number of people who get MRSA skin infections in the community.

Section 42.7

Pseudomonas aeruginosa

This section includes text excerpted from "Healthcare-Associated Infections—*Pseudomonas aeruginosa* in Healthcare Settings," Centers for Disease Control and Prevention (CDC), May 7, 2014.

Pseudomonas Infection

Pseudomonas infection is caused by strains of bacteria found widely in the environment; the most common type causing infections in humans is called *Pseudomonas aeruginosa.*

Pseudomonas Causes Various Types of Infections

Serious *Pseudomonas* infections usually occur in people in the hospital and/or with weakened immune systems. Infections of the blood, pneumonia, and infections following surgery can lead to severe illness and death in these people.

However, healthy people can also develop mild illnesses with *Pseudomonas aeruginosa*, especially after exposure to water. Ear infections, especially in children, and more generalized skin rashes may occur after exposure to inadequately chlorinated hot tubs or swimming pools. Eye infections have occasionally been reported in persons using extended-wear contact lenses.

Risk of Pseudomonas Infection

Patients in hospitals, especially those on breathing machines, those with devices such as catheters, and patients with wounds from surgery or from burns are potentially at risk for serious, life-threatening infections.

Transmission of Pseudomonas Infection

In hospitals, where the most serious infections occur, *Pseudomonas* can be spread on the hands of healthcare workers or by equipment that gets contaminated and is not properly cleaned.

Prevention of Pseudomonas Infection

In the hospital, careful attention to routine infection control practices, especially hand hygiene and environmental cleaning, can substantially lower the risk of infection.

Outside the hospital, avoid hot tubs or pools that may be poorly maintained, and keep contact lenses, equipment, and solutions from becoming contaminated.

Treatment for Pseudomonas Infection

Pseudomonas infections are generally treated with antibiotics. Unfortunately, in hospitalized patients, *Pseudomonas* infections, like those caused by many other hospital bacteria, are becoming more difficult to treat because of increasing antibiotic resistance. Selecting the right antibiotic usually requires that a specimen from a patient be sent to a laboratory to test to see which antibiotics might still be effective for treating the infection.

Multidrug-resistant Pseudomonas can be deadly for patients in critical care. An estimated 51,000 healthcare-associated *P. aeruginosa* infections occur in the United States each year. More than 6,000 (13%) of these are multidrug-resistant, with roughly 400 deaths per year attributed to these infections. *Multidrug-resistant Pseudomonas* was given a threat level of serious threat in the CDC AR Threat report.

Section 42.8

Carbapenem-Resistant Enterobacteriaceae (CRE) Infection

This section includes text excerpted from "Healthcare-Associated Infections—Carbapenem-Resistant Enterobacteriaceae (CRE) Infection: Patient FAQs," Centers for Disease Control and Prevention (CDC), May 7, 2014.

CRE, which stands for Carbapenem-resistant Enterobacteriaceae, are a family of germs that are difficult to treat because they have high levels of resistance to antibiotics. CRE are an important emerging threat to public health.

Common Enterobacteriaceae include *Klebsiella* species and *Escherichia coli (E. coli)*. These germs are found in normal human intestines (gut). Sometimes these bacteria can spread outside the gut and cause serious infections, such as urinary tract infections, bloodstream infections, wound infections, and pneumonia. Enterobacteriaceae can cause infections in people in both healthcare and community settings.

Carbapenems are a group of antibiotics that are usually reserved to treat serious infections, particularly when these infections are caused by germs that are highly resistant to antibiotics. Sometimes carbapenems are considered antibiotics of last resort for some infections. Some Enterobacteriaceae can no longer be treated with carbapenems because they have developed resistance to these antibiotics (i.e., CRE); resistance makes the antibiotics ineffective in killing the resistant germ. Resistance to carbapenems can be due to a few different mechanisms. One of the more common ways that Enterobacteriaceae become resistant to carbapenems is due to production of *Klebsiella pneumoniae* carbapenemase (KPC). KPC is an enzyme that is produced by some CRE that was first identified in the United States around 2001. KPC breaks down carbapenems making them ineffective. Other enzymes, in addition to KPC, can breakdown carbapenems and lead to the development of CRE, but they are uncommon in the United States.

Transmission of Carbapenem-Resistant Enterobacteriaceae (CRE) Infection

To get a CRE infection, a person must be exposed to CRE germs. CRE germs are usually spread person to person through contact with infected or colonized people, particularly contact with wounds or stool. CRE can cause infections when they enter the body, often through medical devices like ventilators, intravenous catheters, urinary catheters, or wounds caused by injury or surgery.

Risk of CRE Infection

Healthy people usually don't get CRE infections. CRE primarily affect patients in acute and long-term healthcare settings, who are being treated for another condition. CRE are more likely to affect those patients who have compromised immune systems or have invasive devices like tubes going into their body. Use of certain types of antibiotics might also make it more likely for patients to get CRE. CRE have been spread during ERCP (endoscopic retrograde cholangiopancreatography), a medical procedure that involves inserting a specialized endoscope commonly called a duodenoscope into the mouth and down to the intestine where the bile duct attaches.

Treatment of CRE Infection

Many people with CRE will have the germ in or on their body without it producing an infection. These people are said to be colonized with CRE, and they do not need antibiotics for the CRE. If the CRE are causing an infection, the antibiotics that will work against it are limited but some options are often available. In addition, some infections might be able to be treated with other therapies, like draining the infection. Strains that have been resistant to all antibiotics are very rare but have been reported.

Hospitals Role in Preventing CRE infections

To prevent the spread of CRE, healthcare personnel and facilities can follow infection-control precautions provided by CDC. These include:

- Washing hands with soap and water or an alcohol-based hand sanitizer before and after caring for a patient.

619

- Carefully cleaning and disinfecting rooms and medical equipment.
- Wearing gloves and a gown before entering the room of a CRE patient.
- Keeping patients with CRE infections in a single room or sharing a room with someone else who has a CRE infection.
- Whenever possible, dedicating equipment and staff to CRE patients.
- Removing gloves and gown and washing hands before leaving the room of a CRE patient.
- Only prescribing antibiotics when necessary.
- Removing temporary medical devices as soon as possible.
- Sometimes, hospitals will test patients for these bacteria to identify them early to help prevent them from being passed on to other patients.

Prevention of CRE infections

Patients should:

- Tell your doctor if you have been hospitalized in another facility or country.
- Take antibiotics only as prescribed.
- Expect all doctors, nurses, and other healthcare providers wash their hands with soap and water or an alcohol-based hand rub before and after touching your body or tubes going into your body. If they do not, ask them to do so.
- Clean your own hands often, especially:
  - Before preparing or eating food
  - Before and after changing wound dressings or bandages
  - After using the bathroom
  - After blowing your nose, coughing, or sneezing
- Ask questions. Understand what is being done to you, the risks and benefits.

Having CRE?

Follow your healthcare provider's instructions. If your provider prescribes you antibiotics, take them exactly as instructed and finish the full course, even if you feel better. Wash your hands, especially after you have contact with the infected area and after using the bathroom. Follow any other hygiene advice your provider gives you.

Precautionary Measures for Caretakers

CRE have primarily been a problem among people with underlying medical problems, especially those with medical devices like urinary catheters or those with chronic wounds. Otherwise healthy people are probably at relatively low risk for problems with CRE. People providing care at home for patients with CRE should be careful about washing their hands, especially after contact with wounds or helping the CRE patient to use the bathroom or after cleaning up stool. Caregivers should also make sure to wash their hands before and after handling the patient's medical device (e.g., urinary catheters). This is particularly important if the caregiver is caring for more than one ill person at home. In addition, gloves should be used when anticipating contact with body fluids or blood.

CRE Infection Related to Medical Care Abroad

A variety of enzymes produced by Enterobacteriaceae make them resistant to carbapenems. Several of these enzymes appear to be more common in other countries than they are in the United States. As with medical care in the United States, medical care abroad can be associated with healthcare–associated infections and/or resistant bacteria.

Section 42.9

Ventilator-Associated Pneumonia (VAP)

This section includes text excerpted from "Healthcare-Associated Infections—Frequently Asked Questions about Ventilator-Associated Pneumonia," Centers for Disease Control and Prevention (CDC), December 14, 2010. Reviewed June 2017.

What Is a Ventilator-Associated Pneumonia (VAP)?

Ventilator-associated pneumonia (VAP) is a lung infection that develops in a person who is on a ventilator. A ventilator is a machine that is used to help a patient breathe by giving oxygen through a tube placed in a patient's mouth or nose, or through a hole in the front of the neck. An infection may occur if germs enter through the tube and get into the patient's lungs.

Why Do Patients Need a Ventilator?

A patient may need a ventilator when he or she is very ill or during and after surgery. Ventilators can be life-saving, but they can also increase a patient's chance of getting pneumonia by making it easier for germs to get into the patient's lungs.

What Are Some of the Things That Hospitals Are Doing to Prevent VAP?

To prevent ventilator-associated pneumonia, doctors, nurses, and other healthcare providers can do the following things:

- Keep the head of the patient's bed raised between 30 and 45 degrees unless other medical conditions do not allow this to occur.

- Check the patient's ability to breathe on his or her own every day so that the patient can be taken off of the ventilator as soon as possible.

- Clean their hands with soap and water or an alcohol-based hand rub before and after touching the patient or the ventilator.

- Clean the inside of the patient's mouth on a regular basis.

- Clean or replace equipment between use on different patients.

What Can I Do to Help Prevent VAP?

Patients and family members can do the following things to help prevent VAP:

Patients

- Quit smoking. Patients who smoke get more infections. Seek information about how to quit before surgery.

- If healthcare providers do not clean their hands, ask them to do so.

Patients and family members

- Ask about raising the head of the bed.

- Ask when the patient will be allowed to try breathing on his or her own.

- If healthcare providers do not clean their hands, ask them to do so.

- Ask about how often healthcare providers clean the patient's mouth.

Can VAP Be Treated?

Most of the time, these infections can be treated with antibiotics. The choice of antibiotics depends on which specific germs are causing the infection. The healthcare provider will decide which antibiotic is best.

Section 42.10

Sepsis

This section contains text excerpted from the following sources: Text beginning with the heading "What Is Sepsis?" is excerpted from "Sepsis Fact Sheet," National Institute of General Medical Sciences (NIGMS), January 2017; Text under the heading "Life after Sepsis" is excerpted from "Life after Sepsis Fact Sheet," Centers for Disease Control and Prevention (CDC), September 1, 2015.

What Is Sepsis?

Sepsis is a serious medical condition caused by an overwhelming immune response to infection. Immune chemicals released into the blood to combat the infection trigger widespread inflammation, which leads to blood clots and leaky vessels. This results in impaired blood flow, which damages the body's organs by depriving them of nutrients and oxygen.

In severe cases, one or more organs fail. In the worst cases, blood pressure drops, the heart weakens and the patient spirals toward septic shock. Once this happens, multiple organs—lungs, kidneys, liver—may quickly fail and the patient can die.

Sepsis is a major challenge in the intensive care unit, where it's one of the leading causes of death. It is also a leading cause of people being readmitted to the hospital. Sepsis arises unpredictably and can progress rapidly.

What Causes Sepsis?

Sepsis does not arise on its own. It stems from another medical condition such as an infection in the lungs, urinary tract, skin, abdomen (such as appendicitis) or other part of the body. Invasive medical procedures like the insertion of a vascular catheter can introduce bacteria into the bloodstream and bring on the condition.

Many different types of microbes can cause sepsis, including bacteria, fungi, and viruses, but bacteria are the most common culprits. Severe cases often result from a body-wide infection that spreads through the bloodstream, but sepsis can also stem from a localized infection.

Who Gets Sepsis?

Anyone can get sepsis, but people with weakened immune systems, children, infants and the elderly are most vulnerable. People with chronic illnesses, such as diabetes, AIDS, cancer, and kidney or liver disease, are also at increased risk, as are those who have experienced a severe burn or physical trauma.

How Many People Get Sepsis?

Every year, severe sepsis strikes more than a million Americans. It's been estimated that between 28 and 50 percent of these people die—far more than the number of U.S. deaths from prostate cancer, breast cancer and AIDS combined.

The number of sepsis cases per year has been on the rise in the United States. This is likely due to a combination of factors, including increased awareness and tracking of the condition, an aging population, the increased longevity of people with chronic diseases, the spread of antibiotic-resistant organisms, an upsurge in invasive procedures and broader use of immunosuppressive and chemotherapeutic agents.

What Are the Symptoms of Sepsis?

Common symptoms of sepsis are fever, chills, rapid breathing and heart rate, rash, confusion, and disorientation. Many of these symptoms, such as fever and difficulty breathing, mimic other conditions, making sepsis hard to diagnose in its early stages.

How Is Sepsis Diagnosed?

Doctors diagnose sepsis by examining patients for fever, increased heart rate and increased respiratory rate. They often perform a blood test to see if a patient has an abnormal number of white blood cells, a common sign of sepsis; or an elevated lactate level, which correlates with severity of the condition. Doctors may also test blood and other bodily fluids such as urine and sputum for the presence of infectious agents.

In addition, a chest X-ray or a CT scan can help identify the site of infection.

How Is Sepsis Treated?

People with sepsis are usually treated in hospital intensive care units. Doctors try to quell the infection, sustain the vital organs and prevent a drop in blood pressure.

The first step is often treatment with broad-spectrum antibiotics, medicines that kill many types of bacteria. Once lab tests identify the infectious agent, doctors can select medicine that specifically targets the microbe. Many patients receive oxygen and intravenous fluids to maintain normal blood oxygen levels and blood pressure.

Depending on the patient's status, other types of treatment, such as mechanical ventilation or kidney dialysis, may be necessary. Sometimes, surgery is required to clear a local site of infection.

Many other drugs, including vasopressors and corticosteroids, may be used to treat sepsis or to revive those who have gone into septic shock. Despite years of research, scientists have not yet succeeded in developing a medicine that specifically targets the aggressive immune response that characterizes sepsis.

Life after Sepsis

What Are the First Steps in Recovery?

After you have had sepsis, rehabilitation usually starts in the hospital by slowly helping you to move around and look after yourself: bathing, sitting up, standing, walking, taking yourself to the restroom, etc. The purpose of rehabilitation is to restore you back to your previous level of health or as close to it as possible. Begin your rehabilitation by building up your activities slowly, and rest when you are tired.

How Will I Feel When I Get Home?

You have been seriously ill, and your body and mind need time to get better. You may experience the following physical symptoms upon returning home:

- General to extreme weakness and fatigue
- Breathlessness
- General body pains or aches
- Difficulty moving around
- Difficulty sleeping
- Weight loss, lack of appetite, food not tasting normal
- Dry and itchy skin that may peel
- Brittle nails
- Hair loss

It is also not unusual to have the following feelings once you're at home:

- Unsure of yourself
- Not caring about your appearance
- Wanting to be alone, avoiding friends and family
- Flashbacks, bad memories
- Confusing reality (e.g., not sure what is real and what isn't)
- Feeling anxious, more worried than usual
- Poor concentration
- Depressed, angry, unmotivated
- Frustration at not being able to do everyday tasks

What Can I Do to Help Myself Recover at Home?

- Set small, achievable goals for yourself each week, such as taking a bath, dressing yourself, or walking up the stairs
- Rest and rebuild your strength
- Talk about what you are feeling to family and friends
- Record your thoughts, struggles, and milestones in a journal
- Learn about sepsis to understand what happened
- Ask your family to fill in any gaps you may have in your memory about what happened to you
- Eat a balanced diet
- Exercise if you feel up to it
- Make a list of questions to ask your doctor when you go for a check up

Are There Any Long-Term Effects of Sepsis?

Many people who survive sepsis recover completely and their lives return to normal. However, as with some other illnesses requiring intensive medical care, some patients have long-term effects. These problems may not become apparent for several weeks (post-sepsis), and may include such consequences as:

- Insomnia, difficulty getting to or staying asleep

- Nightmares, vivid hallucinations, panic attacks
- Disabling muscle and joint pains
- Decreased mental (cognitive) functioning
- Loss of self-esteem and self-belief
- Organ dysfunction (kidney failure, respiratory problems, etc.)
- Amputations (loss of limb(s))

Chapter 43

Other Surgical Complications

Chapter Contents

Section 43.1

Abdominal Adhesions

This section includes text excerpted from "Abdominal Adhesions," National Digestive Diseases, National Institute of Diabetes and Digestive and Kidney Diseases (NIDDK), September 2013. Reviewed June 2017.

Abdominal adhesions are bands of fibrous tissue that can form between abdominal tissues and organs. Normally, internal tissues and organs have slippery surfaces, preventing them from sticking together as the body moves. However, abdominal adhesions cause tissues and organs in the abdominal cavity to stick together.

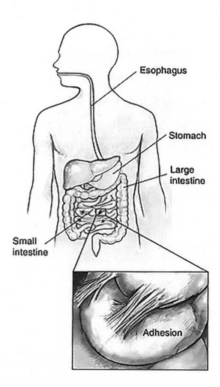

Figure 43.1. *Abdominal Adhesions*

Abdominal Cavity

The abdominal cavity is the internal area of the body between the chest and hips that contains the lower part of the esophagus, stomach, small intestine, and large intestine. The esophagus carries food and liquids from the mouth to the stomach, which slowly pumps them into the small and large intestines. Abdominal adhesions can kink, twist, or pull the small and large intestines out of place, causing an intestinal obstruction. Intestinal obstruction, also called a bowel obstruction, results in the partial or complete blockage of movement of food or stool through the intestines.

Causes of Abdominal Adhesions

Abdominal surgery is the most frequent cause of abdominal adhesions. Surgery-related causes include:

- cuts involving internal organs
- handling of internal organs
- drying out of internal organs and tissues
- contact of internal tissues with foreign materials, such as gauze, surgical gloves, and stitches
- blood or blood clots that were not rinsed away during surgery

Abdominal adhesions can also result from inflammation not related to surgery, including:

- appendix rupture
- radiation treatment
- gynecological infections
- abdominal infections

Rarely, abdominal adhesions form without apparent cause.

Prevalence and Risk of Abdominal Adhesions

Of patients who undergo abdominal surgery, 93 percent develop abdominal adhesions. Surgery in the lower abdomen and pelvis, including bowel and gynecological operations, carries an even greater chance of abdominal adhesions. Abdominal adhesions can become larger and tighter as time passes, sometimes causing problems years after surgery.

631

Symptoms of Abdominal Adhesions

In most cases, abdominal adhesions do not cause symptoms. When symptoms are present, chronic abdominal pain is the most common.

Complications of Abdominal Adhesions

Abdominal adhesions can cause intestinal obstruction and female infertility—the inability to become pregnant after a year of trying.

Abdominal adhesions can lead to female infertility by preventing fertilized eggs from reaching the uterus, where fetal development takes place. Women with abdominal adhesions in or around their fallopian tubes have an increased chance of ectopic pregnancy—a fertilized egg growing outside the uterus. Abdominal adhesions inside the uterus may result in repeated miscarriages—a pregnancy failure before 20 weeks.

Seek Help for Emergency Symptoms

A complete intestinal obstruction is life threatening and requires immediate medical attention and often surgery. Symptoms of an intestinal obstruction include:

- severe abdominal pain or cramping
- nausea
- vomiting
- bloating
- loud bowel sounds
- abdominal swelling
- the inability to have a bowel movement or pass gas
- constipation—a condition in which a person has fewer than three bowel movements a week; the bowel movements may be painful

A person with these symptoms should seek medical attention immediately.

Diagnosis of Abdominal Adhesions and Intestinal Obstructions

Abdominal adhesions cannot be detected by tests or seen through imaging techniques such as X-rays or ultrasound. Most abdominal adhesions are found during surgery performed to examine the abdomen. However, abdominal X-rays, a lower gastrointestinal (GI) series, and computerized tomography (CT) scans can diagnose intestinal obstructions.

- **Abdominal X-rays** use a small amount of radiation to create an image that is recorded on film or a computer. An X-ray is performed at a hospital or an outpatient center by an X-ray technician, and the images are interpreted by a radiologist—a doctor who specializes in medical imaging. An X-ray does not require anesthesia. The person will lie on a table or stand during the X-ray. The X-ray machine is positioned over the abdominal area. The person will hold his or her breath as the picture is taken so that the picture will not be blurry. The person may be asked to change position for additional pictures.

- A **lower GI series** is an X-ray exam that is used to look at the large intestine. The test is performed at a hospital or an outpatient center by an X-ray technician, and the images are interpreted by a radiologist. Anesthesia is not needed. The healthcare provider may provide written bowel prep instructions to follow at home before the test. The person may be asked to follow a clear liquid diet for 1 to 3 days before the procedure. A laxative or an enema may be used before the test. A laxative is medication that loosens stool and increases bowel movements. An enema involves flushing water or laxative into the rectum using a special squirt bottle.

  For the test, the person will lie on a table while the radiologist inserts a flexible tube into the person's anus. The large intestine is filled with barium, making signs of underlying problems show up more clearly on X-rays.

- **CT scans** use a combination of X-rays and computer technology to create images. The procedure is performed at a hospital or an outpatient center by an X-ray technician, and the images are interpreted by a radiologist. Anesthesia is not needed. A CT scan may include the injection of a special dye, called contrast medium. The person will lie on a table that slides into a tunnel-shaped device where the X-rays are taken.

Treatment for Abdominal Adhesions

Abdominal adhesions that do not cause symptoms generally do not require treatment. Surgery is the only way to treat abdominal adhesions that cause pain, intestinal obstruction, or fertility problems. More surgery, however, carries the risk of additional abdominal adhesions. People should speak with their healthcare provider about the best way to treat their abdominal adhesions.

Complete intestinal obstructions usually require immediate surgery to clear the blockage. Most partial intestinal obstructions can be managed without surgery.

Abdominal adhesions are difficult to prevent; however, certain surgical techniques can minimize abdominal adhesions.

Laparoscopic surgery decreases the potential for abdominal adhesions because several tiny incisions are made in the lower abdomen instead of one large incision. The surgeon inserts a laparoscope—a thin tube with a tiny video camera attached—into one of the small incisions. The camera sends a magnified image from inside the body to a video monitor. Patients will usually receive general anesthesia during this surgery.

If laparoscopic surgery is not possible and a large abdominal incision is required, at the end of surgery a special film-like material can be inserted between organs or between the organs and the abdominal incision. The film-like material, which looks similar to wax paper and is absorbed by the body in about a week, hydrates organs to help prevent abdominal adhesions.

Other steps taken during surgery to reduce abdominal adhesions include:

• using starch-and latex-free gloves

• handling tissues and organs gently

• shortening surgery time

• using moistened drapes and swabs

• occasionally applying saline solution

Eat, Diet, and Nutrition

Researchers have not found that eating, diet, and nutrition play a role in causing or preventing abdominal adhesions. A person with a partial intestinal obstruction may relieve symptoms with a liquid or low-fiber diet, which is more easily broken down into smaller particles by the digestive system.

Section 43.2

Deep Vein Thrombosis

This section contains text excerpted from the following sources: Text in this section begins with excerpts from "How to Spot and Prevent Deep Vein Thrombosis," *NIH News in Health*, National Institutes of Health (NIH), January 2017; Text beginning with the heading "How Is Deep Vein Thrombosis Treated?" is excerpted from "Deep Vein Thrombosis," National Heart, Lung, and Blood Institute (NHLBI), October 28, 2011. Reviewed June 2017.

Lots of things can cause pain and swelling in your leg. But if your symptoms stem from a blood clot deep in your leg, it can be dangerous. Blood clots can happen to anyone, anytime. But some people are at increased risk. Taking steps to reduce your chances of a blood clot forming in your veins can help you avoid potentially serious problems.

Blood clots can arise anywhere in your body. They develop when blood thickens and clumps together. When a clot forms in a vein deep in the body, it's called deep vein thrombosis (DVT). Deep vein blood clots typically occur in the lower leg or thigh.

"Deep vein thrombosis has classic symptoms—for example swelling, pain, warmth, and redness on the leg," says Dr. Andrei Kindzelski, a National Institutes of Health (NIH) blood disease expert. "But about 30–40 percent of cases go unnoticed, since they don't have typical symptoms." In fact, some people don't realize they have a deep vein clot until it causes a more serious condition.

Deep vein clots—especially those in the thigh—can break off and travel through the bloodstream. If a clot lodges in an artery in the lungs, it can block blood flow and lead to a sometimes-deadly condition called pulmonary embolism. This disorder can damage the lungs and reduce blood oxygen levels, which can harm other organs as well.

Some people are more at risk for DVT than others. "Usually people who develop DVT have some level of thrombophilia, which means their blood clots more rapidly or easily," Kindzelski says. Getting a blood clot is usually the first sign of this condition because it's hard to notice otherwise. In these cases, lifestyle can contribute to a blood clot forming—if you don't move enough, for example. Your risk is higher if you've recently had surgery or broken a bone, if you're ill and in bed for a long time, or if you're traveling for a long time (such as during long car or airplane rides).

Having other diseases or conditions can also raise your chances of a blood clot. These include a stroke, paralysis (an inability to move), chronic heart disease, high blood pressure, surgical procedure, or having been recently treated for cancer. Women who take hormone therapy pills or birth control pills, are pregnant, or within the first 6 weeks after giving birth are also at higher risk. So are those who smoke or who are older than 60. But DVT can happen at any age.

You can take simple steps to lower your chances for a blood clot. Exercise your lower leg muscles if you're sitting for a long time while traveling. Get out of bed and move around as soon as you're able after having surgery or being ill. The more active you are, the better your chance of avoiding a blood clot. Take any medicines your doctor prescribes to prevent clots after some types of surgery.

A prompt diagnosis and proper treatment can help prevent the complications of blood clots. See your doctor immediately if you have any signs or symptoms of DVT or pulmonary embolism. A physical exam and other tests can help doctors determine whether you've got a blood clot.

Clues of a Clot

Seek treatment if you have these symptoms. They may signal a deep vein clot or pulmonary embolism:

- swelling of the leg or along a vein in the leg
- pain or tenderness in the leg, which you may feel only when standing or walking
- increased warmth in the area of the leg that's swollen or painful
- red or discolored skin on the leg
- unexplained shortness of breath
- pain with deep breathing
- coughing up blood

How Is Deep Vein Thrombosis Treated?

Doctors treat DVT with medicines and other devices and therapies. The main goals of treating DVT are to:

- Stop the blood clot from getting bigger.

- Prevent the blood clot from breaking off and moving to your lungs.

- Reduce your chance of having another blood clot.

Medicines

Your doctor may prescribe medicines to prevent or treat DVT.

Anticoagulants

Anticoagulants are the most common medicines for treating DVT. They're also known as blood thinners. These medicines decrease your blood's ability to clot. They also stop existing blood clots from getting bigger. However, blood thinners can't break up blood clots that have already formed. (The body dissolves most blood clots with time). Blood thinners can be taken as a pill, an injection under the skin, or through a needle or tube inserted into a vein (called intravenous, or IV, injection).

Warfarin and heparin are two blood thinners used to treat DVT. Warfarin is given in pill form. (Coumadin® is a common brand name for warfarin.) Heparin is given as an injection or through an IV tube. There are different types of heparin. Your doctor will discuss the options with you. Your doctor may treat you with both heparin and warfarin at the same time. Heparin acts quickly. Warfarin takes 2 to 3 days before it starts to work. Once the warfarin starts to work, the heparin is stopped. Pregnant women usually are treated with just heparin because warfarin is dangerous during pregnancy.

Treatment for DVT using blood thinners usually lasts for 6 months. The following situations may change the length of treatment:

- If your blood clot occurred after a short-term risk (for example, surgery), your treatment time may be shorter.

- If you've had blood clots before, your treatment time may be longer.

- If you have certain other illnesses, such as cancer, you may need to take blood thinners for as long as you have the illness.

The most common side effect of blood thinners is bleeding. Bleeding can happen if the medicine thins your blood too much. This side effect can be life threatening. Sometimes the bleeding is internal (inside your body). People treated with blood thinners usually have regular blood tests to measure their blood's ability to clot. These tests are called PT (prothrombin time) and partial thromboplastin time (PTT) tests. These tests also help your doctor make sure you're taking the right amount of medicine. Call your doctor right away if you have easy bruising or bleeding. These may be signs that your medicines have thinned your blood too much.

Thrombin Inhibitors

These medicines interfere with the blood clotting process. They're used to treat blood clots in patients who can't take heparin.

Thrombolytics

Doctors prescribe these medicines to quickly dissolve large blood clots that cause severe symptoms. Because thrombolytics can cause sudden bleeding, they're used only in life-threatening situations.

Other Types of Treatment

Vena Cava Filter

If you can't take blood thinners or they're not working well, your doctor may recommend a vena cava filter. The filter is inserted inside a large vein called the vena cava. The filter catches blood clots before they travel to the lungs, which prevents pulmonary embolism. However, the filter doesn't stop new blood clots from forming.

Graduated Compression Stockings

Graduated compression stockings can reduce leg swelling caused by a blood clot. These stockings are worn on the legs from the arch of the foot to just above or below the knee. Compression stockings are tight at the ankle and become looser as they go up the leg. This creates gentle pressure up the leg. The pressure keeps blood from pooling and clotting.

There are three types of compression stockings. One type is support pantyhose, which offer the least amount of pressure. The second type is over-the-counter compression hose. These stockings give a little more pressure than support pantyhose. Over-the-counter compression hose are sold in medical supply stores and pharmacies. Prescription-strength compression hose offers the greatest amount of pressure. They also are sold in medical supply stores and pharmacies. However, a specially trained person needs to fit you for these stockings.

Talk with your doctor about how long you should wear compression stockings.

Section 43.3

Headache after Lumbar Puncture

This section contains text excerpted from the following sources:
Text beginning with the heading "What Is Lumbar Puncture?" is
excerpted from "Lumbar Puncture Fact Sheet," National
Institute on Aging (NIA), National Institutes of Health (NIH),
June 11, 2010. Reviewed June 2017; Text under the heading
"Headaches after Surgery" is excerpted from "Headache: Hope
through Research," National Institute of Neurological
Disorders and Stroke (NINDS), April 2016.

What Is Lumbar Puncture?

A lumbar puncture (spinal tap) test is a procedure to remove a small sample of cerebral spinal fluid from the lower spine. A needle is inserted between the vertebrae (backbones) in the lower back and into the space containing the spinal fluid which surrounds and cushions the brain and spinal cord.

How Long Does It Take?

About 20 to 30 minutes. There is an additional recovery period of about 30 minutes after the test, when you will remain at the clinic.

Why Is the Lumbar Puncture Test Performed?

To obtain a specimen of fluid for testing. Cerebrospinal fluid (CSF) bathes the brain and contains proteins that can provide clues about disorders such as Alzheimer disease or changes in the brain that accompany aging.

Does It Hurt?

You may experience pressure when the needle is inserted. You may also feel some very brief leg pain while the needle is positioned because it may briefly touch a floating nerve ending.

How Is It Performed?

- You will lie on your side with your knees drawn up toward your chin as far as possible or you will sit on the edge of an exam table, in a hunched forward position.

- The doctor will cleanse the skin over your spinal column with iodine.

- An injection of local anesthetic may be given at the puncture site.

- A needle is inserted into your spinal fluid space.

- Spinal fluid is collected into specimen tubes for laboratory testing.

- The needle is withdrawn, your back is cleaned, and a band-aid is placed over the spot.

After the Test

- You will be asked to lie down for about 30 minutes.

- You will be given something to eat and drink.

- While you are recovering, please report any of the following symptoms to the doctor or nurse:

  - Headache

  - Tingling

  - Numbness or pain in your lower back and legs

  - Problems with urination

- You will return home after the recovery period.

Instructions to follow at home:

- Drink at least 6 glasses of fluid (no alcohol) in the next 12 hours.

- Remain quiet for the next 24 hours.

- Avoid any strenuous physical activity for 48 hours – no exercising, heavy lifting, or repeated bending.

- A mild headache may follow a lumbar puncture. It is often relieved by caffeine, aspirin or tylenol, and drinking plenty of fluids.

- If you develop a headache that persists more than 24 hours, in particular one that is worse on sitting or standing, and better when lying down, then call the doctor or study coordinator at the clinic.

Headaches after Surgery

About one-fourth of people who undergo a lumbar puncture develop a headache due to a leak of cerebrospinal fluid following the procedure. Since the headache occurs only when the individual stands up, the "cure" is to lie down until the headache runs its course-anywhere from a few hours to several days. Severe postdural headaches may be treated by injecting a small amount of the individual's own blood into the low back to stop the leak (called an epidural blood patch). Occasionally spinal fluid leaks spontaneously, causing this "low pressure headache."

Section 43.4

Lung Function Tests Help Identify Lung Complications after Surgery

This section includes text excerpted from "Pulmonary Function Tests," National Heart, Lung, and Blood Institute (NHLBI), December 9, 2016.

Pulmonary function tests, or PFTs, also known as lung function tests, measure how well your lungs work. They include tests that measure lung size and airflow, such as spirometry and lung volume tests. Other tests measure how well gases such as oxygen get in and out of your blood. These tests include pulse oximetry and arterial blood gas tests. Another pulmonary function test, called fractional exhaled nitric oxide (FeNO), measures nitric oxide, which is a marker for inflammation in the lungs. You may have one or more of these tests to diagnose lung and airway diseases, compare your lung function to expected levels of function, monitor if your disease is stable or worsening, and see if your treatment is working.

The purpose, procedure, discomfort, and risks of each test will vary.

- **Spirometry measures the rate of airflow and estimates lung size.** For this test, you will breathe multiple times, with regular and maximal effort, through a tube that is connected to a computer. Some people feel lightheaded or tired from the required breathing effort.

- **Lung volume tests are the most accurate way to measure how much air your lungs can hold.** The procedure is similar to spirometry, except that you will be in a small room with clear walls. Some people feel lightheaded or tired from the required breathing effort.

- **Lung diffusion capacity assesses how well oxygen gets into the blood from the air you breathe.** For this test, you will breathe in and out through a tube for several minutes without having to breathe intensely. You also may need to have blood drawn to measure the level of hemoglobin in your blood.

- **Pulse oximetry estimates oxygen levels in your blood.** For this test, a probe will be placed on your finger or another skin surface such as your ear. It causes no pain and has few or no risks.

- **Arterial blood gas tests directly measure the levels of gases, such as oxygen and carbon dioxide, in your blood.** Arterial blood gas tests are usually performed in a hospital, but may be done in a doctor's office. For this test, blood will be taken from an artery, usually in the wrist where your pulse is measured. You may feel brief pain when the needle is inserted or when a tube attached to the needle fills with blood. It is possible to have bleeding or infection where the needle was inserted.

- **Fractional exhaled nitric oxide tests measure how much nitric oxide is in the air that you exhale.** For this test, you will breathe out into a tube that is connected to the portable device. It requires steady but not intense breathing. It has few or no risks.

Other tests may be needed to assess lung function in infants, children, or patients who are not able to perform spirometry and lung volume tests. Before your tests, you may be asked to not eat some foods or take certain medicines that can affect some pulmonary function test results.

Section 43.5

Cardiogenic Shock

This section includes text excerpted from "Cardiogenic Shock," National Digestive Diseases, National Heart, Lung, and Blood Institute (NHLBI), July 1, 2011. Reviewed June 2017.

What Is Shock?

The medical term "shock" refers to a state in which not enough blood and oxygen reach important organs in the body, such as the brain and kidneys. Shock causes very low blood pressure and may be life threatening. Shock can have many causes.

Cardiogenic shock is only one type of shock. Other types of shock include hypovolemic shock and vasodilatory shock. Hypovolemic shock is a condition in which the heart can't pump enough blood to the body because of severe blood loss. In vasodilatory shock, the blood vessels suddenly relax. When the blood vessels are too relaxed, blood pressure drops and blood flow becomes very low. Without enough blood pressure, blood and oxygen don't reach the body's organs.

A bacterial infection in the bloodstream, a severe allergic reaction, or damage to the nervous system (brain and nerves) may cause vasodilatory shock. When a person is in shock (from any cause), not enough blood and oxygen are reaching the body's organs. If shock lasts more than a few minutes, the lack of oxygen starts to damage the body's organs. If shock isn't treated quickly, it can cause permanent organ damage or death.

Some of the signs and symptoms of shock include:

- Confusion or lack of alertness

- Loss of consciousness

- A sudden and ongoing rapid heartbeat

643

- Sweating

- Pale skin

- A weak pulse

- Rapid breathing

- Decreased or no urine output

- Cool hands and feet

If you think that you or someone else is in shock, call 9–1–1 right away for emergency treatment. Prompt medical care can save your life and prevent or limit damage to your body's organs.

What Causes Cardiogenic Shock?

Immediate Causes

Cardiogenic shock occurs if the heart suddenly can't pump enough oxygen-rich blood to the body. The most common cause of cardiogenic shock is damage to the heart muscle from a severe heart attack. This damage prevents the heart's main pumping chamber, the left ventricle, from working well. As a result, the heart can't pump enough oxygen-rich blood to the rest of the body. In about 3 percent of cardiogenic shock cases, the heart's lower right chamber, the right ventricle, doesn't work well. This means the heart can't properly pump blood to the lungs, where it picks up oxygen to bring back to the heart and the rest of the body.

Without enough oxygen-rich blood reaching the body's major organs, many problems can occur. For example:

- Cardiogenic shock can cause death if the flow of oxygen-rich blood to the organs isn't restored quickly. This is why emergency medical treatment is required.

- If organs don't get enough oxygen-rich blood, they won't work well. Cells in the organs die, and the organs may never work well again.

- As some organs stop working, they may cause problems with other bodily functions. This, in turn, can worsen shock. For example:

  - If the kidneys aren't working well, the levels of important chemicals in the body change. This may cause the heart and other muscles to become even weaker, limiting blood flow even more.

644

- If the liver isn't working well, the body stops making proteins that help the blood clot. This can lead to more bleeding if the shock is due to blood loss.

How well the brain, kidneys, and other organs recover will depend on how long a person is in shock. The less time a person is in shock, the less damage will occur to the organs. This is another reason why emergency treatment is so important.

Underlying Causes

The underlying causes of cardiogenic shock are conditions that weaken the heart and prevent it from pumping enough oxygen-rich blood to the body.

Heart Attack

Most heart attacks occur as a result of coronary heart disease (CHD). CHD is a condition in which a waxy substance called plaque (plak) narrows or blocks the coronary (heart) arteries. Plaque reduces blood flow to your heart muscle. It also makes it more likely that blood clots will form in your arteries. Blood clots can partially or completely block blood flow.

Conditions Caused by Heart Attack

Heart attacks can cause some serious heart conditions that can lead to cardiogenic shock. One example is ventricular septal rupture. This condition occurs if the wall that separates the ventricles (the heart's two lower chambers) breaks down. The breakdown happens because cells in the wall have died due to a heart attack. Without the wall to separate them, the ventricles can't pump properly. Heart attacks also can cause papillary muscle infarction or rupture. This condition occurs if the muscles that help anchor the heart valves stop working or break because a heart attack cuts off their blood supply. If this happens, blood doesn't flow correctly between the heart's chambers. This prevents the heart from pumping properly.

Other Heart Conditions

Serious heart conditions that may occur with or without a heart attack can cause cardiogenic shock. Examples include:

- **Myocarditis.** This is inflammation of the heart muscle.

645

- **Endocarditis.** This is an infection of the inner lining of the heart chambers and valves.

- **Life-threatening arrhythmias.** These are problems with the rate or rhythm of the heartbeat.

- **Pericardial tamponade.** This is too much fluid or blood around the heart. The fluid squeezes the heart muscle so it can't pump properly.

Pulmonary Embolism

Pulmonary embolism (PE) is a sudden blockage in a lung artery. This condition usually is caused by a blood clot that travels to the lung from a vein in the leg. PE can damage your heart and other organs in your body.

Who Is at Risk for Cardiogenic Shock?

The most common risk factor for cardiogenic shock is having a heart attack. If you've had a heart attack, the following factors can further increase your risk for cardiogenic shock:

- Older age

- A history of heart attacks or heart failure

- Coronary heart disease that affects all of the heart's major blood vessels

- High blood pressure

- Diabetes

Women who have heart attacks are at higher risk for cardiogenic shock than men who have heart attacks.

What Are the Signs and Symptoms of Cardiogenic Shock?

A lack of oxygen-rich blood reaching the brain, kidneys, skin, and other parts of the body causes the signs and symptoms of cardiogenic shock.

Some of the typical signs and symptoms of shock usually include at least two or more of the following:

- Confusion or lack of alertness

- Loss of consciousness

- A sudden and ongoing rapid heartbeat

- Sweating

- Pale skin

- A weak pulse

- Rapid breathing

- Decreased or no urine output

- Cool hands and feet

Any of these alone is unlikely to be a sign or symptom of shock.

If you or someone else is having these signs and symptoms, call 9–1–1 right away for emergency treatment. Prompt medical care can save your life and prevent or limit organ damage.

How Is Cardiogenic Shock Diagnosed?

The first step in diagnosing cardiogenic shock is to identify that a person is in shock. At that point, emergency treatment should begin. Once emergency treatment starts, doctors can look for the specific cause of the shock. If the reason for the shock is that the heart isn't pumping strongly enough, then the diagnosis is cardiogenic shock.

Tests and Procedures to Diagnose Shock and Its Underlying Causes

Blood Pressure Test

Medical personnel can use a simple blood pressure cuff and stethoscope to check whether a person has very low blood pressure. This is the most common sign of shock. A blood pressure test can be done before the person goes to a hospital. Less serious conditions also can cause low blood pressure, such as fainting or taking certain medicines, such as those used to treat high blood pressure.

EKG (Electrocardiogram)

An EKG is a simple test that detects and records the heart's electrical activity. The test shows how fast the heart is beating and its rhythm (steady or irregular). An EKG also records the strength and timing of electrical signals as they pass through each part of the heart.

Doctors use EKGs to diagnose severe heart attacks and monitor the heart's condition.

Echocardiography

Echocardiography (echo) uses sound waves to create a moving picture of the heart. The test provides information about the size and shape of the heart and how well the heart chambers and valves are working. Echo also can identify areas of poor blood flow to the heart, areas of heart muscle that aren't contracting normally, and previous injury to the heart muscle caused by poor blood flow.

Chest X-ray

A chest X-ray takes pictures of organs and structures in the chest, including the heart, lungs, and blood vessels. This test shows whether the heart is enlarged or whether fluid is present in the lungs. These can be signs of cardiogenic shock.

Cardiac Enzyme Test

When cells in the heart die, they release enzymes into the blood. These enzymes are called markers or biomarkers. Measuring these markers can show whether the heart is damaged and the extent of the damage.

Coronary Angiography

Coronary angiography is an X-ray exam of the heart and blood vessels. The doctor passes a catheter (a thin, flexible tube) through an artery in the leg or arm to the heart. The catheter can measure the pressure inside the heart chambers. Dye that can be seen on an X-ray image is injected into the bloodstream through the tip of the catheter. The dye lets the doctor study the flow of blood through the heart and blood vessels and see any blockages.

Pulmonary Artery Catheterization

For this procedure, a catheter is inserted into a vein in the arm or neck or near the collarbone. Then, the catheter is moved into the pulmonary artery. This artery connects the right side of the heart to the lungs. The catheter is used to check blood pressure in the pulmonary artery. If the blood pressure is too high or too low, treatment may be needed.

Blood Tests

Some blood tests also are used to help diagnose cardiogenic shock, including:

- Arterial blood gas measurement. For this test, a blood sample is taken from an artery. The sample is used to measure oxygen, carbon dioxide, and pH (acidity) levels in the blood. Certain levels of these substances are associated with shock.

- Tests that measure the function of various organs, such as the kidneys and liver. If these organs aren't working well, they may not be getting enough oxygen-rich blood. This could be a sign of cardiogenic shock.

How Is Cardiogenic Shock Treated?

Cardiogenic shock is life threatening and requires emergency medical treatment. The condition usually is diagnosed after a person has been admitted to a hospital for a heart attack. If the person isn't already in a hospital, emergency treatment can start as soon as medical personnel arrive. The first goal of emergency treatment for cardiogenic shock is to improve the flow of blood and oxygen to the body's organs. Sometimes both the shock and its cause are treated at the same time. For example, doctors may quickly open a blocked blood vessel that's damaging the heart. Often, this can get the patient out of shock with little or no additional treatment.

Emergency Life Support

Emergency life support treatment is needed for any type of shock. This treatment helps get oxygen-rich blood flowing to the brain, kidneys, and other organs. Restoring blood flow to the organs keeps the patient alive and may prevent long-term damage to the organs. Emergency life support treatment includes:

- Giving the patient extra oxygen to breathe so that more oxygen reaches the lungs, the heart, and the rest of the body.

- Providing breathing support if needed. A ventilator might be used to protect the airway and provide the patient with extra oxygen. A ventilator is a machine that supports breathing.

- Giving the patient fluids, including blood and blood products, through a needle inserted in a vein (when the shock is due to blood loss). This can help get more blood to major organs and the rest of the body. This treatment usually isn't used for cardiogenic shock because the heart can't pump the blood that's already in the body. Also, too much fluid is in the lungs, making it hard to breathe.

Medicines

During and after emergency life support treatment, doctors will try to find out what's causing the shock. If the reason for the shock is that the heart isn't pumping strongly enough, then the diagnosis is cardiogenic shock.

Treatment for cardiogenic shock will depend on its cause. Doctors may prescribe medicines to:

- prevent blood clots from forming

- increase the force with which the heart muscle contracts

- treat a heart attack

Medical Devices

Medical devices can help the heart pump and improve blood flow. Devices used to treat cardiogenic shock may include:

- **An intra-aortic balloon pump.** This device is placed in the aorta, the main blood vessel that carries blood from the heart to the body. A balloon at the tip of the device is inflated and deflated in a rhythm that matches the heart's pumping rhythm. This allows the weakened heart muscle to pump as much blood as it can, which helps get more blood to vital organs, such as the brain and kidneys.

- **A left ventricular assist device (LVAD).** This device is a battery-operated pump that takes over part of the heart's pumping action. An LVAD helps the heart pump blood to the body. This device may be used if damage to the left ventricle, the heart's main pumping chamber, is causing shock.

Medical Procedures and Surgery

Sometimes medicines and medical devices aren't enough to treat cardiogenic shock. Medical procedures and surgery can restore blood flow to the heart and the rest of the body, repair heart damage, and help keep a patient alive while he or she recovers from shock. Surgery also can improve the chances of long-term survival. Surgery done within 6 hours of the onset of shock symptoms has the greatest chance of improving survival.

The types of procedures and surgery used to treat underlying causes of cardiogenic shock include:

- Percutaneous coronary intervention (PCI) and stents. PCI, also known as coronary angioplasty, is a procedure used to open narrowed or blocked coronary (heart) arteries and treat an ongoing heart attack. A stent is a small mesh tube that's placed in a coronary artery during PCI to help keep it open.

- Coronary artery bypass grafting. For this surgery, arteries or veins from other parts of the body are used to bypass (that is, go around) narrowed coronary arteries. This creates a new passage for oxygen-rich blood to reach the heart.

- Surgery to repair damaged heart valves.

- Surgery to repair a break in the wall that separates the heart's chambers. This break is called a septal rupture.

- Heart transplant. This type of surgery rarely is done during an emergency situation like cardiogenic shock because of other available options. Also, doctors need to do very careful testing to make sure a patient will benefit from a heart transplant and to find a matching heart from a donor. Still, in some cases, doctors may recommend a transplant if they feel it's the best way to improve a patient's chances of long-term survival.

How Can Cardiogenic Shock Be Prevented?

The best way to prevent cardiogenic shock is to lower your risk for coronary heart disease (CHD) and heart attack. If you already have CHD, it's important to get ongoing treatment from a doctor who has experience treating heart problems.

If you have a heart attack, you should get treatment right away to try to prevent cardiogenic shock and other possible complications.

- Act in time. Know the warning signs of a heart attack so you can act fast to get treatment. Many heart attack victims wait 2 hours or more after their symptoms begin before they seek medical help. Delays in treatment increase the risk of complications and death.

- If you think you're having a heart attack, call 9–1–1 for help. Don't drive yourself or have friends or family drive you to the hospital. Call an ambulance so that medical personnel can begin life-saving treatment on the way to the emergency room.

Section 43.6

Breast Implant Complications

This section includes text excerpted from "Breast Implants," U.S. Food and Drug Administration (FDA), March 23, 2017.

This section highlights the most common problems associated with silicone gel-filled and saline-filled breast implants: those that occur in the breast or chest area, known as "local complications." The most common local complications and adverse outcomes are capsular contracture (hardening of breast area around the implant), reoperation (additional surgeries), implant removal and rupture or deflation of the implant. Other local complications include implant wrinkling, asymmetry, scarring, pain, and infection at the incision site. These local complications often result in reoperation or implant removal.

Local Complications and Adverse Outcomes

The following is a list of local complications and adverse outcomes that occur in one percent or more of patients at any time after breast implant surgery. They are listed in alphabetical order—not in order of prevalence.

- Asymmetry—when breasts are uneven in appearance in terms of size, shape, or breast level
- Breastfeeding difficulties
- Breast pain
- Breast sagging, also called "ptosis"
- Calcium buildup in breast tissue, also called "calcification"

- Capsular contracture—hardening of the breast area around the implant

- Chest wall deformity—when the chest wall or underlying rib cage appears deformed

- Deflation of the breast implant—when filler material leaks from the breast implant often due to a valve leak or a tear or cut in the implant shell

- Delayed wound healing

- Extrusion—when the skin breaks down and the implant appears through the skin

- Hematoma—collection of blood near the surgical site

- Iatrogenic injury or damage—when new injury or damage occurs to the tissue or implant as a result of implant surgery

- Implant displacement or malposition—when the implant is not in the correct position in the breast

- Implant palpability or visibility—when the implant can be felt through the skin

- Implant removal—with or without implant replacement

- Implant visibility—when the implant can be seen through the skin

- Implant wrinkling or rippling

- Infection, including Toxic Shock Syndrome—when during breast implant surgery, wounds are contaminated with microorganisms, such as bacteria or fungi

- Inflammation or irritation

- Necrosis—when there is dead skin or tissue around the breast

- Nipple or breast changes, including change in or loss of nipple sensation

- Redness or bruising

- Reoperation—additional surgeries

- Rupture of the breast implant—when there is a tear or hole in the implant's outer shell

- Scarring

- Seroma—the collection of fluid around the breast implant

- Skin rash

- Swollen or enlarged lymph nodes, also called "lymphedema or lymphadenopathy"

- Thinning and shrinking of the skin, also called "breast tissue atrophy"

- Unsatisfactory appearance due to implant style or size

If you experience any of the local complications listed above after breast implant surgery, you may need specific treatments, including additional surgery. Maintain an active role in your healthcare and inform your doctor immediately if you experience any new health issues.

Things to Consider, before You Get Breast Implants

There are several important things to consider before deciding to undergo breast implant surgery, including understanding your own personal expectations and reasons for having the surgery. Below are some things the U.S. Food and drug administration (FDA) thinks you should consider before undergoing breast augmentation, reconstruction or revision surgery.

- Breast implants are not lifetime devices; the longer you have your implants, the more likely it will be for you to have them removed.

- The longer you have breast implants, the more likely you are to experience local complications and adverse outcomes.

- The most common local complications and adverse outcomes are capsular contracture, reoperation, implant removal, and rupture or deflation of the implant. Other complications include wrinkling, asymmetry, scarring, pain, and infection at the incision site.

- You should assume that you will need to have additional surgeries (reoperations).

- Many of the changes to your breast following implantation may be cosmetically undesirable and irreversible.

- If you have your implants removed but not replaced, you may experience changes to your natural breasts such as dimpling, puckering, wrinkling, breast tissue loss or other undesirable cosmetic changes.

- If you have breast implants, you will need to monitor your breasts for the rest of your life. If you notice any abnormal changes in your breasts, you will need to see a doctor promptly.

- If you have silicone gel-filled breast implants, you will need to undergo periodic magnetic resonance imaging (MRI) examinations in order to detect ruptures of the implant that do not cause symptoms ("silent ruptures"). For early detection of silent rupture, the FDA and breast implant manufacturers recommend that women with silicone gel-filled breast implants receive MRI screenings 3 years after they receive a new implant and every 2 years after that. MRI screening for implant rupture is costly and may not be covered by your insurance.

- If you have breast implants, you have a low risk of developing a rare type of cancer called breast implant-associated anaplastic large cell lymphoma (BIA-ALCL) in the breast tissue surrounding the implant. BIA-ALCL is not breast cancer. Women diagnosed with BIA-ALCL may need to be treated with surgery, chemotherapy and/or radiation therapy.

Part Five

Recovering from Surgery

Chapter 44

What to Expect after Surgery

Chapter Contents

Section 44.1

What to Expect in the Postanesthesia Care Unit (PACU)

Text in this section is from "What to Expect in the Postanesthesia Care Unit (PACU)," © 2017 American Society of PeriAnesthesia Nurses (ASPAN). Reprinted with permission.

Where Do I Go after Surgery?

Right after surgery, you will be taken to the postanesthesia care unit (PACU) or directly to the intensive care unit where nurses will take care of you and watch you closely. A nurse will check your temperature, blood pressure and pulse often, look at your bandages, regulate your intravenous (IV) and give you pain medication as you need it.

What Do I Need to Tell the PACU Nurse?

Please tell the nurse if you are having pain. The nurse will ask you to give your pain a number on a scale of 0 to 10, with 0 meaning you have no pain, and 10 you have the worst pain. The nurse will check your pain and continue to help you manage it until you are as comfortable as possible.

What Do I Need to Do with My Nausea (Feeling Sick to Your Stomach)?

Some patients feel very sick to their stomach (nausea). It is important to tell your nurse about it right away, so it can be treated with medication. If you have had problems with nausea in the past, the anesthesia care provider knows this before surgery.

What Other Feelings May I Experience after Surgery?

You may feel sleepy, dizzy and/or forgetful from the medication given to you during your surgery.

When Will I See My Family after Surgery?

The facility determines visitation in the PACU. Check with the nursing staff to find out if your family will be allowed to visit you.

What Type of Information Do I Need to Know before Going Home?

If you are going home that same day, you will be given printed discharge instructions for your care at home. The nursing staff will go over all the information with you and a family member or friend. Your instructions will include:

- Activity restrictions

- Diet

- Pain medication

- Follow up instructions with your surgeon

- Signs to watch for if you need to call the doctor

You might be given a prescription depending on your doctor's orders and what kind of surgery you had done.

Section 44.2

What to Expect If You Are Going Home the Day of Surgery

Text in this section is from "What to Expect If You Are Going Home on the Day of Surgery," © 2017 American Society of PeriAnesthesia Nurses (ASPAN). Reprinted with permission.

Once your surgery is over and you have been moved from the postanesthesia care unit (PACU), you will either be sent to an inpatient bed or taken to the area where the nurses will get you ready to go home.

What Do I Need to Know before Going Home?

Before leaving the building, you must meet certain discharge criteria. You may be asked to urinate before going home after certain surgical procedures. If you had a spinal anesthetic, you may be sent home with special instructions about what you should do if you cannot urinate within a certain time period.

Your nurse will go over your postoperative/after surgery instructions with you and your family/friend. The goal is to teach you several things about going home. These things include:

- Pain medicines

- Special diet plans

- Special instructions related to your surgery

- Follow up with your surgeon

- Signs to watch for infection

- When you should report to your surgeon

If you have stopped taking medications before your surgery, your nurse or doctor will let you know when you can start taking them again. You may also be given a prescription from your doctor at this time.

How Long Will It Take Me to Feel Normal Again?

Be prepared at home to continue your recovery. Plan to take it easy for a few days until you feel back to normal. Patients often feel minor effects following surgery due to anesthesia, which might include:

- Being very tired

- Muscle aches

- A sore throat

- Dizziness

- Headaches

Sometimes patients can feel very sick to their stomach and may throw up. These side effects usually go away quickly in the first few hours after surgery, but it can take several days before they are completely gone. Due to feeling tired or having some discomfort, most patients do not feel up to their normal activities for several days.

Can I Drive Myself Home?

Patients who have outpatient/same day surgery must have someone drive them home and stay with for 24 hours following their surgery. The medications you were give during your surgery may affect your memory and mental judgment for the next 24 hours. During that time frame, do not use alcoholic beverages and tobacco products. It is also advised for you not to make any important business or personal decisions and do not use machinery or electrical equipment.

In a day or two after surgery, a nurse may call to check to see how you are feeling. It is important that you provide the staff with a correct working phone number so they can contact you.

Section 44.3

What to Expect after Hip Replacement Surgery

This section includes text excerpted from "Hip Replacement—What to Expect in Recovery," NIHSeniorHealth, National Institute on Aging (NIA), February 2015.

To prepare for recovery, you should learn what to expect in the days and weeks following surgery, including what you will and won't be able to do. It also means arranging for social support and arranging your house to make everyday tasks easier and help speed your recovery.

Before leaving the hospital, talk with your doctor about activities you should avoid as well as any other special instructions for your recovery. By preparing for surgery and recovery and following your doctor's advice, you can get achieve the greatest benefits from your new hip with the least risk of complications.

You Will Need Help

Because you will not be able to drive for several weeks after surgery, you will need someone to take you home from the hospital and be on hand to run errands or take you to appointments until you can drive yourself.

In your first week or two home from the hospital you will likely need someone to stay with you or at least be close by and available in case you need help. If you don't live with a family member who can stay home with you, you should plan to stay with someone or have someone come and stay with you.

If you do not have a family member close by, a friend or neighbor may be able to help. Other options include staying in an extended-care facility during your recovery or hiring someone to come to your home and help you. Your hospital social worker should be able to help you make arrangements.

Prepare Your Home Beforehand

To prepare your home for your recovery, stock up on needed items before you leave for the hospital. Make sure you have plenty of non-perishable foods on hand. Prepare meals and freeze them to put in the microwave when you need an easy meal.

In the first weeks after surgery you should avoid going up and down stairs. If your bedroom is on the second floor of your home, consider moving to a downstairs bedroom temporarily or sleeping on the sofa.

Set up a "recovery station" at home. Place the television remote control, radio, telephone, medicine, tissues, wastebasket, and pitcher and glass next to the spot where you will spend the most time while you recover.

Place items you use every day at arm's level to avoid reaching up or bending down. Ask your doctor or physical therapist about devices and tips that may make daily activities easier once you get home.

Devices you may find helpful include long-handled reachers to retrieve items placed on high shelves or dropped on the floor, aprons with pockets that allow you to carry items while leaving your hands free for crutches, shower benches that let you sit while you shower, and dressing sticks to help you get dressed without bending your new hip excessively.

Make Your Home Fall Proof

Because a fall can damage your new hip, making your home a safe place is crucial. Before your surgery, look for and correct hazards, including cluttered floors, loose electrical cords, unsecured rugs, and dark hallways.

Bathrooms are likely places to fall, so particular attention is needed there. A raised toilet seat can make it easier to get up and down. Grab bars in the tub can keep you steady. Textured shapes on the shower floor can minimize slipping.

Exercise Appropriately

It is also important to exercise to get stronger while avoiding any activities that can damage or dislocate your new joint. Talk to your doctor or physical therapist about developing an appropriate exercise program. Proper exercise can reduce stiffness and increase flexibility and muscle strength.

Most programs begin with safe range-of-motion activities and muscle-strengthening exercises. Activity should include a walking program that gradually increases in time and distance and specific exercises several times a day to restore movement and strengthen your hip joint. Other recommended exercises are stationary bicycling, swimming, and cross-country skiing. These exercises can increase muscle strength and cardiovascular fitness without injuring the new hip.

The doctor or therapist will decide when you can move on to more demanding activities. Many doctors recommend avoiding high-impact activities, such as basketball, jogging, and tennis. These activities can damage the new hip or cause loosening of its parts.

Section 44.4

What to Expect after Knee Replacement Surgery

This section includes text excerpted from "Knee Replacement—What to Expect in Recovery," NIHSeniorHealth, National Institute on Aging (NIA), February 2015.

Recovery from knee replacement extends long after you leave the hospital. Preparing for recovery requires learning what to expect in the days and weeks following surgery. It requires understanding what you will and won't be able to do—and when. It also means arranging for social support and arranging your house to make everyday tasks easier and to help speed your recovery.

Find Someone to Stay with You

Because you will not be able to drive for several weeks after surgery, you will need someone to take you home from the hospital and be on hand to run errands or take you to appointments until you can drive yourself.

If you live with someone, you should have them plan to stay home with you or at least stay close by, in case you need help. If you don't live with a family member or have one close by, a friend or neighbor may be able to help. Other options include staying in an extended-care facility during your recovery or hiring someone to come to your home and help you. Your hospital social worker should be able to help you make arrangements.

Prepare Your Home for Your Recovery

To prepare your home for your recovery, stock up on needed items before you leave for the hospital. Make sure you have plenty of non-perishable foods on hand. Prepare meals and freeze them to put in the microwave when you need an easy meal.

In the first weeks after surgery, you should avoid going up and down stairs. If your bedroom is on the second floor of your home, consider moving to a downstairs bedroom temporarily or sleeping on the sofa.

Set Up a "Recovery Station"

Set up a "recovery station" at home. Place a sturdy chair where you plan to spend most of your time sitting during the first weeks after surgery. The chair should be 18 to 20 inches high and should have two arms and a firm seat and back. Place a foot stool in front of the chair so you can elevate your legs, and place items you will need—such as the television remote control, telephone, medicine, and tissues—where you can reach them easily from the chair.

Place items you use every day at arm's level to avoid reaching up or bending down. Ask your doctor or physical therapist about devices and tips that may make daily activities easier once you get home.

Devices you may find helpful include long-handled reachers to retrieve items placed on high shelves or dropped on the floor, aprons with pockets that allow you to carry items while leaving your hands free for crutches, shower benches that let you sit while you shower, and dressing sticks to help you get dressed without bending your new knee excessively.

Safeguard against Falls

Because a fall can damage your new knee, making your home a safe place is crucial. Before your surgery, look for and correct hazards, including cluttered floors, loose electrical cords, unsecured rugs, and dark hallways.

Bathrooms are likely places to fall, so particular attention is needed there. A raised toilet seat can make it easier to get up and down. Grab bars in the tub can keep you steady. Textured shapes on the shower floor can minimize slipping.

Gradually Increase Activity

It is also important to exercise to get stronger while avoiding any activities that can damage or dislocate your new joint. Activity should include a graduated walking program (where you slowly increase the time, distance, and pace that you walk) and specific exercises several times a day to prevent scarring, restore movement, and stabilize and strengthen your new knee.

Remember Follow-Ups

Your surgeon will let you know about follow-up visits. Even after you have healed from surgery, you will need to see your surgeon periodically for examinations and X-rays to detect any potential problems with your knee.

By preparing for surgery and recovery and following your doctor's advice, you can get the greatest benefits from your new knee with the least risk of complications for many years to come.

Chapter 45

Hospital Discharge Planning

During your stay, your doctor and the staff will work with you to plan for your discharge. You and your caregiver (a family member or friend who may be helping you) are important members of the planning team. You and your caregiver can use this checklist to prepare for your discharge.

What's Ahead?

- Ask where you'll get care after you leave (after you're discharged). Do you have options (like home healthcare)? Be sure you tell the staff what you prefer.

- If a caregiver will be helping you after discharge, write down their name and phone number.

Your Health

- Ask the staff about your health condition and what you can do to help yourself get better.

- Ask about problems to watch for and what to do about them. Write down a name and phone number of a person to call if you have problems.

This chapter includes text excerpted from "Your Discharge Planning Checklist," Centers for Medicare and Medicaid Services (CMS), February 2017.

- Use a drug list to write down your prescription drugs, over-the-counter drugs, vitamins, and herbal supplements.

- Review the list with the staff.

- Tell the staff what drugs, vitamins, or supplements you took before you were admitted. Ask if you should still take these after you leave.

- Write down a name and phone number of a person to call if you have questions.

Recovery and Support

- Ask if you'll need medical equipment (like a walker). Who will arrange for this? Write down a name and phone number of a person you can call if you have questions about equipment.

- Ask if you're ready to do the activities below. Note the ones you need help with, and tell the staff:

  - Bathing, dressing, using the bathroom, climbing stairs

  - Cooking, food shopping, house cleaning, paying bills

  - Getting to doctor's appointments, picking up prescription drugs

- Make sure you have support (like a caregiver) in place that can help you.

- Ask the staff to show you and your caregiver any other tasks that require special skills (like changing a bandage or giving a shot). Then, show them you can do these tasks. Write down a name and phone number of a person you can call if you need help.

- Ask to speak to a social worker if you're concerned about how you and your family are coping with your illness. Write down information about support groups and other resources.

- Talk to a social worker or your health plan if you have questions about what your insurance will cover and how much you'll have to pay. Ask about possible ways to get help with your costs.

- Ask for written discharge instructions (that you can read and understand) and a summary of your current health status. Bring this information and your completed drug list to your follow-up appointments.

- Write down any appointments and tests you'll need in the next several weeks.

For the Caregiver

- Do you have any questions about the items on this checklist or on the discharge instructions? Write them down, and discuss them with the staff.

- Can you give the patient the help he or she needs?

- What tasks do you need help with?

- Do you need any education or training?

- Talk to the staff about getting the help you need before discharge.

- Write down a name and phone number of a person you can call if you have questions.

- Get prescriptions and any special diet instructions early, so you won't have to make extra trips after discharge.

More Information for People with Medicare

If you need help choosing a home health agency or nursing home:

- Talk to the staff.

- Visit Medicare.gov to compare the quality of home health agencies, nursing homes, dialysis facilities, and hospitals in your area.

- Call 800-MEDICARE (800-633-4227). TTY users can call 877-486-2048.

If you think you're being asked to leave a hospital or other healthcare setting (discharged) too soon, you may have the right to ask for a review of the discharge decision by the Beneficiary and Family Centered Care Quality Improvement Organization (BFCC-QIO) before you leave.

A BFCC-QIO is a type of quality improvement organization (a group of doctors and other healthcare experts under contract with Medicare) that reviews complaints and quality of care for people with Medicare. To get the phone number for your BFCC-QIO, visit www.medicare.gov/contacts, or call 800-MEDICARE (800-633-4227). You can also ask the staff for this information. If you're in a hospital, the staff should give you a notice called "Important Message from Medicare," which contains information on your BFCC-QIO. If you don't get this notice, ask for it.

671

Chapter 46

Moving to a Nursing Home

Nursing Home

A nursing home, also known as a skilled nursing facility, is a place for people who don't need to be in a hospital but can no longer be cared for at home. This can include people needing care after surgery, or those with critical injuries or serious illnesses. Most nursing homes have aides and skilled nurses on hand 24 hours a day. Talk to your healthcare provider to find out if a nursing home is the best choice for you or a member of your family.

Nursing homes can be:

- **Hospital-like.** This type of nursing home is often set up like a hospital. Members of the staff give medical care, as well as physical, speech, and occupational therapy. There can be a nurses' station on each floor. As a rule, one or two people live in a room. A number of nursing homes will let couples live together. Things that make a room special, like family photos, are often welcome.

- **Household-like.** These facilities are designed to be more like homes, and the day-to-day routine is not fixed. Teams of staff and residents try to create a relaxed feeling. Kitchens are often open to residents, decorations give a sense of home, and the staff is encouraged to develop relationships with residents.

This chapter includes text excerpted from "Nursing Homes: Making the Right Choice," National Institute on Aging (NIA), National Institutes of Health (NIH), July 22, 2016.

- **Combination.** Some nursing homes have a combination of hospital-like and household-like units.

Many nursing homes have visiting doctors who see their patients on site. Other nursing homes have patients visit the doctor's office. Nursing homes sometimes have separate areas called "Special Care Units" for people with serious memory problems, like dementia.

Tips to Keep in Mind

If you need to go to a nursing home after a hospital stay, the hospital staff can help you find one that will provide the kind of care that's best for you. Most hospitals have social workers who can help you with these decisions. If you are looking for a nursing home, ask your doctor's office for some recommendations. Once you know what choices you have, it's a good idea to:

- **Consider.** What is important to you—nursing care, meals, physical therapy, a religious connection, hospice care, or Special Care Units for dementia patients? Do you want a place close to family and friends so they can easily visit?

- **Ask.** Talk with friends, relatives, social workers, and religious groups to find out what places they suggest. Check with healthcare providers about which nursing homes they feel provide good care. Use their suggestions to make a list of homes that offer the types of services you want.

- **Call.** Get in touch with each place on your list. Ask questions about how many people live there and what it costs. Find out about waiting lists.

- **Visit.** Make plans to meet with the director and the nursing director. The Medicare Nursing Home Checklist (www.medicare. gov/nursinghomecompare/search.html) has some good ideas to consider when visiting. For example, look for:
  - Medicare and Medicaid certification
  - Handicap access
  - Residents who look well cared for
  - Warm interaction between staff and residents

- **Talk.** Don't be afraid to ask questions. For example, you can ask the staff to explain any strong odors. Bad smells might indicate a problem; good ones might hide a problem. You might want to find out how long the director and heads of nursing, food, and social services departments have worked at the nursing home. If key members of the staff change often, that could mean there's something wrong.

- **Visit again.** Make a second visit without calling ahead. Try another day of the week or time of day so you will meet other staff members and see different activities. Stop by at mealtime. Is the dining room attractive and clean? Does the food look tempting?

- **Understand.** Once you select a nursing home, carefully read the contract. Question the director or assistant director about anything you don't understand. Ask a good friend or family member to read over the contract before you sign it.

Do Nursing Homes Have to Meet Standards?

The Centers for Medicare and Medicaid Services (CMS) requires each state to inspect any nursing home that gets money from the government. Homes that don't pass inspection are not certified. Ask to see the current inspection report and certification of any nursing home you are considering.

Paying for Nursing Home Care

It's important to check with Medicare, Medicaid, and any private insurance provider you have to find out their current rules about covering the costs of long-term care. You can pay for nursing home care in several ways. Here are some examples:

- **Medicare.** For someone who needs special care, Medicare, a Federal program, will cover part of the cost in a skilled nursing home approved by Medicare. Check with Medicare for details.

- **Medicaid.** Medicaid is a State/Federal program that provides health benefits to some people with low incomes. Contact your county family services department to see if you qualify.

- **Private pay.** Some people pay for long-term care with their own savings for as long as possible. When that is no longer possible, they may apply for help from Medicaid. If you think you may need to apply for Medicaid at some point, make sure the nursing home you're interested in accepts Medicaid payments. Not all do.

- **Long-term care insurance.** Some people buy private long-term care insurance. It can pay part of the costs for a nursing home or other long-term care for the length of time stated in your policy. This type of insurance is sold by many different companies and benefits vary widely. Look carefully at several policies before making a choice.

When thinking about nursing home costs, keep in mind that you can have extra out-of-pocket charges for some supplies or personal care, for instance, hair appointments, laundry, and services that are outside routine care.

Chapter 47

Nutrition and Exercise Concerns after Surgery

Chapter Contents

Section 47.1

Postsurgical Physical Activity Recommendations

This section includes text excerpted from "Chronic Fatigue
Syndrome (CFS)," Centers for Disease Control and
Prevention (CDC), February 14, 2013. Reviewed June 2017.

Developing an Activity Program

Start Slow

It is very important that any activity plan be started slowly and
increased gradually. When beginning an activity program, some
patients may only be able to exercise for as little as a few minutes.
Patients who are severely deconditioned or who are caught in the
push-crash cycle should limit themselves to the basic activities of
daily living—getting up, personal hygiene, dressing, and necessary
tasks—until they have stabilized.

Light, Low-Impact Activity

Several daily sessions of brief, low-impact (light) activity can then
be added. Simple stretching and strengthening exercise using only
body weight for resistance is a good starting place for most people. All
exercise needs to be followed by a rest period at a 1:3 ratio, exercising
for one minute then resting for three minutes. These sessions can be
slowly increased by one to five minutes a week as tolerance develops.

Daily exercise can be divided into two or more sessions to avoid
symptom flare-ups. Activity should be alternating and brief, spread
throughout the day and followed by rest. If patients experience a worsening of symptoms, they should return to the most recent manageable
level of activity.

Strength and Conditioning Exercises

Strength and conditioning exercises are an important component
of the overall activity program. Standard rehabilitative methods, such

as resistance training and flexibility exercises, may help improve stamina and function, increase strength and flexibility, reduce pain, and increase range of motion.

Activity should begin slowly with simple stretching and strengthening exercises. Examples of functional exercises include repeated hand stretches, sitting and standing, wall push-ups, and picking up and grasping objects. Patients can begin with a set of two to four repetitions, building to a maximum of eight repetitions. Once this stage is mastered, resistance band exercises (using bands for strength training) can be added to build strength and flexibility. Patients should be careful to adhere to the principle of brief intervals of exercise, followed by adequate rest, to avoid postexertion malaise.

Graded Exercise Therapy (GET)

GET is a type of physical activity therapy that starts very slowly and gradually increases over time. A GET program that includes active stretching followed by range-of-motion contractions and extensions is usually an effective start. Five minutes per day is a typical starting point for an individual who has been totally inactive. When beginning a GET program, it is important for patients to avoid extremes and instead balance physical activity and rest. Gradual, guided physical activity can help some patients manage the illness. Appropriate rest is an important element of GET, and patients should learn to stop activity before illness and fatigue are worsened.

The end point of each GET session should be preset by the clock or number of repetitions, and these endpoints should be reached before the patient becomes tired. Each patient will have to determine their individual limits by trial and error; limits by time or repetition assist in this goal. Appropriate goals are to prevent tiredness, to avoid activating the syndrome, and to increase overall fitness. GET may be summarized by the adage that no exercise is bad, some is good, but too much is not helpful.

Modifying Exercises for Severely Ill Patients

A subset of people are so severely ill that they're largely housebound or bedbound. They require special attention, including a modified approach to exercise. Hand stretches and picking up and grasping objects may be all that can be managed at first. Gradually increasing activity to the point patients can handle essential activities of daily living—getting up, personal hygiene and dressing—is the next step.

A realistic goal with severely ill patients is focusing on improving flexibility and minimizing the impact of deconditioning so they can increase function enough to manage basic activities.

Section 47.2

Tube Feeding

This section contains text excerpted from the following sources: Text under the heading "Tube Feeding and Its Requirement" is excerpted from "End of Life: Helping with Comfort and Care," National Institute on Aging (NIA), National Institutes of Health (NIH), July 2016; Text under the heading "Gastrostomy (G-tube)" is excerpted from "Home Bolus Tube Feeding Instructions," U.S. Department of Veterans Affairs (VA), June 4, 2012. Reviewed June 2017; Text under the heading "Nasogastric Tube" is excerpted from "Where's the Feeding Tube?" Agency for Healthcare Research and Quality (AHRQ), U.S. Department of Health and Human Services (HHS), September 2008. Reviewed June 2017; Text under the heading "Getting Ready for Tube Feeding" is excerpted from "GCVA Patient Education Handout Tube Feeding Guidelines," U.S. Department of Veterans Affairs (VA), December 2013. Reviewed June 2017.

Tube Feeding and Its Requirement

If a patient can't or won't eat or drink, the doctor might suggest a feeding tube. While a patient recovers from an illness, getting nutrition temporarily through a feeding tube can be helpful. But, at the end of life, a feeding tube might cause more discomfort than not eating. For people with dementia, tube feeding does not prolong life or prevent aspiration.

As death approaches, loss of appetite is common. Body systems start shutting down, and fluids and food are not needed as before. Some experts believe that at this point few nutrients are absorbed from any type of nutrition, including those received through a feeding tube. Further, after a feeding tube is inserted, the family might need to make a difficult decision about when, or if, to remove it.

If tube feeding will be tried, there are two methods that could be used. In the first, a feeding tube, known as a nasogastric or NG tube, is threaded through the nose down to the stomach to give nutrition for a short time. Sometimes, the tube is uncomfortable. Someone with an NG tube might try to remove it. This usually means the person has to be restrained, which could mean binding his or her hands to the bed.

If tube feeding is required for an extended time, then a gastric or G-tube is put directly into the stomach through an opening made in the side or abdomen. This second method is sometimes called a PEG (percutaneous endoscopic gastrostomy) tube. It carries risks of infection, pneumonia, and nausea.

Hand feeding (sometimes called assisted oral feeding) is an alternative to tube feeding. This approach may have fewer risks, especially for people with dementia.

Gastrostomy (G-Tube)

For some people, eating, drinking, and swallowing become impossible. They cannot eat enough, or at all, so they get their nutrition through a feeding tube. Unlike regular eating, the mouth and esophagus are bypassed.

Tube feeding through the stomach is accomplished by using a gastrostomy (also called a G-tube). Tube feeding can also be done through the jejunum (a section of the small intestine) using a jejunostomy (J-tube).

Formulas for Tube Feeding

With tube feeding, you can get the nutrition you need when you can't eat or are unable to eat enough. The special medical nutritional product that is given through the tube is called a formula. It contains all of the nutrients you need—just like a well balanced diet. There are many different types of formulas designed for particular diet needs. Your medical team will select the formula that will best meet your nutritional needs.

Giving Medicine through the Feeding Tube

- Most medicine that your doctor orders for you will be in liquid form and may be given through your feeding tube using a syringe.

- Some medicine does not come in liquid form. It must be crushed and placed in warm water before taking.

- Some medicine will not work if crushed. So be sure to ask first before crushing any of your medications.

- Do not dilute your medicine with formula.

- Do not add your medicine to the formula in the feeding set.

- Always flush tube with water before and after taking the medicine so that it does not plug up the tube

Nasogastric Tube

Patients who require short-term (less than 1 month) feeding often have tubes placed directly through the nose into the gastrointestinal tract. These feeding tubes are thin (often less than 2 mm in diameter) and flexible to maximize patient comfort. As described in this case, these tubes can either end in the stomach (nasogastric tube) or in the small intestine (nasojejunal tube).

Getting Ready for Tube Feeding

1. If your work surface is washable, clean it with soap and water and dry it with a clean towel or paper towel. If your work surface is not washable, wipe it free of dust. Spread a clean towel or paper towels over the surface.

2. Wash your hands with soap and water.

3. Check placement of your feeding tube.

4. Check feeding tube residuals if your nurse, dietitian or doctor told you to do so. Your initial feeding will not require checking for residuals.

5. Shake the formula well. Wipe off the top of the can with a clean, damp paper towel.

6. Always use room temperature feeding formula.

Feeding

1. Draw approximately 30 mL of water into the syringe. Attach it to the end of the feeding tube. Flush the tube free of stomach contents. Clamp the feeding tube. Remove the syringe.

2. Pour the proper amount of formula into a clean, empty container such as a glass measuring cup.

3. Draw formula into the syringe. Attach the tip of the syringe to the feeding tube or adaptor. Make sure the tip of the syringe is firmly inserted into the tube or adaptor. Unclamp the feeding tube.

4. Slowly push the plunger down. Clamp the feeding tube between each bolus to prevent leakage. Refill the syringe with formula. Repeat the procedure until the desired amount of formula is given. If you feel full, wait 10 to 15 minutes before you continue the feeding.

5. After the desired amount of formula has been given, flush the feeding tube with approximately 30 mL of water, clamp and detach.

6. Clean, rinse, and dry your feeding equipment after each feeding.

7. Stay in an upright position for 30 to 60 minutes after your feeding to prevent stomach upset.

Checking the Residual

The residual is the contents left in your stomach since your last feeding. Once you are stable on your goal amount of tube feeding and have no symptoms of excessive fullness, bloating or upset stomach, your healthcare provider may tell you to stop checking residuals before each feeding. If these symptoms return, check your residual before giving the next feeding.

How to check your residual:

1. Flush tube with 30 mL of water before checking residual.

2. Using a 60 mL syringe, push the plunger all the way in. Insert the syringe into the end of the feeding tube. Unclamp.

3. Gently draw back the plunger to withdraw stomach contents. Clamp.

4. Check the amount of fluid in the syringe. If the entire syringe is filled, put the fluid in a measuring cup. Continue to withdraw stomach contents until no more can be withdrawn. Measure and record the total volume.

5. Unless you were told differently, if the residual measures less than one cup (240 mL), return the residual to your stomach. This fluid contains things your body needs. If the residual is

more than 250 mL or if you feel nauseous or full, do not return the residual to your stomach. Wait one hour and recheck the residual. Do not give tube feeding if the residual is still high or if you still feel nauseous or full.

6. Flush tube with 30 mL of water after checking residual clamp.

How to Store Your Formula

1. Store all unopened cans or containers of formula in a clean, dry location.

2. Do not store formula on the floor, near the stove, above the refrigerator or in the garage. Store the formula at a temperature of 50 to 70 degrees Fahrenheit.

3. Check the expiration date on the can before you use it. Discard the can if it is out of date.

4. Store opened, unused formula in the refrigerator. Keep it covered. Throw it away if it is not used in 24 hours.

Preventing a Clogged Feeding Tube

1. Flush your feeding tube with 30 mL of water before and after:

    *   feeding

    *   medicines

    *   checking residuals

2. Do not use the following items to unclog your tube. They may make the clog worse.

    *   meat tenderizer

    *   fruit or vegetable juice

    *   Colas

    *   ginger ale

    *   root beer

    *   any other sodas or soda pops

3. If your tube clogs, pull out excess water with your syringe. Add 15 mL of warm water. Clamp the tube for 10 minutes. Then flush with 15 mL or warm water. Call your healthcare provider if the tube is still clogged.

General Tips and Guidelines

1. Never set up or do the feeding in the bathroom.

2. Remain in an upright position during the feeding and for 30 to 60 minutes after the feeding. Always sit in a chair, propped up in a bed or on a couch in a half-sitting position. You should be sitting at about 30 to 45 degrees (for example, when using two pillows).

3. Store all unopened cans of formula in a clean, dry location. Do not store formula on the floor, near a stove, above the refrigerator or in the garage. Store your formula at a temperature of 50 to 70 degrees.

4. Check the expiration date on the can before using the formula. Discard the can if it is out of date.

5. Store any opened, unused formula in the refrigerator. Keep it covered. Throw it away if not used within 24 hours.

6. Check your tube daily. If you have a skin disk that is not sutured in place, gently rotate the feeding tube daily by 360 degrees. Call your healthcare provider if the tube has moved more than one inch from where it comes out of your abdomen.

7. Do not add medicine, juices or any other substances to the tube feeding formula.

Calling Your Primary Care Physician or Home Care Nurse

1. Your feeding tube comes out and is no longer in place.

2. Anything makes you stop tube feedings for more than 24 hours.

3. A weight loss or gain of more than two to three pounds over two to three days.

4. A feeling of choking, coughing or difficulty breathing.

5. Swelling, redness or draining from the feeding tube site.

6. Nausea, vomiting or heartburn that lasts for more than 24 hours.

7. Diarrhea (more than three loose stools a day for more than two days)

8. Constipation that lasts for more than three days.

9. Blood in or around your feeding tube.

10. Signs of dehydration:

    • fever

    • thirst

    • decreased urine output

    • mouth dryness

Section 47.3

Nutrition Considerations after Weight-Loss (Bariatric) Surgery

This section includes text excerpted from "Nutrition Management after Bariatric Surgery," Federal Bureau of Prisons (BOP), October 2013. Reviewed June 2017.

Weight-Loss (Bariatric) Surgery

Bariatric surgery refers to a variety of surgical procedures whose primary goal is weight loss through malabsorption, restriction, or a combination of the two, depending on the type of procedure performed. Malabsorptive procedures (biliopancreatic diversion and duodenal switch) work by bypassing the intestinal lumen where most nutrient absorption occurs. Restrictive procedures (laparoscopic adjustable gastric banding [LAGB], sleeve gastrectomy, and vertical banded gastroplasty) primarily limit the volume of food ingested. Roux-en-Y gastric bypass (gastrojejunostomy) achieves weight loss through a combination of malabsorption and restriction.

Nutrition Management

Nutrition management following bariatric surgery requires both behavioral modification of eating habits and modifications to the content and quality of food items consumed. All bariatric surgery patients are at risk for nutrition deficiencies. Dietary management is based on the amount of time since the surgery was performed, and may be divided into early (up to six months postoperative) and long-term maintenance. Nutrition therapy and nutrition needs of postoperative bariatric surgery patients can be met through texture-modified special diets, self-selection of food items, food service supplemental feeding, and nutrition supplementation.

During the early postoperative period, the initial goals are healing of the surgery site, adequate fluid and protein intake, and avoidance of certain complications such as food impaction and vomiting.

- Immediately following surgery, all oral intake is liquid and the diet is advanced gradually to solid foods as tolerated by the patient.

- During the transition from liquid to solid food, it is common to provide nutrition using blenderized solid food and mechanically soft diets.

- In patients with LAGB, diet usually can be advanced more quickly from liquid to solid foods because the band typically is not inflated at the time it is applied intraoperatively.

Diet

Once the diet has been advanced to regular solid food, patients should be encouraged to self-select heart healthy diet. Patients should also be encouraged to:

- Eat protein foods first at meals, followed by soft vegetables and fruits, and then starchy foods last.

- Wait at least 30 minutes after a meal to drink fluids; do not use a straw, which can result in swallowing air.

- Thoroughly chew food before swallowing.

- Stop eating or drinking when full.

- Avoid sugar and sweets.

- Avoid high-fat and starchy foods that may cause dumping syndrome, including fried meats, French fries, pastries, rolls, desserts, and chips.

- Avoid carbonated beverages.

- Avoid alcoholic beverages (prohibited in correctional environment)

Nutrition Supplementation

Postoperative bariatric surgery patients are required to take certain vitamin and mineral supplements for the remainder of their life. These include:

- Multivitamin and mineral supplement, either two regular or chewable tablets per day or liquid equivalent, based on patient preference and tolerance

- Calcium with vitamin D, either calcium citrate 1,200–1,500 mg per day in divided doses, or calcium carbonate 2,000 mg per day in divided doses, taken at least two hours before or after supplements with iron

- Vitamin B12 supplement, for all cases of Roux-en-Y gastric bypass only

Some vitamin and mineral supplements are taken only if clinically indicated for specific deficiencies:

- Iron, 325 mg iron (with 250 mg Vitamin C to increase absorption)

- Vitamin B12 supplement, when needed after bariatric procedures other than Roux-en-Y

Nutrition supplementation for additional protein is indicated routinely during the early postoperative period.

Chapter 48

Caring for Surgical Incisions and Drains

Chapter Contents

Section 48.1

Caring for Your Incision

This section contains text excerpted from the following sources: Text
in this section begins with excerpts from "Surgical Site Infection
(SSI) Event," Centers for Disease Control and Prevention (CDC),
January 1, 2017; Text beginning with the heading "Surgical Site
Care" is excerpted from "Post-Op Instructions: Taking Care of
Yourself after Surgery," National Institutes of Health (NIH),
February 1, 2016.

A prevalence study found that surgical site infections (SSIs) were
the most common healthcare-associated infection, accounting for 31
percent of all HAIs among hospitalized patients. The Centers for Disease Control and Prevention (CDC) healthcare-associated infection
(HAI) prevalence survey found that there were an estimated 157,500
surgical site infections associated with inpatient surgeries in 2011. The
National Healthcare Safety Network (NHSN) data included 16,147
SSIs following 849,659 operative procedures in all groups reported,
for an overall SSI rate of 1.9 percent between 2006–2008. A 19 percent
decrease in SSI related to 10 select procedures was reported between
2008 and 2013.

While advances have been made in infection control practices,
including improved operating room ventilation, sterilization methods, barriers, surgical technique, and availability of antimicrobial
prophylaxis, SSIs remain a substantial cause of morbidity, prolonged
hospitalization, and death. SSI is associated with a mortality rate of
3 percent, and 75 percent of SSI associated deaths are directly attributable to the SSI.

Wounds are divided into four classes:

1. **Clean.** An uninfected operative wound in which no inflammation is encountered and the respiratory, alimentary, genital, or uninfected urinary tracts are not entered. In addition,
clean wounds are primarily closed and, if necessary, drained
with closed drainage. Operative incisional wounds that follow

nonpenetrating (blunt) trauma should be included in this category if they meet the criteria.

2. **Clean-Contaminated.** Operative wounds in which the respiratory, alimentary, genital, or urinary tracts are entered under controlled conditions and without unusual contamination. Specifically, operations involving the biliary tract, appendix, vagina, and oropharynx are included in this category, provided no evidence of infection or major break in technique is encountered.

3. **Contaminated.** Open, fresh, accidental wounds. In addition, operations with major breaks in sterile technique (e.g., open cardiac massage) or gross spillage from the gastrointestinal tract, and incisions in which acute, nonpurulent inflammation is encountered including necrotic tissue without evidence of purulent drainage (e.g., dry gangrene) are included in this category.

4. **Dirty or Infected.** Includes old traumatic wounds with retained devitalized tissue and those that involve existing clinical infection or perforated viscera. This definition suggests that the organisms causing postoperative infection were present in the operative field before the operation.

Surgical Site Care

Follow your doctor's instructions about caring for your surgical site or incision area. Watch for any separation, bleeding, or signs of infection which include:

- Redness

- Pain

- Swelling

- Drainage of fluid or pus

- Heat at incision site

- Fever (which is usually a temperature of 101°F or higher)

If you notice any of these problems, call your nurse or doctor right away.

691

Care of Your Incision

Wash your hands before and after touching your incision(s). Hand washing is the best way to prevent infection. It is normal to have some numbness around the incision for some time after surgery. This may subside as the incision heals. If you have been sent home with staples in your incision, then see your regular doctor to have your staples removed. You may shower with staples in place, unless your doctor has told you not to.

If you have been sent home with sterile tape over your incision, you may shower, but be gentle around the tape. Use regular soap and water. Wash your incision gently, and then pat the incision dry. Do not pull, tug, or rub the tape. If the tape has not fallen off 2 weeks after surgery, then you may peel the tape off gently. Check with your doctor about applying creams or lotions to your incisions. Apply these only after the tape has fallen off or has been removed.

Avoid exposing your incision to the sun. This can cause the incision to become red. Scars turn white over time without exposure to the sun. You will receive information from your doctor about any dressing changes or suture removal.

Section 48.2

Caring for a Surgical Drain

This section includes text excerpted from "How to Care for the Jackson-Pratt Drain," National Institute on Aging (NIA), National Institutes of Health (NIH), July 2008. Reviewed June 2017.

Jackson-Pratt (JP) Drain

The Jackson-Pratt (JP) drain is a special tube that prevents body fluid from collecting near the site of your surgery. The drain pulls this fluid (by suction) into a bulb. The bulb can then be emptied and the fluid inside measured.

At first, this fluid is bloody. Then, as your wound heals, the fluid changes to light pink, light yellow, or clear. The drain will stay in place until less than 30 cc (about 2 tablespoons) of fluid can be collected in a 24 hour period.

Caring for the JP drain is easy. Depending on how much fluid drains from your surgical site, you will need to empty the bulb every 8 to 12 hours. The bulb should be emptied when it is half full. Before you are discharged from the hospital, your nurse will show you how to:

- empty the collection bulb

- record the amount of fluid collected

- squeeze the bulb flat and plug so that the suction works again

- keep the drain site clean and free of infection

How to Empty the Drain

1. Wash your hands well with soap and water.

2. Pull the plug out of the bulb.

3. Pour the fluid inside the bulb into a measuring cup.

4. Clean the plug with alcohol. Then squeeze the bulb flat. While the bulb is flat, put the plug back into the bulb. The bulb should stay flat after it is plugged so that the vacuum suction can restart. If you can't squeeze the bulb flat and plug it at the same time, use a hard, flat surface (such as a table) to help you press the bulb flat while you replug it.

5. Measure how much fluid you collected. Write the amount of drainage, and the date and time you collected it, on the JP drainage chart.

6. Flush the fluid down the toilet.

7. Wash your hands.

How to Care for the Skin and the Drain Site

1. Wash your hands well with soap and water.

2. Remove the dressing from around the drain. Use soap and water or 0.9 percent normal saline (on a gauze or cotton swab) to clean the drain site and the skin around it. Clean this area once a day.

3. When the drain site is clean and dry, put a new dressing around the drain. Put surgical tape on the dressing to hold it down against your skin.

4. Place the old dressing into the trash. If it is bloody, wrap it in a small plastic bag (like a sandwich bag).

5. Wash your hands.

Complications of the Drain

Sometimes, a large amount of fluid may leak from around the drain site, making the gauze dressing completely wet. If this happens, use soap and water to clean the area. Verify that the bulb drain is secured and "flat" to provide the needed suction.

Another potential side effect is the development of a clot within the drain. This appears as a dark, stringy lining. It could prevent the drainage from flowing through the tube. Be sure to notify your doctor if either of these complications occurs.

How to Check for Infection

Watch the skin around the drain for these signs of infection:

-   increased redness

-   increased pain

-   increased swelling

Other signs of infection:

-   fever greater than 101°F

-   cloudy yellow, tan, or foul-smelling drainage

Report any of these symptoms to your doctor as soon as possible. If you have questions, please call your patient care unit.

Chapter 49

Caring for an Ostomy Pouch after Surgery

During the recovery in the hospital and at home, a person will learn to care for the ostomy. The type of care required depends on the type of ostomy surgery. A Wound, Ostomy, and Continence (WOC) nurse or an enterostomal therapist will teach a person about special care after ostomy surgery.

Ileostomy and colostomy. People with an ileostomy or a colostomy will to learn how to attach, drain, and change their ostomy pouch and care for the stoma and the surrounding skin. Ostomy pouches, or pouching systems, may be one piece or two pieces. They include a barrier, also called a wafer or flange, and a disposable plastic pouch. In a two-piece system, the pouch can be detached or replaced without removing the barrier. For both systems, the barrier attaches to the skin around the stoma and protects it from stool. The length of time the barrier stays sealed to the skin depends on many things, such as:

- how well the barrier fits
- the condition of the skin around the stoma
- the person's level of physical activity
- the shape of the body around the stoma

This chapter includes text excerpted from "Ostomy Surgery of the Bowel," National Institute of Diabetes and Digestive and Kidney Diseases (NIDDK), July 2014.

Most people can leave the barrier on for 3 to 7 days. However, a person should change the barrier as soon as stool starts to go underneath it and onto the skin.

Most ostomy pouches empty through an opening in the bottom. Emptying the pouch several times a day reduces the chance of leakage and bulges underneath the person's clothing. A person should empty the pouch when it is about one-third full. He or she should rinse the pouch in a two-piece system before reattaching it to the skin barrier. How often a person needs to change his or her pouching system depends on the type of system. Many pouching systems may be worn for 3 to 7 days. Some pouching systems are made to be changed every day. When changing a pouch system, the person should:

- wipe away any mucus on the stoma

- clean the skin around the stoma with warm water and a washcloth

- rinse the skin thoroughly

- dry the skin completely

People may use mild soap to clean the skin. However, the soap should not have oils, perfumes, or deodorants, which may cause skin problems or keep the skin barrier from sticking. A WOC nurse or an enterostomal therapist can give advice if a person has problems attaching the skin barrier or keeping it attached.

When changing the pouching system, people should inspect the stoma and contact a healthcare provider about any dramatic changes in stoma size, shape, or color. People should look for blood and signs of skin irritation around the stoma. Sensitivities or allergies to ostomy products such as adhesives, skin barriers, pastes, tape, or pouch materials can cause skin irritation. People with pouching systems can test different products to see if their skin reacts to them. People should use only ostomy products recommended by their healthcare provider.

Ileoanal reservoir. People with an ileoanal reservoir will learn how to care for irritated skin around the anus resulting from frequent stools or fecal incontinence. A WOC nurse or an enterostomal therapist may recommend pelvic floor exercises to help strengthen the muscles around the anus.

Continent ileostomy. People with a continent ileostomy will learn how to insert a catheter through the stoma to drain the internal pouch. They can drain the pouch by standing in front of the toilet or by sitting on the toilet and then emptying the catheter. During the first few weeks after a continent ileostomy, the person needs to drain the internal pouch about every 2 hours. After a few weeks, the person is able to go 4 to 6 hours between pouch drainings. The person should wash his or her hands with soap and water after using a catheter. The person should clean the skin around the stoma with warm water and a washcloth and let the skin dry completely.

Chapter 50

Blood Clot Risks and Travel

More than 300 million people travel on long-distance flights (generally more than four hours) each year. Blood clots, also called deep vein thrombosis (DVT), can be a serious risk for some long-distance travelers. Most information about blood clots and long-distance travel comes from information that has been gathered about air travel. However, anyone traveling more than four hours, whether by air, car, bus, or train, can be at risk for blood clots.

Blood clots can form in the deep veins (veins below the surface that are not visible through the skin) of your legs during travel because you are sitting still in a confined space for long periods of time. The longer you are immobile, the greater is your risk of developing a blood clot. Many times the blood clot will dissolve on its own. However, a serious health problem can occur when a part of the blood clot breaks off and travels to the lungs causing a blockage. This is called a pulmonary embolism, and it may be fatal. The good news is there are things you can do to protect your health and reduce your risk of blood clots during a long-distance trip.

Understand What Can Increase Your Risk for Blood Clots

Even if you travel a long distance, the risk of developing a blood clot is generally very small. Your level of risk depends on the duration

This chapter includes text excerpted from "Venous Thromboembolism (Blood Clots)—Blood Clots and Travel: What You Need to Know," Centers for Disease Control and Prevention (CDC), December 19, 2016.

of travel as well as whether you have any other risks for blood clots. Most people who develop travel-associated blood clots have one or more other risks for blood clots, such as:

- Recent surgery or injury (within 3 months)

- Older age (risk increases after age 40)

- Obesity (body mass index (BMI) greater than 30 kg/m2)

- Use of estrogen-containing contraceptives (for example, birth control pills, rings, patches)

- Hormone replacement therapy (medical treatment in which hormones are given to reduce the effects of menopause)

- Pregnancy and the postpartum period (up to 6 weeks after childbirth)

- Previous blood clot or a family history of blood clots

- Active cancer or recent cancer treatment

- Limited mobility (for example, a leg cast)

- Catheter placed in a large vein

- Varicose veins

The combination of long-distance travel with one or more of these risks may increase the likelihood of developing a blood clot. The more risks you have, the greater your chances of experiencing a blood clot. If you plan on traveling soon, talk with your doctor to learn more about what you can do to protect your health. The most important thing you can do is to learn and recognize the symptoms of blood clots.

Protect Yourself and Reduce Your Risk of Blood Clots during Travel

- Know what to look for. Be alert to the signs and symptoms of blood clots.

- Talk with your doctor if you think you may be at risk for blood clots. If you have had a previous blood clot, or if a family member has a history of blood clots or an inherited clotting disorder, talk with your doctor to learn more about your individual risks.

- Move your legs frequently when on long trips and exercise your calf muscles to improve the flow of blood. If you've been sitting for a long time, take a break to stretch your legs. Extend your legs straight out and flex your ankles (pulling your toes toward you). Some airlines suggest pulling each knee up toward the chest and holding it there with your hands on your lower leg for 15 seconds, and repeat up to 10 times. These types of activities help to improve the flow of blood in your legs.

- If you are at risk, talk with your doctor to learn more about how to prevent blood clots. For example, some people may benefit by wearing graduated compression stockings.

- If you are on blood thinners, also known as anticoagulants, be sure to follow your doctor's recommendations on medication use.

Part Six

Additional Help and Information

Chapter 51

Glossary of Terms Related to Surgery

amputation: Removal of part or all of a body part, except for organs in the body. It usually takes place during surgery in a hospital operating room.

aneurysm: A thin or weak spot in an artery that balloons out and can burst.

antibiotic: Drugs used to fight bacteria in the body.

antibodies: Blood proteins made by certain white blood cells called B cells in response to germs or other foreign substances that enter the body. Antibodies help the body fight illness and disease by attaching to germs and marking them for destruction.

atherosclerosis: A disease in which fatty material is deposited on the wall of the arteries. This fatty material causes the arteries to become narrow and it eventually restricts blood flow.

bacteria: Microorganisms that can cause infections.

benign: A tumor or cells that are not cancerous.

biopsy: The removal of body tissues for examination under a microscope or for other tests on the tissue.

This glossary contains terms excerpted from documents produced by several sources deemed reliable.

bladder: The organ in the human body that stores urine. It is found in the lower part of the abdomen.

blood transfusion: A procedure in which a person is given an infusion of whole blood or parts of blood. The blood may be donated by another person, or it may have been taken from the patient earlier and stored until needed.

body mass index (BMI): BMI is a measure of body weight relative to height. The BMI tool uses a formula that produces a score often used to determine if a person is underweight, at a normal weight, overweight, or obese.

bone marrow: The soft, sponge-like tissue in the center of most bones. Bone marrow makes all kinds of blood cells: white blood cells, red blood cells, and platelets (clotting cells).

carbohydrate: A "carb" is a major source of energy for your body. Your digestive system changes carbohydrates into blood glucose (sugar).

cataracts: Cloudy or thick areas in the lens of the eye.

chiropractic: An occupational discipline based on the relationship of the spine to health and disease. The spine is analyzed by X-rays and palpation, and vertebrae are adjusted manually to relieve pressures on the spinal cord.

cholesterol: Cholesterol is a fat-like substance that is made by your body and found naturally in animal foods such as dairy products, eggs, meat, poultry, and seafood.

chronic illness: An illness that persists over a long period of time.

colonoscopy: A colonoscopy is a procedure that allows your doctor to look inside your large intestine using an instrument with a tiny camera called a scope.

critical care: A subspecialty of medicine concerned with the diagnosis, treatment, and support of patients with multiple organ dysfunction (i.e., critically ill) during a medical emergency or crisis.

Crohn's disease: An ongoing condition that causes inflammation of the digestive tract, also called the GI tract. It can affect any part of the GI tract from the mouth to the anus.

elective surgery: A surgery that is optional and not required.

endoscope: A thin illuminated flexible or rigid tube-like optical system used to examine the interior of a hollow organ or body cavity by direct insertion. Instruments can be attached for biopsy and surgery.

epilepsy: A physical disorder that involves recurrent seizures. It is caused by sudden changes in how the brain works.

episiotomy: This is a procedure where an incision is made in the perineum (area between the vagina and the anus) to make the vaginal opening larger in order to prevent the area from tearing during delivery.

estrogen: A type of hormone made by the body that helps develop and maintain female sex characteristics and the growth of long bones.

exercise: A type of physical activity that is planned and structured. Exercise is done on purpose to improve or maintain health, physical fitness, and/or physical performance.

fat: A major source of energy in the diet, fat helps the body absorb fat-soluble vitamins, such as vitamins A, D, E, and K.

gallbladder: A sac that stores a fluid called bile, which is produced by the liver. After eating, bile is secreted into the small intestine, where it helps digest fats.

gastrointestinal: A term that refers to the stomach and the intestines or bowels.

glucose: Glucose is a major source of energy for our bodies and a building block for many carbohydrates. The food digestion process breaks down carbohydrates in foods and drinks into glucose.

hormone: Substance produced by one tissue and conveyed by the bloodstream to another to effect a function of the body, such as growth or metabolism.

hypnosis: A focused state of concentration used to reduce pain. With self-hypnosis, you repeat a positive statement over and over. With guided imagery, you create relaxing images in your mind.

hysterectomy: Surgery to remove the uterus and, sometimes, the cervix. When the uterus and the cervix are removed, it is called a total hysterectomy. When only the uterus is removed, it is called a partial hysterectomy.

immune system: The body's natural defense system against getting an infection and disease. White blood cells are the main part of your immune system that fight infections.

incision: A cut made in the body to perform surgery.

infection: When germs enter a person's body and multiply, causing disease. The germs may be bacteria, viruses, yeast, or fungi. When the body's natural defense system is strong, it can often fight the germs and prevent infection. Some cancer treatments can weaken the natural defense system.

kidney stones: Hard mass developed from crystals that separate from the urine and build up on the inner surfaces of the kidney.

larynx: Valve structure between the trachea (windpipe) and the pharynx (the upper throat) that is the primary organ of voice production.

malignant: A tumor or cells that are cancerous.

mammography: An X-ray imaging method used to image the breast for the early detection of cancer and other breast diseases. It is used as both a diagnostic and screening tool.

medical error: An unintended but preventable adverse effect of care, whether or not it is evident or harmful to the patient.

mortality: Mortality refers to the death rate, or the number of deaths in a certain group of people in a certain period of time.

nasogastric tube: A tube that is inserted through the nose, down the throat and esophagus, and into the stomach. It can be used to give drugs, liquids, and liquid food, or used to remove substances from the stomach. Giving food through a nasogastric tube is a type of enteral nutrition. Also called gastric feeding tube and NG tube.

nonsteroidal anti-inflammatory drugs (NSAIDs): Pain relievers such as aspirin, ibuprofen, and naproxen. These medicines are safe and effective when taken as directed, but they can cause stomach bleeding or kidney problems in some people.

photon: A particle of light or electromagnetic radiation. The energies of photons range from high-energy gamma rays and X-rays to low-energy radio waves.

prescription: A direction written by the physician to the pharmacist for the preparation and use of a medicine or remedy.

prognosis: The likely outcome or course of a disease; the chance of recovery or recurrence.

radiation: The emission of energy as electromagnetic waves or as moving subatomic particles, especially high-energy particles that cause ionization.

radiologist: Doctors who specialize in diagnosing and treating diseases and injuries using medical imaging techniques, such as X-rays, computed tomography (CT), magnetic resonance imaging (MRI), nuclear medicine, positron emission tomography (PET), and ultrasound.

radiology: The specialty concerned with the use of X-ray and other forms of radiant energy in the diagnosis and treatment of disease.

side effect: An effect of a drug, chemical, or other medicine that is in addition to its intended effect, especially an effect that is harmful or unpleasant.

spinal block: A small dose of medicine given as a shot into the spinal fluid in the lower back.

surveillance (medical): Closely watching a patient's condition, but not treating it unless there are changes in test results. Surveillance is also used to find early signs that a disease has come back.

tracheostomy: Surgical opening into the trachea (windpipe) to help someone breathe who has an obstruction or swelling in the larynx (voice box) or upper throat or who has had the larynx surgically removed.

tumor: A tumor is an abnormal growth of body tissue. Tumors can be cancerous (malignant) or noncancerous (benign). Cancerous tumors can have uncontrolled growth and may spread to other parts of the body. Noncancerous tumors do not grow or spread.

tympanometry: Technique that varies air pressure in the ear canal to test how well the middle-ear functions.

ventilator: In medicine, a machine used to help a patient breathe. Also called a respirator.

viruses: Small microscopic organisms that often cause disease.

Chapter 52

Directory of Organizations That Provide Information about Surgery

Government Agencies That Provide Information about Surgery

Agency for Healthcare Research and Quality (AHRQ)
Office of Communications and Knowledge Transfer
5600 Fishers Ln.
7th Fl.
Rockville, MD 20857
Phone: 301-427-1364
Website: www.ahrq.gov

Centers for Medicare and Medicaid Services (CMS)
7500 Security Blvd.
Baltimore, MD 21244
Toll-Free: 800-MEDICARE (800-633-4227)
Phone: 410-786-3000
Toll-Free TTY: 877-486-2048
Website: www.cms.gov

Resources in this chapter were compiled from several sources deemed reliable; all contact information was verified and updated in June 2017.

Centers for Disease Control and Prevention (CDC)
1600 Clifton Rd.
Atlanta, GA 30329-4027
Toll-Free: 800-CDC-INFO
(800-232-4636)
Phone: 404-639-3311
Toll-Free TTY: 888-232-6348
Website: www.cdc.gov

Eunice Kennedy Shriver National Institute of Child Health and Human Development (NICHD)
P.O. Box 3006, Rockville, MD 20847
Phone: 301-496-5133
Toll Free: 800-370-2943
TTY: 888-320-6942
Fax: 866-760-5947
Website: www.nichd.nih.gov
Email: NICHDInformationResource Center@mail.nih.gov

Federal Trade Commission (FTC)
600 Pennsylvania Ave. N.W.
Washington, DC 20580
Toll-Free: 877-FTC-HELP
(877-382-4357)
Phone: 202-326-2222
Website: www.ftc.gov

Healthfinder®
National Health Information Center (NHIC)
1101 Wootton Pkwy
Rockville, MD 20852
Website: www.healthfinder.gov
E-mail: healthfinder@hhs.gov

National Cancer Institute (NCI)
Public Inquiries Office
9609 Medical Center Dr.
Bethesda, MD 20892-9760
Toll-Free: 800-4-CANCER
(800-422-6237)
Website: www.cancer.gov
E-mail: cancergovstaff@mail.nih.gov

National Center for Health Statistics (NCHS)
3311 Toledo Rd.
Hyattsville, MD 20782-2064
Toll-Free: 800-CDC-INFO
(800-232-4636)
Phone: 301-458-4000
Website: www.cdc.gov/nchs

National Eye Institute (NEI)
Information Office
31 Center Dr. MSC 2510
Bethesda, MD 20892-2510
Phone: 301-496-5248
Website: www.nei.nih.gov
E-mail: 2020@nei.nih.gov

National Heart, Lung, and Blood Institute (NHLBI)
P.O. Box 30105
Bethesda, MD 20824-0105
Phone: 301-592-8573
Website: www.nhlbi.nih.gov
E-mail: nhlbiinfo@nhlbi.nih.gov

712

National Institute of Neurological Disorders and Stroke (NINDS)
NIH Neurological Institute
P.O. Box 5801
Bethesda, MD 20824
Toll-Free: 800-352-9424
Phone: 301-496-5751
Website: www.ninds.nih.gov

National Institute of Arthritis and Musculoskeletal and Skin Diseases (NIAMS)
1 AMS Cir.
Bethesda, MD 20892-3675
Toll-Free: 877-22-NIAMS
(877-226-4267)
Phone: 301-495-4484
TTY: 301-565-2966
Fax: 301-718-6366
Website: www.niams.nih.gov
E-mail: NIAMSinfo@mail.nih.gov

National Institute of Diabetes and Digestive and Kidney Diseases (NIDDK)
National Institutes of Health (NIH)
31 Center Dr. MSC 2560
Bldg. 31, Rm. 9A06
Bethesda, MD 20892-2560
Phone: 301-496-3583
Website: www.niddk.nih.gov

National Institute on Aging (NIA)
31 Center Dr. MSC 2292
Bldg. 31, Rm. 5C27
Bethesda, MD 20892
Toll-Free: 800-222-2225
Phone: 301-496-1752
Toll-Free TTY: 800-222-4225
Website: www.nia.nih.gov
E-mail: niaic@nia.nih.gov

National Institutes of Health (NIH)
9000 Rockville Pike
Bethesda, MD 20892
Phone: 301-496-4000
Website: www.nih.gov
E-mail: NIHinfo@od.nih.gov

National Women's Health Information Center (NWHIC)
Office on Women's Health (OWH)
200 Independence Ave. S.W. Rm. 712E
Washington, DC 20201
Toll-Free: 800-994-9662
Phone: 202-690-7650
Toll-Free TDD: 888-220-5446
Fax: 202-205-2631
Website: www.womenshealth.gov

U.S. Department of Health and Human Services (HHS)
200 Independence Ave. S.W.
Washington, DC 20201
Toll-Free: 877-696-6775
Website: www.hhs.gov

U.S. Food and Drug Administration (FDA)
10903 New Hampshire Ave.
Silver Spring, MD 20993
Toll-Free: 888-INFO-FDA
(888-463-6332)
Website: www.fda.gov

U.S. National Library of Medicine (NLM)
8600 Rockville Pike
Bethesda, MD 20894
Toll-Free: 888-FIND-NLM
(888-346-3656)
Phone: 301-594-5983
Website: www.nlm.nih.gov
E-mail: custserv@nlm.nih.gov

Private Agencies That Provide Information about Surgery

Accreditation Association for Ambulatory Health Care (AAAHC)
5250 Old Orchard Rd., Ste. 200
Skokie, IL 60077
Phone: 847-853-6060
Fax: 847-853-9028
Website: www.aaahc.org
E-mail: info@aaahc.org

American Academy of Dermatology (AAD)
930 E. Woodfield Rd.
Schaumburg, IL 60173
Toll-Free: 866-503-SKIN
(866-503-7546)
Phone: 847-240-1280
Fax: 847-240-1859
Website: www.aad.org

American Academy of Facial Plastic and Reconstructive Surgery (AAFPRS)
310 S. Henry St.
Alexandria, VA 22314
Phone: 703-299-9291
Fax: 703-299-8898
Website: www.aafprs.org
E-mail: info@aafprs.org

American Academy of Family Physicians (AAFP)
11400 Tomahawk Creek Pkwy
Leawood, KS 66211-2680
Toll-Free: 800-274-2237
Phone: 913-906-6000
Fax: 913-906-6075
Website: www.aafp.org

American Academy of Ophthalmology (AAO)
655 Beach St.
San Francisco, CA 94109
Phone: 415-561-8500
Fax: 415-561-8533
Website: www.aao.org

American Academy of Orthopaedic Surgeons (AAOS)
9400 W. Higgins Rd.
Rosemont, IL 60018
Phone: 847-823-7186
Fax: 847-823-8125
Website: www.aaos.org

714

American Academy of Otolaryngology–Head and Neck Surgery (AAO-HNS)
1650 Diagonal Rd.
Alexandria, VA 22314
Phone: 703-836-4444
Website: www.entnet.org

American Association of Endodontists (AAE)
211 E. Chicago Ave.
Ste. 1100
Chicago, IL 60611-2691
Toll-Free: 800-872-3636
Phone: 312-266-7255
Fax: 312-266-9867
Toll-Free Fax: 866-451-9020
Website: www.aae.org
E-mail: info@aae.org

American Association of Hip and Knee Surgeons (AAHKS)
9400 W. Higgins Rd.
Ste. 230
Rosemont, IL 60018-4976
Phone: 847-698-1200
Fax: 847-698-0704
Website: www.aahks.org
E-mail: helpdesk@aahks.org

American Association of Nurse Anesthetists (AANA)
222 S. Prospect Ave.
Park Ridge, IL 60068-4037
Toll-Free: 855-526-2262
Phone: 847-692-7050
Fax: 847-692-6968
Website: www.aana.com

American Cancer Society (ACS)
250 Williams St. N.W.
Atlanta, GA 30303
Toll-Free: 800-227-2345
Website: www.cancer.org

American College of Chest Physicians (CHEST)
2595 Patriot Blvd.
Glenview, IL 60026
Phone: 224-521-9800
Fax: 224-521-9801
Website: www.chestnet.org

American College of Obstetricians and Gynecologists (ACOG)
409 12th St. S.W.
Washington, DC 20024-2188
Toll-Free: 800-673-8444
Phone: 202-638-5577
Website: www.acog.org
E-mail: resources@acog.org

American College of Radiology (ACR)
1891 Preston White Dr.
Reston, VA 20191
Toll-Free: 800-227-5463
Phone: 703-648-8900
Website: www.acr.org
E-mail: info@acr.org

American College of Surgeons (ACS)
633 N. Saint Clair St.
Chicago, IL 60611-3211
Toll-Free: 800-621-4111
Phone: 312-202-5000
Fax: 312-202-5001
Website: www.facs.org
E-mail: postmaster@facs.org

American Dental Association (ADA)
211 E. Chicago Ave.
Chicago, IL 60611-2678
Phone: 312-440-2500
Website: www.ada.org

American Heart Association (AHA)
7272 Greenville Ave.
Dallas, TX 75231
Toll-Free: 800-AHA-USA-1
(800-242-8721)
Website: www.heart.org

American Medical Association (AMA)
AMA Plaza 330 N. Wabash Ave.
Ste. 39300
Chicago, IL 60611-5885
Toll-Free: 800-621-8335
Website: www.ama-assn.org

American Optometric Association (AOA)
243 N. Lindbergh Blvd.
First Fl.
St. Louis, MO 63141
Toll-Free: 800-365-2219
Phone: 314-991-4100
Website: www.aoa.org

American Pediatric Surgical Association (APSA)
1 Parkview Plaza
Ste. 800
Oakbrook Terrace, IL 60181
Phone: 847-686-2237
Fax: 847-686-2253
Website: www.eapsa.org
E-mail: eapsa@eapsa.org

American Pregnancy Association
3007 Skyway Cir. N.
Ste. 800
Irving, TX 75038
Toll-Free: 800-672-2296
Website: americanpregnancy.org
E-mail: info@
americanpregnancy.org

American Psychological Association (APA)
750 First St. N.E.
Washington, DC 20002-4242
Toll-Free: 800-374-2721
Phone: 202-336-5500
TDD/TTY: 202-336-6123
Website: www.apa.org

American Rhinologic Society (ARS)
P.O. Box 269
Oak Ridge, NJ 07438
Phone: 845-988-1631
Fax: 845-986-1527
Website: www.american-rhinologic.org

American Society for Dermatologic Surgery (ASDS)
5550 Meadowbrook Dr.
Ste. 120
Rolling Meadows, IL 60008
Phone: 847-956-0900
Website: www.asds.net

716

American Society for Laser Medicine and Surgery (ASLMS)
2100 Stewart Ave., Ste. 240
Wausau, WI 54401
Toll-Free: 877-258-6028
Phone: 715-845-9283
Fax: 715-848-2493
Website: www.aslms.org
E-mail: information@aslms.org

American Society for Metabolic and Bariatric Surgery (ASMBS)
100 S.W. 75th St., Ste. 201
Gainesville, FL 32607
Phone: 352-331-4900
Fax: 352-331-4975
Website: asmbs.org
E-mail: info@asmbs.org

American Society for Radiation Oncology (ASTRO)
251 18th St. S.
Eighth Fl.
Arlington, VA 22202
Toll-Free: 800-962-7876
Phone: 703-502-1550
Fax: 703-502-7852
Website: www.astro.org

American Society for Reproductive Medicine (ASRM)
1209 Montgomery Hwy
Birmingham, AL 35216-2809
Phone: 205-978-5000
Fax: 205-978-5005
Website: www.reproductivefacts.org
E-mail: asrm@asrm.org

American Society for Surgery of the Hand (ASSH)
822 W. Washington Blvd.
Chicago, IL 60607
Phone: 312-880-1900
Fax: 847-384-1435
Website: www.assh.org
E-mail: info@assh.org

American Society of Anesthesiologists (ASA)
1061 American Ln.
Schaumburg, IL 60173-4973
Phone: 847-825-5586
Fax: 847-825-1692
Website: www.asahq.org

American Society of Colon and Rectal Surgeons (ASCRS)
85 W. Algonquin Rd.
Ste. 550
Arlington Heights, IL 60005
Phone: 847-290-9184
Fax: 847-427-9656
Website: www.fascrs.org
E-mail: ascrs@fascrs.org

American Society of Ophthalmic Plastic and Reconstructive Surgery (ASOPRS)
1043 Grand Ave.
Ste. 132
St Paul, MN 55105
Phone: 612-601-3168
Fax: 952-545-6073
Website: www.asoprs.org
E-mail: info@asoprs.org

American Society of PeriAnesthesia Nurses (ASPAN)
90 Frontage Rd.
Cherry Hill, NJ 08034-1424
Toll-Free: 877-737-9696
Fax: 856-616-9601
Website: www.aspan.org
E-mail: aspan@aspan.org

American Society of Plastic Surgeons (ASPS)
444 E. Algonquin Rd.
Arlington Heights, IL 60005
Toll-Free: 800-514-5058
Phone: 847-228-9900
Website: www.plasticsurgery.org
E-mail: memserv@
plasticsurgery.org

American Society of Transplantation (AST)
1120 Route 73
Ste. 200
Mt. Laurel, NJ 08054
Phone: 856-439-9986
Fax: 856-581-9604
Website: www.myast.org

American Thoracic Society (ATS)
25 Bdwy.
New York, NY 10004
Phone: 212-315-8600
Fax: 212-315-6498
Website: www.thoracic.org
E-mail: atsinfo@thoracic.org

American Thyroid Association (ATA)
6066 Leesburg Pike
Ste. 550
Falls Church, VA 22041
Phone: 703-998-8890
Fax: 703-998-8893
Website: www.thyroid.org
E-mail: thyroid@thyroid.org

Amputee Coalition of America (ACA)
9303 Center St., Ste. 100
Manassas, VA 20110
Toll-Free: 888-267-5669
TTY: 865-525-4512
Fax: 865-525-7917
Website: www.amputee-coalition.org

Arthritis Foundation
1355 Peachtree St. N.E.
Ste. 600
Atlanta, GA 30309
Toll-Free: 844-571-4357
Phone: 404-872-7100
Website: www.arthritis.org

Cleveland Clinic
9500 Euclid Ave.
Cleveland, OH 44195
Toll-Free: 800-223-2273
Website: my.clevelandclinic.org

General Surgery News
McMahon Publishing
545 W. 45th St.
Eighth Fl.
New York, NY 10036
Phone: 212-957-5300, ext. 262
Website: www.
generalsurgerynews.com

The Joint Commission
1515 W. 22nd St.
Ste. 1300W
Oakbrook Terrace, IL 60523
Phone: 630-268-7400
Website: www.jointcommission.
org

KidsHealth / TeensHealth
The Nemours Foundation
10140 Centurion Pkwy N.
Jacksonville, FL 32256
Phone: 904-697-4100
Website: www.kidshealth.org /
www.teenshealth.org

Mayo Foundation for
Medical Education and
Research (MFMER)
Mayo Clinic
200 First St. S.W.
Rochester, MN 55905
Phone: 507-284-2511
Fax: 507-284-0161
Website: www.mayoclinic.org

National Hospice and
Palliative Care Organization
(NHPCO)
1731 King St.
Alexandria, VA 22314
Toll-Free: 800-658-8898
Phone: 703-837-1500
Fax: 703-837-1233
Website: www.nhpco.org
E-mail: nhpco_info@nhpco.org

Planned Parenthood
Federation of America, Inc.
123 William St.
10th Fl.
New York, NY 10038
Toll-Free: 800-230-PLAN
(800-230-7526)
Phone: 212-541-7800
Fax: 212-245-1845
Website: www.
plannedparenthood.org

Society of Critical Care
Medicine (SCCM)
500 Midway Dr.
Mount Prospect, IL 60056
Phone: 847-827-6869
Fax: 847-439-7226
Website: www.sccm.org
E-mail: info@sccm.org

Society of Interventional
Radiology (SIR)
3975 Fair Ridge Dr.
Ste. 400 N.
Fairfax, VA 22033
Toll-Free: 800-488-7284
Phone: 703-691-1805
Fax: 703-691-1855
Website: www.sirweb.org

Society of Nuclear Medicine
and Molecular Imaging
(SNMMI)
1850 Samuel Morse Dr.
Reston, VA 20190
Phone: 703-708-9000
Fax: 703-708-9015
Website: www.snmmi.org

Society of Thoracic Surgeons (STS)
633 N. Saint Clair St.
Fl. 23
Chicago, IL 60611-3658
Phone: 312-202-5852
Fax: 312-202-5801
Website: www.sts.org

Texas Heart Institute
6770 Bertner Ave.
Houston, TX 77030
Toll-Free: 800-292-2221
Phone: 832-355-3792
Website: www.texasheart.org

United Network for Organ Sharing (UNOS)
700 N. Fourth St.
Richmond, VA 23219
Toll-Free: 804-782-4800
Phone: 804-782-4800
Fax: 804-782-4817
Website: www.unos.org
E-mail: patientservices@unos.org

United Ostomy Associations of America, Inc. (UOAA)
P.O. Box 525
Kennebunk, ME 04043-0525
Toll-Free: 800-826-0826
Website: www.ostomy.org
E-mail: info@ostomy.org

Index

Index

O